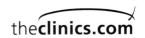

ENDOCRINOLOGY AND METABOLISM CLINICS OF NORTH AMERICA

Endocrinology of Aging

GUEST EDITOR
Johannes D. Veldhuis, MD

CONSULTING EDITOR
Derek LeRoith, MD, PhD

December 2005 • Volume 34 • Number 4

SAUNDERS

An Imprint of Elsevier, Inc.
PHILADELPHIA   LONDON   TORONTO   MONTREAL   SYDNEY   TOKYO

W.B. SAUNDERS COMPANY
A Division of Elsevier Inc.

1600 John F. Kennedy Boulevard • Suite 1800 • Philadelphia, Pennsylvania 19103-2899

http://www.theclinics.com

ENDOCRINOLOGY AND METABOLISM	**Volume 34, Number 4**
CLINICS OF NORTH AMERICA	**ISSN 0889-8529**
December 2005	**ISBN 1-4160-2689-4**
Editor: Joe Rusko	

The ideas and opinions expressed in *Endocrinology and Metabolism Clinics of North America* do not necessarily reflect those of the Publisher. The Publisher does not assume any responsibility for any injury and/or damage to persons or property arising out of or related to any use of the material contained in this periodical. The reader is advised to check the appropriate medical literature and the product information currently provided by the manufacturer of each drug to be administered to verify the dosage, the method and duration of administration, or contraindications. It is the responsibility of the treating physician or other health care professional, relying on independent experience and knowledge of the patient, to determine drug dosages and the best treatment for the patient. Mention of any product in this issue should not be construed as endorsement by the contributors, editors, or the Publisher of the product or manufacturers' claims.

Endocrinology and Metabolism Clinics of North America (ISSN 0889-8529) is published quarterly by Elsevier Inc. Corporate and editorial offices: 1600 John F. Kennedy Boulevard, Suite 1800, Philadelphia, PA 19103-2899. Accounting and circulation offices: 6277 Sea Harbor Drive, Orlando, FL 32887-4800. Periodicals postage paid at Orlando, FL 32862, and additional mailing offices. Subscription prices are USD 175 per year for US individuals, USD 295 per year for US institutions, USD 90 per year for US students and residents, USD 220 per year for Canadian individuals, USD 355 per year for Canadian institutions, USD 240 per year for international individuals, USD 355 per year for international institutions and USD 125 per year for Canadian and foreign students/residents. To receive student/resident rate, orders must be accompanied by name of affiliated institution, date of term, and the *signature* of program/residency coordinator on institution letterhead. Orders will be billed at individual rate until proof of status is received. Foreign air speed delivery is included in all *Clinics* subscription prices. All prices are subject to change without notice. POSTMASTER: Send address changes to *Endocrinology and Metabolism Clinics of North America*, W.B. Saunders Company, Periodicals Fulfillment, Orlando, FL 32887-4800. **Customer Service: (+1) 800-654-2452 (US). From outside of the US, call (+1) 407-345-4000; e-mail: hhspcs@harcourt.com.**

Reprints. For copies of 100 or more, of articles in this publication, please contact the Commercial Rights Department, Elsevier Inc., 360 Park Avenue South, New York, NY 10010-1710; phone: (+1) 212-633-3813; fax: (+1) 212-462-1935; e-mail: reprints@elsevier.com.

Endocrinology and Metabolism Clinics of North America is covered in *Index Medicus, EMBASE/Excerpta Medica, Current Contents/Clinical Medicine, Current Contents/Life Sciences, Science Citation Index, ISI/BIOMED, BIOSIS, and Chemical Abstracts.*

Printed in the United States of America.

CONSULTING EDITOR

DEREK LeROITH, MD, PhD, Chief, Division of Endocrinology, Diabetes, and Bone Diseases, Mount Sinai School of Medicine, New York, NY, USA

GUEST EDITOR

JOHANNES D. VELDHUIS, MD, Professor (Medicine); and Clinical Investigator, Endocrine Research Unit, Department of Internal Medicine, Mayo School of Graduate Education, General Clinical Research Center, Mayo Clinic, Rochester, Minnesota

CONTRIBUTORS

GIANLUCA AIMARETTI, MD, PhD, Division of Endocrinology and Metabolism, Department of Internal Medicine, University of Turin, Turin, Italy

EMANUELA ARVAT, MD, Associate Professor, Division of Endocrinology and Metabolism, Department of Internal Medicine, University of Turin, Turin, Italy

ROBERTO BALDELLI, MD, Division of Endocrinology and Metabolism, Department of Internal Medicine, University of Turin, Turin, Italy

MATTEO BALDI, MD, Division of Endocrinology and Metabolism, Department of Internal Medicine, University of Turin, Turin, Italy

MARIO BO, MD, Assistant Professor, Section of Geriatrics, Department of Medical and Surgical Disciplines, University of Turin, Turin, Italy

CYRIL Y. BOWERS, MD, Professor (Medicine) and Chief, Division of Endocrinology and Metabolism, Department of Internal Medicine, Tulane University Medical Center, New Orleans, Louisiana

FABIO BROGLIO, MD, PhD, Division of Endocrinology and Metabolism, Department of Internal Medicine, University of Turin, Turin, Italy

HENRY G. BURGER, MD, Emeritus Director, Prince Henry's Institute of Medical Research, Monash Medical Centre, Clayton, Victoria, Australia

LISA S. CHOW, MD, Fellow in Endocrinology and Instructor (Medicine), Division of Endocrinology, Nutrition, and Metabolism, Mayo Clinic College of Medicine, Rochester, Minnesota

DANA ERICKSON, MD, Associate Professor (Medicine), Endocrine Research Unit, Department of Internal Medicine, Mayo School of Graduate Medical Education, General Clinical Research Center, Mayo Clinic, Rochester, Minnesota

JAN FRYSTYK, MD, PhD, DMSc, Medical Research Laboratories, Aarhus University Hospital, Aarhus, Denmark

EZIO GHIGO, MD, Full Professor, Division of Endocrinology and Metabolism, Department of Internal Medicine, University of Turin, Turin, Italy

ROBERTA GIORDANO, MD, Division of Endocrinology and Metabolism, Department of Internal Medicine, University of Turin, Turin, Italy

SILVIA GROTTOLI, MD, Division of Endocrinology and Metabolism, Department of Internal Medicine, University of Turin, Turin, Italy

GEORGINA E. HALE, MD, Research Fellow, Department of Obstetrics and Gynaecology, University of Sydney, Sydney, New South Wales, Australia

STEVEN P. HODAK, MD, Endocrinology Fellow, Division of Endocrinology and Metabolism, Georgetown University Medical Center, Washington, DC

ALI IRANMANESH, MD, Chief, Endocrine Section; Coordinator, Research and Development, Endocrine Service, Medical Section Salem, Salem Veterans Affairs Medical Center, Salem; and Associate Professor (Clinical Medicine), University of Virginia School of Medicine, Charlottesville, Virginia

DANIEL M. KEENAN, PhD, Professor (Statistics), Department of Statistics, University of Virginia, Charlottesville, Virginia

SUNDEEP KHOSLA, MD, Professor (Medicine), Division of Endocrinology, Metabolism, and Nutrition, Mayo Clinic College of Medicine, Rochester, Minnesota

FABIO LANFRANCO, MD, Division of Endocrinology and Metabolism, Department of Internal Medicine, University of Turin, Turin, Italy

PETER Y. LIU, MD, PhD, Visiting Scientist, Division of Endocrinology, Department of Medicine, Los Angeles Biomedical Research Institute, Harbor–University of California at Los Angeles Medical Center, Torrance, California

JOHN M. MILES, MD, Professor (Medicine), Endocrine Research Unit, Department of Internal Medicine, Mayo School of Graduate Medical Education, General Clinical Research Center, Mayo Clinic, Rochester, Minnesota

JOHN C. MORRIS, MD, Professor and Chair, Division of Endocrinology, Mayo Clinic College of Medicine, Rochester, Minnesota

K. SREEKUMARAN NAIR, MD, PhD, Professor (Medicine), Division of Endocrinology, Nutrition, and Metabolism, Mayo Clinic College of Medicine, Rochester, Minnesota

AJAY X. NEHRA, MD, Professor (Urology), Department of Urology, Mayo Medical and Graduate Schools of Medicine, Mayo Clinic, Rochester, Minnesota

ROBERT W. REBAR, MD, Executive Director, American Society for Reproductive Medicine; and Volunteer Clinical Professor, Department of Obstetrics and Gynecology, University of Alabama, Birmingham, Birmingham, Alabama

B. LAWRENCE RIGGS, MD, Professor (Medicine), Division of Endocrinology, Metabolism, and Nutrition, Mayo Clinic College of Medicine, Rochester, Minnesota

FERDINAND ROELFSEMA, MD, Associate Professor, Department of Endocrinology, Leiden University Medical Center, Leiden, The Netherlands

MARIUS STAN, MD, Endocrine Fellow, Division of Endocrinology, Mayo Clinic College of Medicine, Rochester, Minnesota

RONALD S. SWERDLOFF, MD, Chief, Division of Endocrinology, Department of Medicine, Los Angeles Biomedical Research Institute, Harbor–University of California at Los Angeles Medical Center, Torrance; and Professor (Medicine), David Geffen School of Medicine, University of California at Los Angeles, Los Angeles, California

JOHANNES D. VELDHUIS, MD, Professor (Medicine) and Clinical Investigator, Endocrine Research Unit, Department of Internal Medicine, Mayo School of Graduate Education, General Clinical Research Center, Mayo Clinic, Rochester, Minnesota

JOSEPH G. VERBALIS, MD, Professor (Medicine) and Chief, Division of Endocrinology and Metabolism, Georgetown University Medical Center, Washington, DC

CHRISTINA WANG, MD, Professor (Medicine), David Geffen School of Medicine, University of California at Los Angeles, Los Angeles; and Director, General Clinical Research Center, Los Angeles Biomedical Research Institute, Harbor–University of California at Los Angeles Medical Center, Torrance, California

CONTENTS

Sarcopenia is a common consequence of aging with onset as early as the fourth decade. At the cellular level, this loss of muscle function is associated with declines in muscle protein synthesis and mitochondrial capacity. Resistance and aerobic exercise enhance mixed muscle protein synthesis, although resistance training has a more profound stimulatory effect. Although increased age and declining muscle function are associated with decreased testosterone levels in men, the role of testosterone supplementation remains controversial. Strong evidence exists for testosterone increasing muscle mass and muscle protein synthesis, yet a clear increase of muscle strength in elderly people by testosterone has not been observed, an observation vulnerable to confounding factors and experimental design.

Dynamic control of the somatotropic axis varies significantly across the human lifespan. Concentrations of growth hormone (GH) decline precipitously after a neonatal surge, stabilize during childhood, increase during puberty, and then fall exponentially as adulthood unfolds. Augmented GH release during adolescence is an appropriate physiologic mechanism to promote normal growth and physical maturity. The importance of adequate GH availability in later life was recognized recently based upon studies of adult hypopituitarism. Organic and age-related hyposomatotropism are marked by decreased bone and muscle mass, increased visceral adiposity, dyslipidemia, insulin resistance, diminished sense of well being, and reduced quality of life. Detailed assessment of the basis of reduced somatotropic function in aging individuals had been impeded by insufficiently sensitive assays to measure low GH concentrations. Ultrasensitive assay methods have unveiled an ensemble of distinct age-related deficits for regulating GH secretion.

Although the insulin-like growth factor binding proteins (IGFBPs) are truly multifactorial proteins, there is little doubt that one of their most important functions is to act in concert to regulate circulating levels of free IGF-I. This article reviews current knowledge on changes in the IGFBPs during aging and discusses how this affects levels of free IGF-I and -II and hence the bioactivity of the circulating IGF system.

Growth hormone (GH) concentrations decline progressively with increasing age. In contrast, the maximal pituitary secretory capacity, plasma elimination kinetics, and hepatic actions of GH are preserved in older people. Reduced availability of GH and thereby insulin-like growth factor in the elderly has significant implications. In particular, epidemiologic investigations correlate hyposomatotropism with reduced insulin sensitivity, dyslipidemia, increased cardiovascular mortality, intra-abdominal adiposity, sarcopenia, osteopenia, and diminished quality of life. Obesity forecasts decreased GH secretion in the adult. In addition, sex steroid depletion after adolescence predicts relative GH deficiency. Conversely, supplementation with estradiol or an aromatizable androgen, such as testosterone, stimulates GH production in aging and hypogonadal adults. Recent developments in this arena allow new clinical perspectives in aging, which are highlighted in this article.

Changes in endocrine function in aging individuals often reflect age-related impairment in animal and human neuroendocrine regulation of pituitary function. This article reviews the age-related variations in somatotroph responsiveness to classical and nonclassical stimulations, with particular attention to the best tools to evaluate somatotroph capacity in aging and to diagnose growth hormone deficiency among aged people suspected for hypopituitarism.

Perimenopausal Reproductive Endocrinology
Georgina E. Hale and Henry G. Burger

Reproductive aging is associated with an acceleration in the decline of ovarian follicle numbers. Menstrual cycles change from regular to irregular when follicle numbers reach a critical level of between 100 and 1000. With the onset of irregular cycles, there is an increased incidence of anovulatory cycles and elongated ovulatory cycles, both of which are characterized by high FSH, low estradiol, low inhibin B, and, in the case of elongated ovulatory cycles, low progesterone. During normal length ovulatory cycles, changes in gonadotropins, sex steroids, and the inhibins remain subtle and reflect preservation of normal menstrual cycle function. These normal cycles occur less often as the final menstrual period approaches, and high FSH levels, low estradiol, and low inhibin levels predominate.

Mechanisms of Premature Menopause
Robert W. Rebar

Premature menopause is characterized by amenorrhea, elevated circulating gonadotropin levels, and low circulating estrogen levels in women under the age of 40 years. Although hormonal values are similar to those found during the menopausal transition and after menopause, it is clear that women with this disorder differ in important ways from normal postmenopausal women. The use of the term "premature menopause" itself is inappropriate because approximately half have eveidene of ovarian function and 6% to 8% will ovulate after the diagnosis is made. This article focuses on what is known about several distinct mechanisms for the ovarian failure and conclusions by briefly offering potential treatment strategies.

Mechanisms of Hypoandrogenemia in Healthy Aging Men
Peter Y. Liu, Ali Iranmanesh, Ajay X. Nehra, Daniel M. Keenan, and Johannes D. Veldhuis

The systemic availability of testosterone is now firmly established to fall by 35% to 50% after the sixth decade of life in healthy men and may contribute to decreased muscular and bone strength and physical frailty. The mechanistic bases and their relative importance for relative hypoandrogenemia remain poorly defined. This article explores the mechanisms of hypoandrogenemia in aging men.

time-delayed signaling among the hypothalamus and the pituitary and adrenal glands.

FORTHCOMING ISSUES

RECENT ISSUES

ELSEVIER
SAUNDERS

Endocrinol Metab Clin N Am
34 (2005) xiii–xv

ENDOCRINOLOGY
AND METABOLISM
CLINICS
OF NORTH AMERICA

Foreword

Endocrinology of Aging

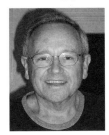

Derek LeRoith, MD, PhD
Consulting Editor

In this issue on aging, Dr. Veldhuis has assembled a number of articles that cover the endocrinopathy of aging. The articles range from dysfunctional aspects of the hypothalamus and pituitary to peripheral organs, particularly those involving sex steroids. In the article by Chow and Nair, the basic and physiologic processes of muscle wasting (sarcopenia) with age are described, and its effect on muscle strength is emphasized. The degree of sarcopenia is dependent on multiple factors, including exercise, and the authors describe the maintenance of muscle by a sustained exercise program and discuss the possible use of testosterone in the elderly man. It has long been noted that growth hormone (GH) and insulin-like growth factor-1 (IGF-1) levels decline with aging, and these changes have been thought to be related to loss of muscle, bone, and other tissue components with aging. The article by Iranmanesh and Veldhuis describes the use of an ultrasensitive GH assay and demonstrate that the reduced GH action is due primarily to a reduction in the size of the pulsatile GH spikes due to reduced GHRH and GHRP/ghrelin drive from the hypothalamus and excessive inhibition by somatostatin. Frystyk's article, on the other hand, discusses the changes in the IGF-binding proteins with aging and suggests that changes in these proteins may also be important in the process of aging. In the article by Veldhuis and colleagues, there is a description of the effects of sex steroids on the GH–IGF-1 axis; testosterone and estrogen are known to stimulate GH secretion. With aging in men and women, there is a decrease in testosterone, estrogen, and GH. How to diagnose pituitary dysfunction, especially

doi:10.1016/j.ecl.2005.08.001   *endo.theclinics.com*

GH-deficiency, is outlined in the article by Giordano. Although the insulin tolerance test (ITT) is still the gold standard for adults according to the GH Research Society, the hypoglycemia is often contraindicated in the elderly and because IGF-1 levels are often not discriminatory; it is suggested that the GHRH combined with arginine test be used when the ITT is to be avoided. Although the alternative 24-hour GH sampling test is an excellent discriminatory test, it is not practical outside of the research setting.

Abnormalities of the reproductive system with aging are covered by a number of articles. Hale and Burger briefly introduce the normal female cycle and its hormonal control and then the changes associated with the menopause. They also discuss the menopausal symptoms usually associated with changes in estrogen levels. Rebar presents the etiology of premature menopause, which ranges from genetic causes and autoimmune etiologies to physical causes, including chemotherapy, and concludes his article with practical suggestions for management of the disorder. In summarizing some very elegant clinical studies, Liu and colleagues describe the mechanisms involved in the hypoandrogenism seen in healthy aging men; the conclusion is impairment of hypothalamic gonadotropin-releasing hormone outflow with reduced pulsatile luteinizing hormone-stimulated testosterone. Clinically, this results in reduced libido, reduced sexual potency, reduced effort tolerance, osteoporosis, muscle mass, and other commonly seen changes. In a companion article, these authors discuss the important clinical question as to whether treatment of this "relative testosterone deficiency in older men" is warranted. As proposed by a number of organizations, they conclude that a sustained reduction in serum testosterone together with significant symptoms warrants a trial of testosterone replacement, after careful consideration of comorbidities.

There are changes in the hypothalamic-pituitary-thyroid axis associated with aging. Stan and Morris suggest in their article that thyroid-stimulating hormone not be used by itself to make the diagnosis of hypothyroidism; rather, the usual full panel of tests should be used. Similarly, the article by Veldhuis and colleagues describes changes in the hypothalamic-pituitary-adrenal axis. Although many of the features of aging, such as visceral adiposity, memory loss, osteopenia, and sarcopenia, could be ascribed to excess cortisol, no hard data are available. With respect to osteoporosis of aging, there are a number of causative agents, as discussed by Khosla and Riggs. These include changes in the sex steroids and GH–IGF-1 axis, reduced vitamin D levels, and increases in parathyroid levels. Furthermore, the parallel in sarcopenia and osteopenia indicates a role for inactivity—a common problem in the aging population. Finally, an important feature of aging is the increased incidence of syndrome of inappropriate secretion of antidiuretic hormone. As explained by Hodak and Verbalis, this is most likely the consequence of excessive arginine vasopressin (AVP) secretion due to lack of negative feedback with fluid intake. Although the renal responsiveness to AVP is reduced with aging, it is still present.

In summary, this issue focuses on the pathophysiologic aspects of the endocrine changes that occur with aging and gives the reader important insights into these processes and some practical suggestions for dealing with this increasing population of patients.

Derek LeRoith, MD, PhD
Chief
Division of Endocrinology, Diabetes, and Bone Diseases
Mount Sinai School of Medicine
New York, NY, USA

ELSEVIER
SAUNDERS

Endocrinol Metab Clin N Am
34 (2005) xvii–xviii

ENDOCRINOLOGY
AND METABOLISM
CLINICS
OF NORTH AMERICA

Preface

Endocrinology of Aging

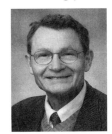

Johannes D. Veldhuis, MD
Guest Editor

Successful aging is an implicit expectation in all cultures. Healthy aging, even in the absence of significant comorbidity, is marked by gradual attrition of muscle and bone mass, reduced physical stamina, increased visceral adiposity, skin fragility, insulin resistance, elevation of blood pressure and detectable cognitive impairment. The concept of successful aging implies a limited pace and severity of deficits that predict frailty, cardiovascular risk, disability, and morbidity.

The fundamental biologic basis of aging is not known. In fact, virtually all measures of somatic structure and function undergo subtle decremental changes. A pivotal contemporary issue is the extent to which the aging-related decline in specific regulatory systems (eg, neurohormonal axes) exacerbates or obviates the impact of the primary aging process.

In this issue of the *Endocrinology and Metabolism Clinics of North America*, scholars in key subdisciplines of endocrinology and metabolism review current knowledge of neuroendocrine adaptations in aging. The focus includes thyroid hormones, water and electrolyte balance, male and female reproductive aging, and somatotropic hormones. Each contribution highlights present understanding and poses questions for further study. For example, more complex multisignal mechanisms of control are emerging in the gonadal, somatotropic, and thyrotropic axes. The enhanced conceptual platform presages the development of nonsteroidal and nonpeptidyl interventions to forestall depletion of anabolic hormones in elderly adults. The putative beneficiaries would be patients at increased risk of frailty, disability, and

0889-8529/05/$ - see front matter © 2005 Elsevier Inc. All rights reserved.
doi:10.1016/j.ecl.2005.07.011   *endo.theclinics.com*

morbidity. A major objective will be to define safety, practicability, benefit, and relevant indications.

Johannes D. Veldhuis, MD
Endocrine Research Unit
Department of Internal Medicine
Mayo School of Graduate Education
General Clinical Research Center
Mayo Clinic
200 First Street SW
Room 5-194 Joseph
Rochester, MN 55905, USA

E-mail address: veldhuis.johannes@mayo.edu

ELSEVIER
SAUNDERS

Endocrinol Metab Clin N Am
34 (2005) 833–852

ENDOCRINOLOGY
AND METABOLISM
CLINICS
OF NORTH AMERICA

Sarcopenia of Male Aging

Lisa S. Chow, MD, K. Sreekumaran Nair, MD, PhD*

*Division of Endocrinology, Nutrition, and Metabolism,
Mayo Clinic College of Medicine, Rochester, MN, USA*

The word "sarcopenia" arises from two components, sarco, meaning muscle, and penia, meaning wasting. Sarcopenia and progressive debilitation are potential complications of aging. Defined as the age-related loss of muscle mass, strength, and function, sarcopenia evokes images of decreased vitality and lost youth. Indeed, sarcopenia has been associated with increased frailty, falls, morbidity, and mortality in the elderly [1,2].

Sarcopenia is not unique to people. The nematode *Caenorhabditis elegans* is an important model for aging, with a mean lifespan of 2 to 3 weeks. Upon reaching adulthood (age 2–3 days), these animals are highly mobile and move vigorously away from a touch stimulus. At the end of its reproductive period (about age 6–7 days), the animals move only when prodded. By age 9 to 10 days, these animals exhibit minimal movement and only twitch when prodded. This progressive loss of locomotion is associated with progressive loss of muscle mass/quality despite an intact nervous system. Electron microscopic analysis has described the muscle damage, demonstrating a loss of myofilament numbers, reduction of cytoplasmic volume, loosening of sarcomere geometry, fraying of individual sarcomeres, and disorganization of individual sarcomeres [3].

In people, sarcopenia onset depends on the measurement modality. Sarcopenia can be described as a loss of muscle mass. Studies of muscle mass as measured indirectly by whole body potassium content have demonstrated decline of lean mass by the fourth decade [4,5]. More recently, muscle mass estimates using muscle cross-sectional area (CSA) measured by CT or MRI have been used. By using 12 subjects per decade in a population

Funding was provided by a Public Health Service Award (RO1AG09531), the Mayo Foundation, a National Institutes of Health Training Grant to Dr. Chow (T32 DK07352), and the Dole-Murdock Professorship to Dr. Nair.

* Corresponding author. Division of Endocrinology, Nutrition, and Metabolism, Mayo Clinic College of Medicine, 200 First Street Southwest, Rochester, MN 55905.

E-mail address: nair.sree@mayo.edu (K.S. Nair).

spanning 18 to 88 years (n = 78), Short and colleagues [6] measured thigh muscle CSA using a single-slice CT scan and reported progressive decline of muscle area, confirming the findings reported by earlier studies using total body potassium (Fig. 1). Because CT and MRI imaging are costly, their role for large-scale population estimates of sarcopenia is limited. Instead, dual-energy x-ray absorptiometry (DXA) has been the most common modality for population studies, with several large studies reporting the decline of skeletal mass in men by age 55 [7,8]. DXA scanning, however, cannot distinguish between muscle and water content and poses the risk of overestimating muscle mass in older people with increased water retention [9]. At the muscle fiber level, an autopsy study of fiber composition in the vastus lateralis muscle showed muscle fiber loss by the third decade with progressive preferential loss of type 2 fibers with increasing age [10]. Structurally, these age-related changes appear to be caused by fiber number decline rather than fiber size shrinkage [11]. As measurement of total body potassium represents total body cell mass, the results from autopsy studies on muscle fibers complement the results previously reported by total body potassium measurements [4,5].

Sarcopenia also can be described as a loss of muscle strength. In a large cross-sectional study of 654 subjects (aged 20–93 years), Lindle and colleagues [12] reported both men and women having age-related declines in knee extensor strength starting in the fourth decade and then continuing to lose strength at a rate of 8% to 10% per decade. Similar findings have been reported by other studies [13,14]. This age-related decline of muscle strength has been demonstrated by several longitudinal studies, with annual rates of decline ranging from 0.5% to 3.1% [15–18]. A 27-year longitudinal study of grip strength in 3680 Japanese American men (baseline age 45–68 years) reported a decline of 1% per year, with a steeper decline (1.5% per

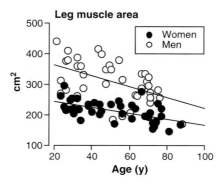

Fig. 1. Age-associated decline in thigh muscle cross-sectional area (CSA). CSA of the midthigh of both legs was measured by CT and reported as cm^2. The rate of decline was 5% per decade in men and 4% per decade in women (both r = −0.55, P < 0.01). (*Data from* Short KR, Vittone JL, Bigelow ML, et al. Age and aerobic exercise training effects on whole body and muscle protein metabolism. Am J Physiol Endocrinol Metab 2004;286(1):E92–101.)

year) associated with older baseline age, greater weight loss, and chronic co-morbid disease [17]. Another 12-year study of 12 men (mean baseline age: 65.4 ± 4.2 years) showed strength declining by 20% to 30% with concurrent loss of muscle mass as determined by CT CSA [18]. Thus, both cross-sectional and longitudinal data document loss of muscle strength with increasing age, particularly after the fourth decade.

Is this loss of strength caused by loss of muscle mass? Or does aging also compromise muscle quality? Although it would be logical to presume that aging compromises muscle quality, the actual data are conflicting. Several studies have found that adjusting for muscle mass minimizes any age-associated loss of strength, with muscle mass estimated by urinary creatinine [19,20], CT CSA [21], or arm circumference [19]. Other studies, however, have noted age-related decreases in muscle strength per unit of muscle mass, with muscle mass measured by bioelectric impedence [22], DXA scan [13], or CT CSA (Kevin Short, PhD, personal communication, 2004). This conflict may be caused by different measuring techniques and equipment in assessing muscle mass and strength. Studies of isolated muscle fibers have shown age-related declines in contractility. Frontera and colleagues measured maximal force in single type I fibers and type IIA fibers isolated from young men (n = 7: age 36.5 ± 3.0 years), older men (n = 12: age 74.4 ± 5.9 years), and older women (n = 12: age 72.1 ± 4.3 years). Comparing muscle fibers from young and old men, the study found young men's type I and type IIA fibers exerting higher force (44% and 37%, respectively), even after correcting for size [21]. Larsson and colleagues [23] isolated muscle fibers from young (n = 4, 25- to 31-year-old) and old (n = 4, 73- to 81-year-old) men. Maximum unloaded shortening velocity and maximum force normalized to cross-sectional fiber area (specific tension) of types I and IIa myosin heavy chain (MHC) fibers in the young control group were significantly higher compared with the old control and old physically active groups [23].

Besides the age-related decline of muscle mass and muscle quality, other changes likely contribute to sarcopenia. At the muscle level, these changes may include fat/connective tissue infiltration [24] and nerve deinervation [25]. Muscle fiber type also appears to change with age, as most, but not all [18], studies of age-related fiber change involving the vastus lateralis muscle have reported the decline of type II (fast-twitch) fibers with age [10,11,26]. This reduction in fast-twitch fibers corresponds to a reduction of fast MHC isoforms [23,27]. Studying a group of sedentary subjects ranging from young (n = 7, mean age 24 ± 1 year), middle aged (n = 12, mean age 52 ± 0.8 years) to old (n = 14, mean age 71 ± 1 year), Balagopal and colleagues showed a significantly lower mRNA level of MHC-IIa and -IIx with increased age and no difference in MHC-I between the groups. With 3 months of resistance exercise, the middle-aged and older group collectively demonstrated an increase in MHC-I by 84%, whereas MHC-IIa mRNA ($P < 0.04$) and MHC-IIx mRNA ($P < 0.01$) levels decreased [28]. At the cellular level, aging is associated with decreased contractile proteins [23], synthesis rate of muscle myosin heavy chain [29], oxidative capacity [26,30,31], muscle mitochondrial protein synthesis [30], and mitochondrial function [30].

Because a delicate balance of protein synthesis and protein breakdown maintains muscle mass, the effects of age on muscle protein synthesis have been studied extensively. In young people, skeletal muscle comprises 45% to 50% of total body mass, and 80% to 85% of fat free mass. In the elderly (> 65 years), skeletal muscle only comprises 35% of body mass and 40% of fat-free mass [32]. Whole body protein synthesis (WBPS) may decline with age, depending on the normalization method [6,33]. Early studies have shown contradictory results of WBPS when normalized for lean body mass [33]. This apparent contradiction may be caused by the low rates of muscle protein synthesis, as skeletal muscle contributes less than 30% to WBPS [34]. A loss of 1 kg of muscle mass will decrease lean body mass more significantly than the consequent decline in protein synthesis; consequently, if WBPS is normalized to lean body mass, a relative proportional increase will occur. Because diet and activity may affect muscle protein metabolism [35], these measures should be standardized in muscle metabolism studies. When these measures are standardized accordingly, age-related decline in WBPS has been demonstrated even when normalizing for lean body mass [29]. As WBPS is a relatively insensitive measure of muscle protein synthesis, techniques have been developed to measure muscle protein-specific metabolism. Studies of mixed muscle protein synthesis measure the aggregate synthesis rate of muscle mitochondrial, sarcoplasmic, and myofibrillar protein and have reported a fractional rate of protein synthesis in the elderly decreasing by 28% to 37% compared with young controls [6,29,36]. Measuring mixed muscle protein synthesis rate has the limitation of representing the average synthesis rate of several proteins with widely varying rates. Thus, the significance of muscle protein synthesis changes on muscle mass can be estimated only by measuring fractional breakdown (proteolysis) of muscle protein subfractions or individual proteins. Studies of individual muscle protein and protein subfractions have shown age-related declines in MHC-I [29] (Fig. 2), mitochondrial [30] and myofibrillar [37] protein synthesis, but not sarcoplasmic protein synthesis [29]. Age has a differential effect on various mRNA transcript levels [28,38] and likely influences the effects of physical activity and diet on individual muscle protein synthesis. The inability of small differences in muscle protein synthesis and breakdown to explain age-associated sarcopenia highlights methodological differences and difficulty in muscle protein measurement [39,40]. To understand the mechanisms underlying age-related sarcopenia, it is important to delineate and distinguish the impact of various factors at multiple molecular levels, a goal yet unattainable by current technology.

Mitochondria power muscle contractility and other muscle functions. Although the effects of habitual physical activity and overall fitness cannot be excluded, age is associated with a reduction in muscle oxidative capacity [30,38,41]. Age-associated mitochondrial decay is seen in animals and

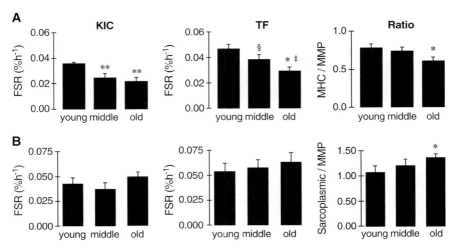

Fig. 2. Age-associated changes in muscle-specific protein synthesis rates. FSR of MHC (*A*) and sarcoplasmic proteins (*B*) in young, middle, and old subjects using α-ketoisocaproate (KIC) and tissue fluid (TF) as precursor for protein synthesis. MHC showed a progressive age-related decline ($P < 0.01$), unlike sarcoplasmic protein. The ratio of MHC and sarcoplasmic protein synthesis rate to mixed muscle protein (MMP) synthesis rate also is shown. These data indicate the contribution of MHC synthesis to mixed muscle protein decreased with age ($P < 0.05$), whereas the contribution of sarcoplasmic protein increased with age ($P < 0.05$). (*$P < 0.05$) denotes significant change from young age group; (**$P < 0.01$) denotes significant change from young age group; ($\ddagger P < 0.01$) denotes significant change from middle age group; and ($\S P = 0.07$) denotes change from young age group. (*From* Balagopal P, Rooyackers OE, Adey DB, et al. Effects of aging on in vivo synthesis of skeletal muscle myosin heavy-chain and sarcoplasmic protein in humans. Am J Physiol 1997;273:E790–800; with permission).

people, likely because of accumulated oxidative damage [42–44]. To examine age effects on mitochondrial function, Rooyackers and colleagues [30] studied muscle mitochondrial protein synthesis rates in three subject groups (young: n = 12, 24 ± 1 year; middle age: n = 12, age 54 ± 1 year; old: n = 16, age 73 ± 2 years). In addition, mitochondrial enzyme activity was measured, specifically citrate synthase, a mitochondrial protein encoded by nuclear DNA, and cytochrome c oxidase, a mitochondrial protein encoded by both nuclear and mitochondrial DNA. With increasing age, maximum oxygen consumption rate (Vo2max) progressively declined. By middle age, declines in the fractional synthesis rate (FSR) of mixed muscle protein (decreased by 12%, $P < 0.05$ versus young) and mitochondrial protein (decreased by 40%, $P < 0.01$ versus young) were seen (Fig. 3). Likewise, muscle homogenates (cytochrome c oxidase: $P = 0.004$ versus young; citrate synthase: $P = 0.01$ versus young) and isolated mitochondria (citrate synthase: $P = 0.035$ versus young) demonstrated declining oxidative capacity with increased age (Fig. 4) [30]. Short and colleagues [38] confirmed these age-related declines in citrate synthase and cytochrome c oxidase activity and also demonstrated declines in mitochondrial mRNA levels encoded by nuclear genes (COX 4

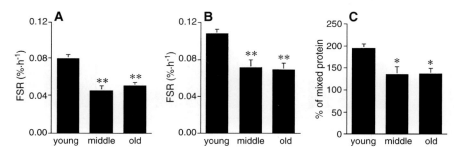

Fig. 3. Age-associated declines in skeletal muscle mitochondrial protein. FSR of skeletal muscle mitochondrial protein using plasma [^{13}C]-KIC (*A*), tissue fluid [^{13}C]-leucine (*B*) as precursor pool enrichment in young, middle-aged, and old human subjects. *Panel C* shows FSR as a percentage of mixed protein synthesis rates. Men and women were presented as one group. *$P < 0.05$, **$P < 0.01$ versus young. (*From* Rooyackers OE, Adey DB, Ades PA, et al. Effect of age on in vivo rates of mitochondrial protein synthesis in human skeletal muscle. Proc Natl Acad Sci USA 1996;93(26):15364–9; with permission.)

mRNA [0.32–0.45, $P < 0.025$]) and by mitochondrial genes (ND4 mRNA [0.45–0.5, $P < 0.025$]) (Fig. 5). These findings suggest changes in mitochondrial protein metabolism may alter muscle function and performance. Using an animal model involving young (6-month-old) and old (27-month-old) rats, Barrazoni and colleagues [44] showed an age-associated decline in skeletal muscle mitochondrial DNA copy number (-23 to -40%, $P < 0.03$). It will be important to see if similar changes occur in human aging muscle, and if present, to determine the underlying mechanism. Both mitochondrial and nuclear encoded gene transcripts of mitochondrial proteins decline with age [38]. The mechanism of age affecting nuclear control of

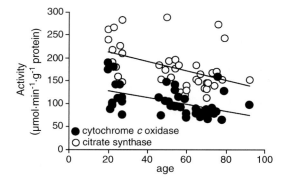

Fig. 4. Age-associated declines in muscle mitochondrial enzymes. An inverse relationship exists between tissue (muscle homogenate) activities of cytochrome c oxidase (y = -0.72x + 142.8; r^2 = 0.22, $P < 0.0017$) and citrate synthase (y = -1.01x + 232.6; r^2 = 0.20, $P < 0.0033$) versus age. For each enzyme, male and female subjects were treated as one group. (*From* Rooyackers OE, Adey DB, Ades PA, et al. Effect of age on in vivo rates of mitochondrial protein synthesis in human skeletal muscle. Proc Natl Acad Sci USA 1996;93(26):15364–9; with permission.)

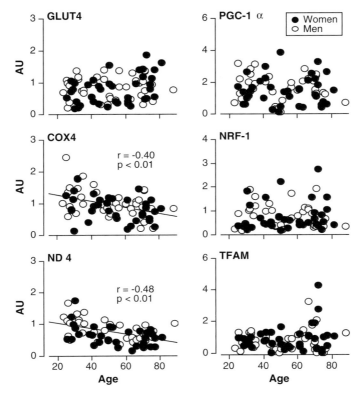

Fig. 5. Age-associated declines in muscle mitochondrial mRNA levels. Effect of age on mRNA levels of muscle mitochondrial genes. Regression lines are given for COX4 and ND4, which declined significantly with age. The other genes did not show an age-related change. Values are given in arbitrary units (AU) after normalization to 28S rRNA. (*From* Short KR, Vittone JL, Bigelow ML, et al. Impact of aerobic exercise training on age-related changes in insulin sensitivity and muscle oxidative capacity. Diabetes 2003;52:1888–96; with permission).

mitochondrial function (ie, PGC-1α) and mitochondrial gene transcription, however, remains undefined.

Reversal of sarcopenia

Given the morbidity associated with sarcopenia, prevention and treatment of sarcopenia are areas of intense interest. Considerable evidence supports the decline of physical activity [45] and testosterone levels [46–48] with aging. Consequently, efforts to counteract age-related sarcopenia have focused on these two areas.

Reversal of sarcopenia with exercise

The effects of physical activity on muscle mass and function are highly variable. Although aerobic activity promotes cardiovascular fitness and improves endurance capacity, muscle mass accumulation appears minimal [49–51]. Recently, Short and colleagues [6,38] studied the effects of aerobic exercise on muscle metabolism on 78 healthy, previously untrained subjects (ages 19–87 years) before and after 4 months of bicycle training (up to 45 minutes at 80% peak heart rate, 3–4 days per week) or placebo (flexibility training). At baseline, an age-associated decline in mixed muscle protein synthesis (3.5% per decade, $P < 0.05$), fat-free mass (3% per decade, $P < 0.001$), resting metabolic rate (2.5% per decade, $P < 0.01$), whole body protein turnover (4%–5% per decade, $P < 0.001$), whole body protein synthesis (4%–5% per baseline, $P < 0.001$) and muscle mitochondrial enzyme activity (cytochrome c oxidase: 5% per decade, $P < 0.025$) were seen. Aerobic exercise training increased VO2 max (9.5%, $P < 0.001$), muscle mitochondrial enzyme activity (citrate synthase 46%, $P < 0.001$; cytochrome c oxidase 87%, $P < 0.001$), muscle mitochondrial mRNA levels (COX4 by 67%, $P < 0.001$; ND4 by 63%, $P < 0.001$), muscle mitochondrial biogenesis mRNA levels (PGC-1α by 55%, $P < 0.001$; NRF-1 by 15%, $P < 0.02$; TFAM by 85%, $P < 0.001$) and mixed muscle protein synthesis (22%, $P < 0.05$) [6,38]. Fat-free mass, whole body protein turnover, and resting metabolic rates were not changed by training. The lack of change in whole body protein turnover was likely caused by the contributions from multiple body protein pools reducing the sensitivity in detecting small increases in leg muscle protein synthesis. An age effect was not observed on the training-induced increase in VO2 max and mixed muscle protein synthesis [6]. The authors demonstrated aerobic exercise increasing muscle protein synthesis regardless of age (Fig. 6). In addition, the authors [38] also demonstrated 4 months of aerobic exercise improving insulin sensitivity (measured 4 days after the last exercise bout) in young people but not in older people (Fig. 7). These studies demonstrate that improvements in muscle mitochondrial function and insulin sensitivity can be disassociated.

Substantial evidence supports resistance training building and maintaining muscle size and strength [49,50]. In particular, resistance exercise has been shown to increase muscle protein synthesis rates in the elderly [28,36,52,53]. Even within 3 hours after resistance exercise, increased muscle protein turnover can be observed. Increased transport of amino acids (leucine, lysine, alanine; $P < 0.05$) into muscle cells is the reported reason for the relatively greater stimulation of protein synthesis compared with protein breakdown [54]. Studies of short-term resistance exercise (~2 weeks) demonstrate age-independent increases in MHC and mixed muscle protein synthesis rates [36,52]. Balagopal and colleagues [28] performed one of the largest studies on the effects of resistance exercise on protein metabolism. Nineteen middle-aged subjects (52 ± 0.8 years) and 20 older subjects (71 ± 1 year) underwent 3 months of resistance training versus nonintervention. At baseline, an age-associated decline in MHC-IIa mRNA and MHC-IIx mRNA was observed. Exercise increased the FSR of MHC (47%, $P < 0.01$) and mixed muscle protein (56%, $P < 0.05$) (Fig. 8); these responses to exercise were age-independent.

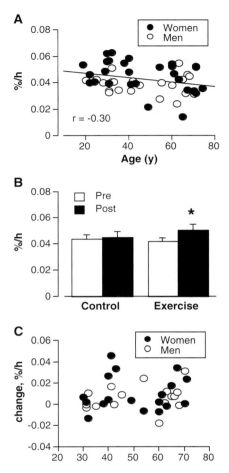

Fig. 6. Effects of age and aerobic exercise training on FSRs of mixed muscle protein. (*A*) shows baseline decline of muscle protein synthesis rate with age. (*B*) shows exercise increasing muscle protein synthesis by 22%. *$P < 0.05$, whereas there was no change in the control group. (*C*) shows the change in muscle protein synthesis rate did not vary with age and was gender-independent. (*From* Short KR, Vittone JL, Bigelow ML, et al. Age and aerobic exercise training effects on whole body and muscle protein metabolism. Am J Physiol Endocrinol Metab 2004;286(1):E92–101; with permission.)

Concurrently, exercise training increased MHC-I mRNA transcript levels (85%, $P < 0.01$) and further decreased mRNA transcript levels of MHC-IIa ($P < 0.04$) and MHC-IIx ($P < 0.01$) (Fig. 9). For the elderly, resistance training improves muscle strength and increases MHC production, although not all MHC isoforms are affected equally. It remains to be determined whether a regular exercise program involving both aerobic and resistance training will prevent or reverse age-related sarcopenia and its subsequent metabolic and functional consequences.

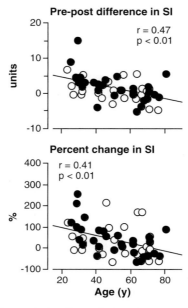

Fig. 7. Effects of age on changes in insulin sensitivity after 4 months of aerobic exercise. The absolute gain in insulin sensitivity with aerobic exercise (SI, measured by intravenous glucose tolerance test: $10^{-5}*min^{-1}*pmoL^{-1}*L^{-1}$) was related inversely to age (*upper panel*, regression line for entire population shown) and persisted when accounting for gender (*closed circles*, women; *open circles*, men). The percent change in SI (*lower panel*, regression line for entire group) also was related inversely to age. When genders were considered separately, women had a significant age-related effect (r = 0.61, $P < 0.01$) but not men (r = 0.16, $P > 0.05$). (*From* Short KR, Vittone JL, Bigelow ML, et al. Impact of aerobic exercise training on age-related changes in insulin sensitivity and muscle oxidative capacity. Diabetes 2003;52:1888–96; with permission).

Reversal of sarcopenia with testosterone supplementation

As aging is associated with sarcopenia, the relationship of hypoandrogenism to sarcopenia remains a key question. Specifically for men, the rationale and effects of testosterone therapy in muscle metabolism remains highly controversial.

Several measures of testosterone exist. Testosterone is bound primarily to sex hormone-binding globulin (SHBG) (50%) but also may be bound to albumin or other proteins. Non–SHBG-bound testosterone, bioavailable testosterone, and non–protein-bound, free testosterone have been considered important indicators of testosterone action, reflecting a hormone that is readily available for cellular membrane passage and nuclear binding. Bioavailable testosterone may be measured by direct assay [55] or by estimation [56]. Likewise, free testosterone may be measured by direct assay [57] or by estimation [56]. Although total testosterone levels remain fairly constant with age, the age-related decline of free testosterone and non-SHBG testosterone is well documented [46–48]. The normal range for serum total

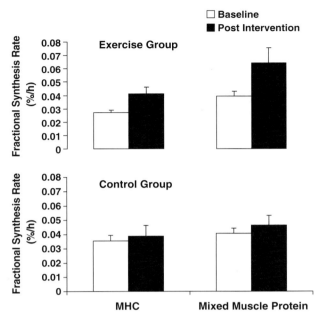

Fig. 8. Effects of resistance exercise (versus control) on the FSR of muscle MHC and mixed muscle protein synthesis in 39 subjects (aged 46–79 years). Exercise increases FSR of MHC ($P < 0.05$) and FSR of mixed muscle protein ($P < 0.05$). (*From* Balagopal P, Schimke JC, Ades P, et al. Age effect on transcript levels and synthesis rate of muscle MHC and response to resistance exercise. Am J Physiol Endocrinol Metab 2001;280(2):E203–8; with permission.)

testosterone in young healthy men (ages 20–40 years) is approximately 300 ng/dL to 1000 ng/dL. Total testosterone levels less than 200 ng/dL generally have been acknowledged as definitively hypogonadal, whereas total testosterone levels greater than 400 ng/dL indicate a very low likelihood of testosterone deficiency [58]. For the male with total testosterone levels between 200 and 400 ng/dL, the diagnosis of androgen deficiency is contingent on the presence of hypogonadism-associated clinical features (Box 1). The Massachusetts Male Aging Study [59] combined testosterone levels and clinical features as criteria to define androgen deficiency and reported an overall prevalence of 12.3% in men ages 48 to 79 years. Using biochemical measures to define testosterone deficiency, Harman and colleagues [46] studied 890 men longitudinally and measured total testosterone and SHBG by radioimmunoassay (RIA). Using total testosterone criteria (total testosterone < 11.3 nmol/L) to define hypogonadism, the study reported the incidence of hypogonadal testosterone levels increasing from 19% in men over age 60 to 49% in men over age 80. Using free testosterone index criteria (free T index < 0.153 nmol/nmol), the study reported the incidence of hypogonadism increasing from 34% in men over age 60 to 91% in men over age 80 [46].

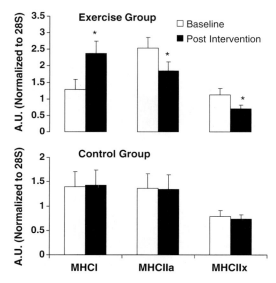

Fig. 9. mRNA response of MHC isoforms to resistance exercise expressed in AU after normalization to 28S rRNA. MHC-I increased after 3 months of resistance exercise ($P < 0.01$), whereas MHC-IIa ($P < 0.04$) and MHC-IIx ($P < 0.01$) decreased after exercise. The control group showed no change in mRNA levels of all MHC isoforms measured. (*From* Balagopal P, Schimke JC, Ades P, et al. Age effect on transcript levels and synthesis rate of muscle MHC and response to resistance exercise. Am J Physiol Endocrinol Metab 2001;280(2):E203–8; with permission.)

Several cross-sectional studies have looked at the specific hypogonadism/sarcopenia relationship. One cross-sectional study of 403 elderly men (mean age 77.8 years) specifically looked for physiological correlates with sarcopenia and found a positive association with non-SHBG testosterone/free testosterone with muscle strength and a negative association of non-SHBG

Box 1. Signs and symptoms of testosterone deficiency in men

Depressed mood
Decreased libido/sexual function/erectile dysfunction
Decreased energy
Decreased strength
Sleep disturbance
Irritability
Sarcopenia
Osteopenia
Decreased hematocrit/Hgb
Regression of secondary sexual characteristics
Decreased memory and/or cognitive function?

testosterone/free testosterone with fat mass [47]. Another cross-sectional study of 845 men (mean age 64 ± 8 years) reported a positive correlation between calculated free testosterone and appendicular skeletal muscle [8]. A positive relationship between free testosterone levels and skeletal muscle MHC synthesis has been observed [29].

Testosterone's direct effects on muscle physiology have been studied with several therapy regimens. Strong evidence exists for testosterone therapy's anabolic ability. Initially, it was demonstrated that testosterone administration in euchnoid men and normal men reduced urinary nitrogen excretion [60]. More recent studies have shown testosterone therapy increasing fat-free mass (FFM) [61–67] and specifically increasing skeletal muscle mass [62,63,67]. Testosterone's increase of lean body mass appears dose-dependent [68]. Recently, Bhasin and colleagues demonstrated increasing serum testosterone from the hypogonadal range to the midnormal range increased FFM by 8% to 10% [62], with further gains in FFM (4.6%) and muscle mass (6.7%–11.8%) seen when supraphysiological testosterone was administered to eugonadal men [63]. Testosterone's effects on fat mass are more controversial, as fat mass reduction [64,67,69] and maintenance [61,62, 66,70] have been observed.

Supporting these observations, several studies have shown testosterone therapy increasing muscle protein synthesis [67,71,72]. One of the earliest studies involved testosterone replacement in five postpubertal hypogonadal men (3 mg/kg testosterone cypionate every 2 weeks). Body composition was measured by DXA and 48-hour urinary creatinine excretion. Muscle protein synthesis was measured by L-[1–carbon-13 (^{13}C)] leucine tracer incorporation into mixed muscle protein and myosin heavy chain. Studies were performed at baseline and 1 week after the last testosterone injection. After 6 months of testosterone therapy, the increase in FFM (average 15%, range 10%–22%, $P = 0.02$) and muscle mass (mean 20%, range 11%–32%, $P = 0.04$) was associated with an increase in the FSR of mixed skeletal muscle proteins (56%, $P = 0.015$) and a trend toward increase in myosin heavy chain (46%, $P = 0.098$) [67]. Another study performed in seven healthy young men also demonstrated short-term testosterone therapy increasing muscle protein synthesis. Upon completion of baseline measurements of muscle protein synthesis/breakdown, the subjects received 200 mg of testosterone enanthate. Five days later, repeat measurements were performed and showed a twofold increase in protein synthesis ($P < 0.05$), nonsignificant changes in protein breakdown, and cessation of the normal fasting-associated muscle protein breakdown [71]. Elderly men also have been shown to increase muscle protein synthesis in response to testosterone. Urban and colleagues studied six elderly men (67 ± SE 2) who received 100 mg of testosterone enanthate weekly for 4 weeks. One week after the last testosterone injection, muscle protein FSR was measured and demonstrated a twofold increase compared with baseline ($P \leq 0.04$) [72]. There are no long-term studies of testosterone replacement in which muscle protein synthesis has been measured, thus testosterone's effects on sustaining muscle protein synthesis are unknown. The long-term effects of testosterone on increasing FFM (1.5%–3.5%) [73,74] have been demonstrated in elderly men by means of DXA studies as shown in Table 1. Because of the limitations of DXA imaging, however, it remains uncertain whether these increases are caused by an accumulation of lean mass, water mass, or other nonfat mass. No long-term studies are available to determine if physiological testosterone administration clearly increases muscle mass by CSA imaging.

In contrast to the strong evidence for testosterone increasing muscle mass and muscle protein synthesis (mostly in younger people), there is conflicting evidence on testosterone's effects on muscle strength. A significant obstacle is the lack of a precise and accurate measure of muscle strength. The variability of muscle strength changes may be caused by several factors, including tested muscle group, measuring equipment, training effect, motivational effect, adequate blinding, and intrinsic intrasubject variation. Clague and colleagues [75] specifically looked at muscle function in 14 elderly men (mean 68.1 $\pm$ 6.6 SD) with low normal testosterone levels (11.3 nmol/L $\pm$ 1.7 SD) treated with testosterone enanthate (200 mg intramuscularly every 2 weeks) or placebo for 12 weeks. Compared with the placebo group, the testosterone-treated group tended to increase muscle strength as measured by handgrip, knee extension, knee flexion, and leg extension. These gains, however, were not significant because of marked measurement variability. The within-day coefficient of variation (CV%) was reported, with knee extension measured by isometric testing (CV% = 2.6%–5.3%), knee flexion measured by isometric testing (CV% = 3.3%–6.0%), handgrip measured by dynamometer (CV% = 3.3%–3.9%) and leg extension measured by the Nottingham power rig (CV% = 2.3%–5.5%) [75]. These findings temper the muscle strength increase reported by some [62,72,76,77], but not all studies [61,69,74,75].

Nevertheless, a common perception of testosterone increasing muscle mass and strength exists, a perception supported by androgen abuse allegations among professional and amateur athletes. Bhasin and colleagues [63] reported the effects of supraphysiological testosterone on muscle size and strength in normal men. Forty-three men were placed into one of four groups categorized by placebo/testosterone, and no-exercise/weight-lifting. A supraphysiological dose of testosterone enanthate (600 mg weekly) was administered for 10 weeks. With the exception of the placebo with no exercise group, the remaining groups demonstrated marked increases in FFM, muscle size (MRI cross-sectional measurement), and muscle strength (bench press). Specifically, the use of testosterone without exercise increased muscle size by 6.7% to 11.8%, FFM by 4.6%, and muscle strength by 9% to 12.6% compared with baseline values. The addition of weight-lifting exercise to the testosterone therapy further enhanced these gains [63].

Because of the increase of sarcopenia with age, elderly men have been the focus of multiple trials of testosterone replacement therapy [70,72–74,76,77].

Table 1
Evidence for testosterone replacement in elderly men

First author, year [Ref.]	Age at treatment ± SD (placebo ± SD)	Completed subjects/placebo	Treatment	Duration (mo)	Lean mass change (%)	Increased strength
Tenover, 1992 [70]	67.5 ± 1.5 y (67.5 ± 1.5 y)	13/13[a]	100 mg IM every wk	3	+3.2% hydrodensitometry	−
Morley, 1993 [77]	77.6 ± 2.3 y (76.0 ± 2.5 y)	8/6	200 mg IM every 2 wk	3	NM	+
Urban, 1995 [72]	67 ± 5 y	6/0	100 mg IM every wk	1	NM	+
Sih, 1997 [76]	65 ± 7 y (68 ± 6 y)	10/12	200 mg IM every 2 wk	12	NM	+
Wittert, 2003 [73]	69 ± 6 y (68 ± 5 y)	35/32	80 mg orally twice daily	12	+1.54% DXA	−
Snyder, 1999 [74]	> 65 y	50/46	Scrotal patch 6 mg/d	36	+3.5% DXA	−

Abbreviations: IM, intramuscular; NM, not measured.
[a] Crossover.

These studies are summarized in Table 1 [70,72–74,76,77]. Initially, several small, short-term studies reported testosterone replacement increasing strength [72,77] and lean body mass [70]. One longer-term study of 12 months in hypogonadal elderly men (mean age 65) treated with testosterone cypionate (200 mg intramuscularly every 2 weeks) reported a significant net positive change in handgrip strength. This study, however, was hampered by a 31% dropout rate, predominantly in the treatment group [76]. Snyder and colleagues [74] performed the largest and longest trial of testosterone replacement in elderly men. One hundred eight elderly men with low normal testosterone levels (total testosterone 367 ± 79 ng/dL) were randomized to receive either placebo or testosterone scrotal patch (~ 6 mg/d) for 3 years. Ninety-six patients completed the entire protocol. Body fat composition was measured by DXA. Testosterone therapy decreased body fat mass (12.3%, $P = 0.001$) and increased only truncal lean mass (3.5%, $P < 0.001$). The lack of increase in appendicular lean mass also was associated with the lack of strength increase in knee extension/flexion or handgrip [74]. The lack of strength change as reported by Snyder and colleagues versus earlier studies may be caused by several factors. Study design may be a factor, as the earlier studies were hampered by unclear randomization [77], absent controls [72], and high dropout [76]. Compared with the earlier studies using intramuscular testosterone injections, Snyder's use of the testosterone patch allows a more continuous administration of testosterone, which may affect muscle protein synthesis. Lastly, the variability associated with strength measurement may obscure small changes in strength. These same reasons also may explain Wittert and colleagues' 1-year study [73] of oral testosterone supplementation reporting no effects on strength.

Summary

Sarcopenia is a common consequence of aging, with onset as early as the fourth decade. The decline in muscle strength is approximately 1% per year and is associated with loss of muscle mass and decreased muscle quality. At the cellular level, this loss of muscle function is associated with declines in muscle protein synthesis and mitochondrial capacity. Resistance strength training has the most substantive evidence in reversing sarcopenia, although aerobic exercise may also be beneficial. Both resistance and aerobic exercise enhance mixed muscle protein synthesis, although resistance training has a more profound stimulatory effect. It is likely that different exercise regimens may have distinctive effects on particular muscle proteins, suggesting the importance of variety in exercise. Although increased age and declining muscle function are associated with decreased testosterone levels in men, the role of testosterone supplementation remains controversial. Strong evidence exists for testosterone increasing muscle mass and muscle protein synthesis. Yet, a clear increase of muscle strength in elderly people by testosterone has not been observed, an observation vulnerable to confounding factors and experimental design. Much has been accomplished in studying the patho-physiology behind sarcopenia. Much still remains in altering its course.

References

[1] Tinetti ME, Speechley M. Prevention of falls among the elderly. N Engl J Med 1989;320(16): 1055–9.

[2] Wolfson L, Judge J, Whipple R, et al. Strength is a major factor in balance, gait, and the occurrence of falls. J Gerontol A Biol Sci Med Sci 1995;50:64–7.

[3] Herndon LA, Schmeissner PJ, Dudaronek JM, et al. Stochastic and genetic factors influence tissue-specific decline in ageing C. elegans. Nature 2002;419(6909):808–14.

[4] Forbes GB, Reina JC. Adult lean body mass declines with age: some longitudinal observations. Metabolism 1970;19(9):653–63.

[5] Kehayias JJ, Fiatarone MA, Zhuang H, et al. Total body potassium and body fat: relevance to aging. Am J Clin Nutr 1997;66(4):904–10.

[6] Short KR, Vittone JL, Bigelow ML, et al. Age and aerobic exercise training effects on whole body and muscle protein metabolism. Am J Physiol Endocrinol Metab 2004;286(1): E92–101.

[7] Melton LJ 3rd, Khosla S, Riggs BL. Epidemiology of sarcopenia. Mayo Clin Proc 2000;75: S10–2.

[8] Szulc P, Duboeuf F, Marchand F, et al. Hormonal and lifestyle determinants of appendicular skeletal muscle mass in men: the MINOS study. Am J Clin Nutr 2004;80(2): 496–503.

[9] Proctor DN, O'Brien PC, Atkinson EJ, et al. Comparison of techniques to estimate total body skeletal muscle mass in people of different age groups. Am J Physiol 1999;277:E489–95.

[10] Lexell J, Taylor CC, Sjostrom M. What is the cause of the ageing atrophy? Total number, size, and proportion of different fiber types studied in whole vastus lateralis muscle from 15- to 83-year-old men. J Neurol Sci 1988;84:275–94.

[11] Lexell J, Henriksson-Larsen K, Winblad B, et al. Distribution of different fiber types in human skeletal muscles: effects of aging studied in whole muscle cross sections. Muscle Nerve 1983;6(8):588–95.

[12] Lindle RS, Metter EJ, Lynch NA, et al. Age and gender comparisons of muscle strength in 654 women and men aged 20–93 yr. J Appl Physiol 1997;83(5):1581–7.

[13] Lynch NA, Metter EJ, Lindle RS, et al. Muscle quality. I. Age-associated differences between arm and leg muscle groups. J Appl Physiol 1999;86(1):188–94.

[14] Kallman DA, Plato CC, Tobin JD. The role of muscle loss in the age-related decline of grip strength: cross-sectional and longitudinal perspectives. J Gerontol 1990;45(3):M82–8.

[15] Hughes VA, Frontera WR, Wood M, et al. Longitudinal muscle strength changes in older adults: influence of muscle mass, physical activity, and health. J Gerontol A Biol Sci Med Sci 2001;56(5):B209–17.

[16] Aniansson A, Hedberg M, Henning GB, et al. Muscle morphology, enzymatic activity, and muscle strength in elderly men: a follow-up study. Muscle Nerve 1986;9(7):585–91.

[17] Rantanen T, Masaki K, Foley D, et al. Grip strength changes over 27 yr in Japanese American men. J Appl Physiol 1998;85(6):2047–53.

[18] Frontera WR, Hughes VA, Fielding RA, et al. Aging of skeletal muscle: a 12-yr longitudinal study. J Appl Physiol 2000;88(4):1321–6.

[19] Metter EJ, Lynch N, Conwit R, et al. Muscle quality and age: cross-sectional and longitudinal comparisons. J Gerontol A Biol Sci Med Sci 1999;54(5):B207–18.

[20] Frontera WR, Hughes VA, Lutz KJ, et al. A cross-sectional study of muscle strength and mass in 45- to 78-yr-old men and women. J Appl Physiol 1991;71(2):644–50.

[21] Frontera WR, Suh D, Krivickas LS, et al. Skeletal muscle fiber quality in older men and women. Am J Physiol Cell Physiol 2000;279(3):C611–8.

[22] Reed RL, Pearlmutter L, Yochum K, et al. The relationship between muscle mass and muscle strength in the elderly. J Am Geriatr Soc 1991;39(6):555–61.

[23] Larsson L, Li X, Frontera WR. Effects of aging on shortening velocity and myosin isoform composition in single human skeletal muscle cells. Am J Physiol 1997;272:C638–49.

[24] Overend TJ, Cunningham DA, Paterson DH, et al. Thigh composition in young and elderly men determined by computed tomography. Clin Physiol 1992;12(6):629–40.

[25] Balice-Gordon RJ. Age-related changes in neuromuscular innervation. Muscle Nerve Suppl 1997;5:S83–7.

[26] Coggan AR, Spina RJ, King DS, et al. Histochemical and enzymatic comparison of the gastrocnemius muscle of young and elderly men and women. J Gerontol 1992;47(3):B71–6.

[27] Klitgaard H, Mantoni M, Schiaffino S, et al. Function, morphology and protein expression of ageing skeletal muscle: a cross-sectional study of elderly men with different training backgrounds. Acta Physiol Scand 1990;140(1):41–54.

[28] Balagopal P, Schimke JC, Ades P, et al. Age effect on transcript levels and synthesis rate of muscle MHC and response to resistance exercise. Am J Physiol Endocrinol Metab 2001; 280(2):E203–8.

[29] Balagopal P, Rooyackers OE, Adey DB, et al. Effects of aging on in vivo synthesis of skeletal muscle myosin heavy-chain and sarcoplasmic protein in humans. Am J Physiol 1997;273: E790–800.

[30] Rooyackers OE, Adey DB, Ades PA, et al. Effect of age on in vivo rates of mitochondrial protein synthesis in human skeletal muscle. Proc Natl Acad Sci USA 1996;93(26):15364–9.

[31] Trounce I, Byrne E, Marzuki S. Decline in skeletal muscle mitochondrial respiratory chain function: possible factor in ageing. Lancet 1989;1(8639):637–9.

[32] Short KR, Nair KS. Mechanisms of sarcopenia of aging. J Endocrinol Invest 1999; 22(Suppl 5):95–105.

[33] Nair KS. Muscle protein turnover: methodological issues and the effect of aging. J Gerontol A Biol Sci Med Sci 1995;50:107–12.

[34] Nair KS, Halliday D, Griggs RC. Leucine incorporation into mixed skeletal muscle protein in humans. Am J Physiol 1988;254:E208–13.

[35] Tipton KD, Wolfe RR. Exercise, protein metabolism, and muscle growth. Int J Sport Nutr Exerc Metab 2001;11(1):109–32.

[36] Yarasheski KE, Zachwieja JJ, Bier DM. Acute effects of resistance exercise on muscle protein synthesis rate in young and elderly men and women. Am J Physiol 1993;265:E210–4.

[37] Welle S, Thornton C, Jozefowicz R, et al. Myofibrillar protein synthesis in young and old men. Am J Physiol 1993;264:E693–8.

[38] Short KR, Vittone JL, Bigelow ML, et al. Impact of aerobic exercise training on age-related changes in insulin sensitivity and muscle oxidative capacity. Diabetes 2003;52(8):1888–96.

[39] Volpi E, Sheffield-Moore M, Rasmussen BB, et al. Basal muscle amino acid kinetics and protein synthesis in healthy young and older men. JAMA 2001;286(10):1206–12.

[40] Yarasheski KE, Welle S, Sreekumaran Nair K. Muscle protein synthesis in younger and older men. JAMA 2002;287(3):317–8.

[41] Russ DW, Kent-Braun JA. Is skeletal muscle oxidative capacity decreased in old age? Sports Med 2004;34(4):221–9.

[42] Melov S, Shoffner JM, Kaufman A, et al. Marked increase in the number and variety of mitochondrial DNA rearrangements in aging human skeletal muscle [erratum appears in Nucleic Acids Res 1995;23(23):4938]. Nucleic Acids Res 1995;23(20):4122–6.

[43] Shigenaga MK, Hagen TM, Ames BN. Oxidative damage and mitochondrial decay in aging. Proc Natl Acad Sci USA 1994;91(23):10771–8.

[44] Barazzoni R, Short KR, Nair KS. Effects of aging on mitochondrial DNA copy number and cytochrome c oxidase gene expression in rat skeletal muscle, liver, and heart. J Biol Chem 2000;275(5):3343–7.

[45] DiPietro L. Physical activity in aging: changes in patterns and their relationship to health and function. J Gerontol A Biol Sci Med Sci 2001;56:13–22.

[46] Harman SM, Metter EJ, Tobin JD, et al. Longitudinal effects of aging on serum total and free testosterone levels in healthy men. Baltimore Longitudinal Study of Aging. J Clin Endocrinol Metab 2001;86(2):724–31.

[47] van den Beld AW, de Jong FH, Grobbee DE, et al. Measures of bioavailable serum testosterone and estradiol and their relationships with muscle strength, bone density, and body composition in elderly men. J Clin Endocrinol Metab 2000;85(9):3276–82.

[48] Ferrini RL, Barrett-Connor E. Sex hormones and age: a cross-sectional study of testosterone and estradiol and their bioavailable fractions in community-dwelling men. Am J Epidemiol 1998;147(8):750–4.

[49] Hurley BF, Hagberg JM. Optimizing health in older persons: aerobic or strength training? Exer Sport Sci Rev 1998;26:61–89.

[50] Rogers MA, Evans WJ. Changes in skeletal muscle with aging: effects of exercise training. Exer Sport Sci Rev 1993;21:65–102.

[51] Meredith CN, Frontera WR, Fisher EC, et al. Peripheral effects of endurance training in young and old subjects. J Appl Physiol 1989;66(6):2844–9.

[52] Hasten DL, Pak-Loduca J, Obert KA, et al. Resistance exercise acutely increases MHC and mixed muscle protein synthesis rates in 78–84 and 23–32-yr-olds. Am J Physiol Endocrinol Metab 2000;278(4):E620–6.

[53] Yarasheski KE, Zachwieja JJ, Campbell JA, et al. Effect of growth hormone and resistance exercise on muscle growth and strength in older men. Am J Physiol 1995;268(2 Pt 1): E268–76.

[54] Biolo G, Maggi SP, Williams BD, et al. Increased rates of muscle protein turnover and amino acid transport after resistance exercise in humans. Am J Physiol 1995;268:E514–20.

[55] Cumming DC, Wall SR. Nonsex hormone-binding globulin-bound testosterone as a marker for hyperandrogenism. J Clin Endocrinol Metab 1985;61(5):873–6.

[56] Vermeulen A, Verdonck L, Kaufman JM. A critical evaluation of simple methods for the estimation of free testosterone in serum. J Clin Endocrinol Metab 1999;84(10):3666–72.

[57] Vermeulen A, Stoica T, Verdonck L. The apparent free testosterone concentration, an index of androgenicity. J Clin Endocrinol Metab 1971;33(5):759–67.

[58] The Endocrine Society. Summary from the 2nd Annual Andropause Consensus Meeting. Chevy Chase (MD): The Endocrine Society; 2001.

[59] Araujo AB, O'Donnell AB, Brambilla DJ, et al. Prevalence and incidence of androgen deficiency in middle-aged and older men: estimates from the Massachusetts Male Aging Study. J Clin Endocrinol Metab 2004;89(12):5920–6.

[60] Kenyon AT, Knowlton K, Sandiford I, et al. A comparative study of the metabolic effects of testosterone propionate in normal men and women and in eunuchoidism. Endocrinology 1940;26:26–45.

[61] Snyder PJ, Peachey H, Berlin JA, et al. Effects of testosterone replacement in hypogonadal men. J Clin Endocrinol Metab 2000;85(8):2670–7.

[62] Bhasin S, Storer TW, Berman N, et al. Testosterone replacement increases fat-free mass and muscle size in hypogonadal men. J Clin Endocrinol Metab 1997;82(2):407–13.

[63] Bhasin S, Storer TW, Berman N, et al. The effects of supraphysiologic doses of testosterone on muscle size and strength in normal men. N Engl J Med 1996;335(1):1–7.

[64] Katznelson L, Finkelstein JS, Schoenfeld DA, et al. Increase in bone density and lean body mass during testosterone administration in men with acquired hypogonadism. J Clin Endocrinol Metab 1996;81(12):4358–65.

[65] Wang C, Swedloff RS, Iranmanesh A, et al. Transdermal testosterone gel improves sexual function, mood, muscle strength, and body composition parameters in hypogonadal men. Testosterone Gel Study Group. J Clin Endocrinol Metab 2000;85(8):2839–53.

[66] Wang C, Eyre DR, Clark R, et al. Sublingual testosterone replacement improves muscle mass and strength, decreases bone resorption, and increases bone formation markers in hypogonadal men—a clinical research center study. J Clin Endocrinol Metab 1996;81(10): 3654–62.

[67] Brodsky IG, Balagopal P, Nair KS. Effects of testosterone replacement on muscle mass and muscle protein synthesis in hypogonadal men—a clinical research center study. J Clin Endocrinol Metab 1996;81(10):3469–75.

[68] Forbes GB. The effect of anabolic steroids on lean body mass: the dose response curve. Metabolism 1985;34(6):571–3.

[69] Wang C, Cunningham G, Dobs A, et al. Long-term testosterone gel (AndroGel) treatment maintains beneficial effects on sexual function and mood, lean and fat mass, and bone mineral density in hypogonadal men. J Clin Endocrinol Metab 2004;89(5):2085–98.

[70] Tenover JS. Effects of testosterone supplementation in the aging male. J Clin Endocrinol Metab 1992;75(4):1092–8.

[71] Ferrando AA, Tipton KD, Doyle D, et al. Testosterone injection stimulates net protein synthesis but not tissue amino acid transport. Am J Physiol 1998;275:E864–71.

[72] Urban RJ, Bodenburg YH, Gilkison C, et al. Testosterone administration to elderly men increases skeletal muscle strength and protein synthesis. Am J Physiol 1995;269:E820–6.

[73] Wittert GA, Chapman IM, Haren MT, et al. Oral testosterone supplementation increases muscle and decreases fat mass in healthy elderly males with low-normal gonadal status. J Gerontol A Biol Sci Med Sci 2003;58(7):618–25.

[74] Snyder PJ, Peachey H, Hannoush P, et al. Effect of testosterone treatment on body composition and muscle strength in men over 65 years of age. J Clin Endocrinol Metab 1999;84(8): 2647–53.

[75] Clague JE, Wu FC, Horan MA. Difficulties in measuring the effect of testosterone replacement therapy on muscle function in older men. Int J Androl 1999;22(4):261–5.

[76] Sih R, Morley JE, Kaiser FE, et al. Testosterone replacement in older hypogonadal men: a 12-month randomized controlled trial. J Clin Endocrinol Metab 1997;82(6):1661–7.

[77] Morley JE, Perry HM 3rd, Kaiser FE, et al. Effects of testosterone replacement therapy in old hypogonadal males: a preliminary study. J Am Geriatr Soc 1993;41(2):149–52.

ELSEVIER
SAUNDERS

Endocrinol Metab Clin N Am
34 (2005) 853–864

ENDOCRINOLOGY
AND METABOLISM
CLINICS
OF NORTH AMERICA

Utility of Ultrasensitive Growth Hormone Assays in Assessing Aging-Related Hyposomatotropism

Ali Iranmanesh, MD[a,b,]*, Johannes D. Veldhuis, MD[c]

[a]*Endocrine Service, Medical Section Salem, Veterans Affairs Medical Center, Salem, VA, USA*
[b]*University of Virginia School of Medicine, Charlottesville, VA, USA*
[c]*Endocrine Research Unit, Department of Internal Medicine, Mayo School of Graduate Medical Education, General Clinical Research Center, Mayo Clinic, Rochester, MN, USA*

Growth hormone (GH) initially was measured by in vivo bioassays of skeletal growth. A hemagglutination–inhibition technique of Boyden was an early in vitro approach [1]. Albeit useful for detecting of GH in purified preparations or crude pituitary extracts, chemical interference imposed by globulins rendered this method unreliable for measuring serum GH concentrations in people. Development of the radioimmunoassay (RIA) allowed more accurate estimates of GH concentrations exceeding 0.4 µg/L [2]. RIAs thus permitted precise evaluation of disorders of GH excess. A typical early assay standard was purified cadaveric pituitary extracts, now replaced by recombinant human 22 kDa GH.

Expanded clinical and research interests in GH dynamics, aging, and hypopituitarism stimulated efforts to develop assays with greater low-end sensitivity. Radioimmunometric assays (IRMA) lowered the detection limit of GH to 0.1 µg/L. IRMA uses two antibodies, each directed to a distinct epitope of the GH molecule [3–5]. Monoclonal antibodies in two-site IRMAs reduced the problem of cross-reactivity with GH fragments and other peptides such as prolactin and somatomammotropin (placental lactogen) [6]. The high specificity of monoclonal antibodies to 22 kDa, however, limits detection of the minor (15%) 20 kDa GH variant [7].

* Corresponding author. Endocrine Service, Medical Section Salem, Veterans Administration Medical Center, 1970 Roanoke Boulevard, Salem, VA 24153.
E-mail address: ali.iranmanesh@med.va.gov (A. Iranmanesh).

0889-8529/05/$ - see front matter. Published by Elsevier Inc.
doi:10.1016/j.ecl.2005.07.005

The demand for more sensitive assays and the problem of radioactive waste disposal prompted the innovation of nonradioactive markers. Major advances in this area include assays based upon ELISA [8], immunofluorometry [9], and immunochemiluminometry [10]. In one ELISA system (Bioclone, Marrickville, Australia), monoclonal GH antibody was used to coat microtiter strips, and biotinylated polyclonal GH antiserum was added to the solution. A biotin–strepavidin capture strategy was used to recover the indicator antibody–antigen complex, and color was generated from peroxidase-catalyzed oxidation of o-phenylenediamine, yielding a sensitivity of 0.05 μg/L GH [8]. Sensitivity was enhanced further by adding GH standards at lower concentrations (0.025 to 0.001 μg/L), increasing the amount of serum added, and incorporating an 18-hour preincubation phase.

Immunofluorometric methodology is illustrated by a solid-phase sandwich assay (Wallac, Turku, Finland) that employs monoclonal antibodies to distinct antigenic loci on 22 kDa GH. Europium serves as the excitable-fluorescing molecule [9,11]. The resultant threshold is approximately 0.0115 μg/L. The utility of high-sensitivity immunofluorometry is illustrated in Fig. 1, in which GH secretion was quantitated accurately, albeit reduced

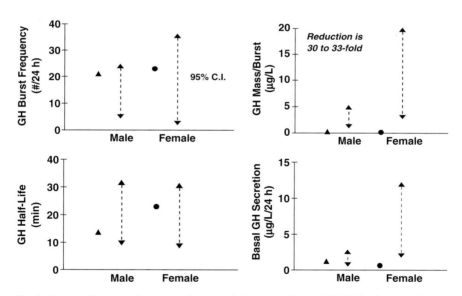

Fig. 1. Immunofluorometric assay and deconvolution analysis reveal 30-fold reductions in pulsatile (GH burst mass) and basal (nonpulsatile) GH secretion with normal GH pulse frequency and half-life in two patients with an inactivating mutation of the GHRH receptor. The solid triangle and circle identify data from the two patients, and vertical interrupted lines mark normal 95% confidence intervals. (*Data from* Roelfsema F, Biermasz NR, Veldman RG, et al. Growth hormone secretion in patients with an inactivating defect of the GH-releasing hormone receptor is pulsatile: evidence for a role for non-GHRH inputs in to the generation of GH pulses. J Clin Endocrinol Metab 2000;86:2459–64.)

by greater than 30-fold, in two patients with genetic truncation of the GH-releasing hormone (GHRH) receptor [12].

Chemiluminometric technology achieves high sensitivity, as indicated initially by the facile detection of GH concentrations as low as 0.02 µg/L (London Diagnostic, London). The commercial reagent was an acridinium ester, which emits light upon alkalinization and hydrolysis (Nichols Institute Diagnostic, San Juan Capistrano, California). The sandwich assay employed a monoclonal capture antibody immobilized on large polystyrene beads and polyclonal indicator antibodies labeled with acridinium ester. Washed GH-bound beads were placed in a luminometer unit designed to inject hydrogen peroxide and sodium hydroxide and quantitate photon emission over a 2-second interval. Raw output was reported in relative light units. Iranmanesh and colleagues modified the procedure by increasing sample volume and labeled antibody concentration, mixing on a rotator at room temperature for 6 hours, and incubating tubes overnight at room temperature, thereby conferring a detection limit of 0.002 to 0.005 µg/L [10,13,14]. The acridinium ester reagent was discontinued in 2003. A comparable dioxetane-based detector system is available, as illustrated in Fig. 2. The latter assay performs well in hyposomatotropic older individuals. Other chemiluminescent approaches achieve similar thresholds [15].

Automated random-access laboratory devices are used to measure multiple hormones, including GH [16,17]. In addition, immunofunctional and

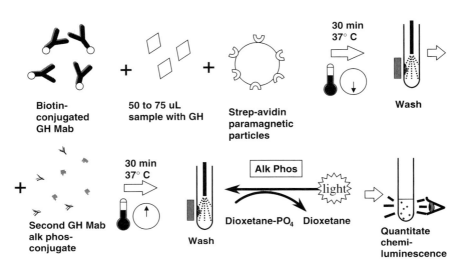

Fig. 2. Immunochemiluminescent GH assay using monoclonal antibodies (Mab) to distinct peptidyl epitopes. One Mab is conjugated to biotin (capture antibody) and the other to alkaline phosphatase (indicator antibody). Avidin-coated paramagnetic particles are used to recover biotinylated Mab bound to GH. Alkaline phosphatase conjugated to the second Mab hydrolyzes the chemiluminescent substrate, phosphorylated dioxetane, to release light. Detection sensitivity approaches 3 to 10 molecules per mL.

monoclonal GH isotype-specific assays have been validated [18,19]. The former monitors the apparent bioactivity of GH by requiring high-affinity association of GH with the cognate plasma-binding protein, whereas the latter detects desired GH isoforms such as placental-variant (GH-V) or 20 kDa GH.

Utility of ultrasensitive growth hormone assays

Dissecting growth hormone secretion and elimination

Normal aging in men and women is associated with a 2 to 30-fold fall in mean GH concentrations measured over 24 hours and following physiologic interventions (fasting, deep sleep, exercise) or pharmacologic stimuli (GHRH and GH-releasing peptide [GHRP], L-dopa, clonidine, propranolol, pyridostigmine, and L-arginine). In contrast, older adults maintain normal responses to either insulin-induced hypoglycemia or threefold combined infusion of GHRH, GHRP, and L-arginine [20–22]. Therefore, maximal somatotrope secretory capacity is preserved in healthy aging.

Understanding the mechanisms of attenuated GH release in healthy aging individuals has been challenging. In this regard, very low GH concentrations (GH less than 0.05) in the awake and fed state in older adults earlier precluded accurate estimates of pulsatile and basal (nonpulsatile) GH secretion. This issue is illustrated by comparing analyses of the same frequently sampled (10-min) 24-hour GH concentration time series by means of an ultrasensitive chemiluminescent assay (sensitivity 0.002 to 0.005 µg/L) and IRMA (sensitivity 0.08 to 0.10 µg/L) in 11 men, two of whom were overweight, three older than age 60, and two hypothyroid [10]. GH concentrations were measurable in all 1595 blood samples by chemiluminometry, whereas 22% to 98% of daytime specimens were undetectable in the IRMA. Deconvolution analysis of chemiluminescent-derived data established the GH secretion occurred in pulses in the awake and fed state in all subjects regardless of age, body mass index (BMI), and thyroid function. The same analysis applied to IRMA data underestimated secretory burst frequency and overestimated burst size by censoring smaller (undetectable) GH pulses, particularly in aging, hypothyroidism, and obesity [10]. The chemiluminescent assay and IRMA predicted comparable GH half-lives and 24-hour GH rhythms, because these measures depend primarily on detecting large GH pulses.

Increasing age is associated with greater relative adiposity, particularly in intra-abdominal visceral depots (eg, hepatic, mesenteric, perinephric regions). For unknown reasons, increased visceral fat represses GH output independently of age [23]. IRMA initially provided insights into possible mechanisms. In one analysis, obese compared with nonobese middle-aged men exhibited smaller GH secretory bursts, a shorter GH half-life, and fewer detectable GH peaks [24,25]. Subsequent chemiluminometric assay in comparable cohorts of men (age and BMI ranges 18 to 73 years and 18 to 39 kg/m^2, respectively) established that:

- There is no decline in GH pulse number in aging or obesity, thus illustrating failure of IRMA technology to identify low-amplitude pulses.
- Concentrations of GH remain detectable between consecutive bursts.
- GH release in both the day and night is predominantly pulsatile.
- Age, testosterone, and percentage body fat jointly determine GH concentrations.
- Pathophysiology specifically modulates the amount of GH released per burst rather than the number of pulses or basal (nonpulsatile) GH secretion [10,13,14].

Investigations in a heterogeneous cohort of 21 men disclosed three major determinants of daily GH production when assessed by chemilumometric assay. These were age, percentage body fat, and testosterone concentrations [10]. Percentage total body fat accounted for approximately 38% of the common variance in 24-hour mean GH concentrations. Comparisons among subjects in the low (12% to 23%), middle (24% to 31%), and high (31% to 47%) tertiles of percentage of body fat revealed that increasing adiposity markedly accentuates the negative association between pulsatile GH secretion and age and reduces the positive correlation between GH secretion and testosterone concentrations. Further analyses indicated that estradiol concentrations predict higher basal (nonpulsatile) GH secretion, especially in lean individuals, and the mass and frequency of GH secretory bursts both increase during

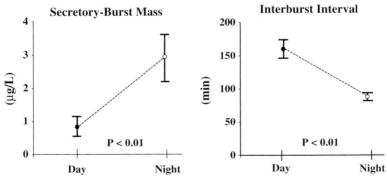

(chemiluminescence assay; N = 21 men)

Fig. 3. Day–night distinctions in pulsatile GH secretion assessed by ultrasensitive chemiluminescent assay in 21 men of varying ages. Secretory burst mass is the amount of GH released in each pulse. The interburst interval (min) is the algebraic reciprocal of frequency (ie, shorter intervals at night denote higher pulse frequency). (*Data from* Veldhuis JD, Liem AY, South S, et al. Differential impact of age, sex steroid hormones, and obesity on basal versus pulsatile growth hormone secretion in men as assessed in ultrasensitive chemiluminescence assay. J Clin Endocrinol Metab 1995;80:3209–22.)

the hours of sleep. Fig. 3 illustrates the day–night contrasts identifiable by high-sensitivity GH assay and recent analytical methods.

Pulsatile and basal modes of growth hormone release

Deconvolution analysis provides a means to quantitate secretion rates without infusing labeled compounds. The technology is applied to frequently sampled hormone concentrations to remove [deconvolve] the otherwise confounding effect of the elimination half-life on measured concentrations [26,27]. Deconvolution methods have unveiled that hormones enter the blood as discrete secretory events superimposed on continuous basal (time-invariant) secretion [28,29]. Distinguishing basal and pulsatile modes of GH secretion becomes important on analytical and physiologic grounds. For example, from an analytical vantage, basal GH release contributes to low daytime, postprandial interpulse GH concentrations that fall as low as 0.015 to 0.050 µg/L. From a physiologic perspective, basal GH availability mediates certain metabolic responses, such as down-regulation of drug-metabolizing enzymes or up-regulation of the hepatic low-density lipoprotein (LDL) receptor [30]. Analysis of the regulated number, amplitude and mass (size) of GH pulses affords indirect insights into how hypothalamic peptides signal to the pituitary gland. In a physiologic context, burst-like elevations in GH concentrations govern the expression of certain growth-related genes [30].

Basal and pulsatile GH secretions are not regulated identically in health or disease. For example, GH and insulin-like growth factor (IGF)-I negative feedback, somatostatin, and octreotide suppress, whereas IGF-I depletion and secretagogues like GHRP-2 and GHRH increase apparent basal GH secretion [31–36]. Fasting, GH secretagogues, puberty, estrogen, testosterone, and female gender amplify the size of GH pulses [11,37], whereas aging, obesity, hypopituitarism, GH and IGF-I feedback, somatostatin, and octreotide suppress GH secretory-burst mass [31–34,38–41]. According to such studies, variations in the amount of GH secreted in each pulse constitute the prime mechanism determining total GH production in healthy adults. Reproducibility analyses indicate that coefficients of variation are 12% to 18% for successive intraindividual estimates of 24-hour pulsatile GH secretion, the mass of GH secreted/burst, and the half-life of endogenous GH [42]. Accordingly, intergroup or interventional differences of at least 30% typically denote significant quantitative distinctions in GH output. Fig. 4 illustrates that the effect of age clearly exceeds this nominal threshold in a two-cohort comparison of GH secretion in young (younger than 30 years) and older (older than 60 years) men.

Orderliness of sample-by-sample growth hormone release

In addition to pulsatile and 24-hour rhythmic features, hormones are released with varying degrees of serial orderliness [43,44]. The sample-by-sample consistency of subpatterns of hormone secretion can be quantified by

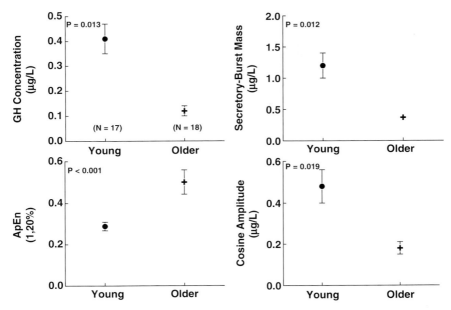

Fig. 4. Comparison of GH secretion in healthy young (N = 17) and older (N = 18) men. Panels (*clockwise*) depict mean 24-hour GH concentrations, GH secretory burst mass, GH ApEn (elevated values signify greater irregularity of GH release), and the amplitude of the 24-hour (cosine) rhythm. (Data compiled from unpublished series, J.D.H.)

means of the regularity statistic, approximate entropy (ApEn), wherein higher values denote reduced orderliness [45]. The orderliness of GH release is reproducible within 15% on consecutive days in healthy young individuals [14,42]. More irregular GH secretion patterns characterize aging, obesity, female gender, and autonomous neuroendocrine tumors [46–48]. Greater randomness of the GH release process is an important marker of altered ensemble control because of heightened feedforward (eg, unopposed GHRH or GHRP stimulation) or reduced negative feedback (GH and IGF-I depletion). In this regard, other investigations suggest that aging-related deterioration of orderly GH secretion (defined by elevated ApEn in Fig. 4) signifies combined defects in feedforward and feedback control.

Effects of secretagogues in age-related hyposomatotropism

Stimulatory or inhibitory interventions are used commonly in the functional assessment of various endocrine systems. The introduction of highly sensitive GH assays has permitted more accurate appraisal of the somatotropic axis in obesity, aging, and organic hyposomatotropism. For example, Friend and colleagues [49] explored the response of GH to putative withdrawal of somatostatin and stimulation of GHRH release induced by the drug pyridostigmine in men aged 29 to 77 years with BMIs of 21 to 47

kg/m^2. Increasing age and obesity singly and jointly reduced pulsatile GH secretion and disrupted orderly GH release. Neither regulatory defect was overcome by the indirect cholinergic agonist, consistent with multi-factorial pathophysiologies. To distinguish between the inferred contributions of GHRH deficiency and somatostatin excess, a comparable group of men received intravenous pulses of GHRH every 90 minutes for 3 days [14]. In this setting, greater age and body fat blunted, whereas higher testosterone concentrations enhanced, GHRH-stimulated GH secretion. The failure of the GHRH clamp to normalize GH pulse amplitude in aging individuals points to diminished GHRH action but does not exclude excessive somatostatin outflow (inhibitory) or deficient GHRP/ghrelin drive (amplifying).

Evidence for reduced GHRH outflow in older adults also was supported by an analysis of GH responses to a GHRH-receptor antagonist [50]. In addition, diminished pulsatile GH secretion in older men can be ameliorated significantly by administration of a high dose of GHRH (1 mg recombinant human peptide subcutaneously twice daily). The foregoing regimen doubled GH and IGF-I concentrations, reduced abdominal visceral fat mass, increased fat-free mass, and enhanced certain measures of physical performance over a 3-month trial [51].

The postulate that endogenous ghrelin/GHRP drive is impaired in healthy older subjects is consistent with the capability of continuous subcutaneous infusion of GHRP-2 to double pulsatile GH secretion and IGF-I concentrations over a 30-day interval in healthy elderly adults [52]. Other observations point to concomitant elevation of somatostatinergic inhibition in aging subjects. For example, GHRH and GHRP stimulation must be combined with pharmacologic reduction of somatostatin release to evoke maximal GH secretion in older volunteers [53]. Thus, available investigations predict tripartite mechanisms of impoverished GH output because of reduced GHRH and GHRP/ghrelin stimulation and heightened somatostatin inhibition.

Discrimination between hyposomatotropism of aging and organic growth hormone deficiency

The distinction between normal aging and organic GH deficiency is important, albeit difficult. The significance arises from the favorable body compositional effects of GH replacement in organically GH-deficient individuals [54–56]. A diagnostic challenge emerges, because integrated GH concentrations are of limited value in distinguishing between hypopituitarism and healthy aging [8,57]. For example, sensitive ELISA documented a 26% overlap between mean GH concentrations in patients with pituitary insufficiency and age-matched healthy subjects [8]. Immunofluorometric assay and deconvolution analysis revealed that organic pituitary disease decreases GH secretory burst amplitude and increases the irregularity of GH release more than aging, but with overlap [39,58]. For these reasons, from a pragmatic viewpoint, insulin-induced hypoglycemia remains a benchmark diagnostic test of GH sufficiency in elderly individuals [59].

Summary

Relative hyposomatotropism in aging is significant, inasmuch as organic GH deficiency and aging have considerable overlap in GH production and clinical phenotype. Ultrasensitive GH assays and biomathematical analyses have established that aging lowers GH concentrations by attenuating the size of GH secretory bursts. This mechanism is important, because pulsatile secretion comprises the predominant (greater than 85%) mode of GH output and correlates with growth and anabolism. Diminutive GH pulses in older adults appear to reflect reduced drive by GHRH and GHRP/ghrelin on the one hand and excessive inhibition by somatostatin on the other. Further studies will be required to identify the precise causes and consequences of GH depletion in various aging populations.

References

[1] Ferguson KA, Boyden SV. Serological evidence of the antigenicity of ox anterior pituitary growth hormone in sheep. J Endocrinol 1953;9:261–6.

[2] Utiger RD, Parker ML, Daughaday WH. Studies on human growth hormone. I. A radio-immunoassay for human growth hormone. J Clin Invest 1962;41:254–61.

[3] Blethen SL, Chasalow FI. Use of a two-site immunoradiometric assay for growth hormone (GH) in identifying children with GH-dependent growth failure. J Clin Endocrinol Metab 1983;57:1031–5.

[4] Iacobello C, Malvano R, Dotti C, et al. Evaluation of IRMA kits using monoclonal antibodies for growth hormone, prolactin and thyrotropin determinations. J Nucl Med Allied Sci 1984;28:271–6.

[5] Rose DP, Berke B, Cohen LA. Serum prolactin and growth hormone determined by radio-immunoassay and a two-site immunoradiometric assay: comparison with the Nb2 cell bioassay. Horm Metab Res 1988;20:49–53.

[6] Celniker AC, Chen AB, Wert RM Jr, et al. Variability in the quantitation of circulating growth hormone using commerical immunoassays. J Clin Endocrinol Metab 1989;68:469–76.

[7] Reiter EO, Morris AH, MacGillivray MH, et al. Variable estimates of serum growth hormone concentrations by different radioassay systems. J Clin Endocrinol Metab 1988;66:68–71.

[8] Reutens AT, Hoffman DM, Leung KC, et al. Evaluation and application of a highly sensitive assay for serum growth hormone (GH) in the study of adult GH deficiency. J Clin Endocrinol Metab 1995;80:480–5.

[9] Andersen M, Petersen PH, Blaabjerg O, et al. Evaluation of growth hormone assays using ratio plots. Clin Chem 1998;44:1032–8.

[10] Iranmanesh A, Grisso B, Veldhuis JD. Low basal and persistent pulsatile growth hormone secretion are revealed in normal and hyposomatotropic men studied with a new ultrasensitive chemiluminescence assay. J Clin Endocrinol Metab 1994;78:526–35.

[11] van den Berg G, Veldhuis JD, Frolich M, et al. An amplitude-specific divergence in the pulsatile mode of GH secretion underlies the gender difference in mean GH concentrations in men and premenopausal women. J Clin Endocrinol Metab 1996;81:2460–6.

[12] Roelfsema F, Biermasz NR, Veldman RG, et al. Growth hormone (GH) secretion in patients with an inactivating defect of the GH-releasing hormone (GHRH) receptor is pulsatile: evidence for a role for non-GHRH inputs into the generation of GH pulses. J Clin Endocrinol Metab 2000;86:2459–64.

[13] Veldhuis JD, Liem AY, South S, et al. Differential impact of age, sex-steroid hormones, and obesity on basal versus pulsatile growth hormone secretion in men as assessed in an ultrasensitive chemiluminescence assay. J Clin Endocrinol Metab 1995;80:3209–22.

[14] Iranmanesh A, South S, Liem AY, et al. Unequal impact of age, percentage body fat, and serum testosterone concentrations on the somatotrophic, IGF-I, and IGF-binding protein responses to a three-day intravenous growth hormone-releasing hormone pulsatile infusion in men. Eur J Endocrinol 1998;139:59–71.

[15] Strassburger CJ, Kohen F. Two-site and competitive chemiluminescent immunoassays. Methods Enzymol 1990;184:481–96.

[16] Veldhuis JD, Iranmanesh A, Mulligan T, et al. Disruption of the young-adult synchrony between luteinizing hormone release and oscillations in follicle-stimulating hormone, prolactin, and nocturnal penile tumescence (NPT) in healthy older men. J Clin Endocrinol Metab 1999;84:3498–505.

[17] Erickson D, Keenan DM, Mielke K, et al. Dual secretagogue drive of burst-like growth hormone secretion in postmenopausal compared with premenopausal women studied under an experimental estradiol clamp. J Clin Endocrinol Metab 2004;89:4746–54.

[18] Wu Z, Bidlingmaier M, Friess SC, et al. A new nonisotopic, highly sensitive assay for the measurement of human placental growth hormone: development and clinical implications. J Clin Endocrinol Metab 2003;88:804–11.

[19] Strassburger CJ, Wu Z, Pflaum CD, et al. Immunofunctional assay of human growth hormone (hGH) in serum: a possible consensus for quantitative hGH measurement. J Clin Endocrinol Metab 1996;81:2613.

[20] Dudl RJ, Ensinck JW, Palmer HE, et al. Effect of age on growth hormone secretion in man. J Clin Endocrinol Metab 1973;37:11–6.

[21] Finkelstein JW, Roffwarg HP, Boyar RM, et al. Age-related change in the twenty-four-hour spontaneous secretion of growth hormone. J Clin Endocrinol Metab 1972;35:665–70.

[22] Ghigo E, Goffi S, Arvat E, et al. Pyridostigmine partially restores the GH responsiveness to GHRH in normal aging. Acta Endocrinol (Copenh) 1990;123:169–74.

[23] Vahl N, Jorgensen JO, Skjaerback C, et al. Abdominal adiposity rather than age and sex predicts the mass and patterned regularity of growth hormone secretion in mid-life healthy adults. Am J Physiol 1997;272:E1108–16.

[24] Iranmanesh A, Lizarralde G, Veldhuis JD. Age and relative adiposity are specific negative determinants of the frequency and amplitude of growth hormone (GH) secretory bursts and the half-life of endogenous GH in healthy men. J Clin Endocrinol Metab 1991;73:1081–8.

[25] Veldhuis JD, Iranmanesh A, Ho KKY, et al. Dual defects in pulsatile growth hormone secretion and clearance subserve the hyposomatotropism of obesity in man. J Clin Endocrinol Metab 1991;72:51–9.

[26] Veldhuis JD, Carlson ML, Johnson ML. The pituitary gland secretes in bursts: appraising the nature of glandular secretory impulses by simultaneous multiple-parameter deconvolution of plasma hormone concentrations. Proc Natl Acad Sci U S A 1987;84:7686–90.

[27] Keenan DM, Roelfsema F, Biermasz N, et al. Physiological control of pituitary hormone secretory burst mass, frequency, and waveform: a statistical formulation and analysis. Am J Physiol 2003;285:R664–73.

[28] Keenan DM, Licinio J, Veldhuis JD. A feedback-controlled ensemble model of the stress-responsive hypothalamo-pituitary-adrenal axis. Proc Natl Acad Sci U S A 2001;98:4028–33.

[29] Keenan DM, Alexander SL, Irvine CHG, et al. Reconstruction of in vivo time-evolving neuroendocrine dose–response properties unveils admixed deterministic and stochastic elements in interglandular signaling. Proc Natl Acad Sci U S A 2004;101:6740–5.

[30] Giustina A, Veldhuis JD. Pathophysiology of the neuroregulation of growth hormone secretion in experimental animals and the human. Endocr Rev 1998;19:717–97.

[31] Calabresi E, Ishikawa E, Bartolini L, et al. Somatostatin infusion suppresses GH secretory burst number and mass in normal men: a dual mechanism of inhibition. Am J Physiol 1996; 270:E975–9.

[32] Shah N, Evans WS, Bowers CY, et al. Tripartite neuroendocrine activation of the human growth hormone (GH) axis in women by continuous 24-hour GH-releasing peptide (GHRP-2) infusion: pulsatile, entropic, and nyctohemeral mechanisms. J Clin Endocrinol Metab 1999;84:2140–50.

[33] Evans WS, Anderson SM, Hull LT, et al. Continuous 24-hour intravenous infusion of recombinant human growth hormone (GH)-releasing hormone-(1, 44)-amide augments pulsatile, entropic, and daily rhythmic GH secretion in postmenopausal women equally in the estrogen-withdrawn and estrogen-supplemented states. J Clin Endocrinol Metab 2001;86: 700–12.

[34] Veldhuis JD, Bidlingmaier M, Anderson SM, et al. Lowering total plasma insulin-like growth factor I concentrations by way of a novel, potent, and selective growth hormone (GH) receptor antagonist, pegvisomant (B2036-peg), augments the amplitude of GH secretory bursts and elevates basal/nonpulsatile GH release in healthy women and men. J Clin Endocrinol Metab 2001;86:3304–10.

[35] Veldhuis JD, Evans WS, Bowers CY. Impact of estradiol supplementation on dual peptidyl drive of growth-hormone secretion in postmenopausal women. J Clin Endocrinol Metab 2002;87:859–66.

[36] Veldhuis JD, Anderson SM, Kok P, et al. Estradiol supplementation modulates growth hormone (GH) secretory-burst waveform and recombinant human insulin-like growth factor-I-enforced suppression of endogenously driven GH release in postmenopausal women. J Clin Endocrinol Metab 2004;89:1312–8.

[37] Gentili A, Mulligan T, Godschalk M, et al. Unequal impact of short-term testosterone repletion on the somatotropic axis of young and older men. J Clin Endocrinol Metab 2002;87: 825–34.

[38] Bray MJ, Vick TM, Shah N, et al. Short-term estradiol replacement in postmenopausal women selectively mutes somatostatin's dose-dependent inhibition of fasting growth hormone secretion. J Clin Endocrinol Metab 2001;86:3143–9.

[39] Roelfsema F, Biermasz NR, Veldhuis JD. Pulsatile, nyctohemeral and entropic characteristics of GH secretion in adult GH-deficient patients: selectively decreased pulsatile release and increased secretory disorderliness with preservation of diurnal timing and gender distinctions. Clin Endocrinol (Oxf) 2002;56:79–87.

[40] Veldhuis JD, Evans WS, Bowers CY. Estradiol supplementation enhances submaximal feedforward drive of growth hormone (GH) secretion by recombinant human GH-releasing hormone-1,44-amide in a putatively somatostatin-withdrawn milieu. J Clin Endocrinol Metab 2003;88:5484–9.

[41] Veldhuis JD, Evans WS, Iranmanesh A, et al. Short-term testosterone supplementation relieves growth hormone autonegative feedback in men. J Clin Endocrinol Metab 2004;89: 1285–90.

[42] Friend K, Iranmanesh A, Veldhuis JD. The orderliness of the growth hormone (GH) release process and the mean mass of GH secreted per burst are highly conserved in individual men on successive days. J Clin Endocrinol Metab 1996;81:3746–53.

[43] Pincus SM. Irregularity and asynchrony in biologic network signals. Methods Enzymol 2000;321:149–82.

[44] Veldhuis JD, Straume M, Iranmanesh A, et al. Secretory process regularity monitors neuroendocrine feedback and feedforward signaling strength in humans. Am J Physiol 2001;280: R721–9.

[45] Pincus SM. Approximate entropy as a measure of system complexity. Proc Natl Acad Sci U S A 1991;88:2297–301.

[46] Hartman ML, Pincus SM, Johnson ML, et al. Enhanced basal and disorderly growth hormone secretion distinguish acromegalic from normal pulsatile growth hormone release. J Clin Invest 1994;94:1277–88.

[47] van den Berg G, Pincus SM, Veldhuis JD, et al. Greater disorderliness of ACTH and cortisol release accompanies pituitary-dependent Cushing's Disease. Eur J Endocrinol 1997;136: 394–400.

[48] Pincus SM, Mulligan T, Iranmanesh A, et al. Older males secrete luteinizing hormone and testosterone more irregularly, and jointly more asynchronously, than younger males. Proc Natl Acad Sci U S A 1996;93:14100–5.

[49] Friend K, Iranmanesh A, Login IS, et al. Pyridostigmine treatment selectively amplifies the mass of GH secreted per burst without altering the GH burst frequency, half-life, basal GH secretion or the orderliness of the GH release process. Eur J Endocrinol 1997;137:377–86.

[50] Russell-Aulet M, Jaffe CA, DeMott-Friberg R, et al. In vivo semiquantification of hypothalamic growth hormone-releasing hormone (GHRH) output in humans: evidence for relative GHRH deficiency in aging. J Clin Endocrinol Metab 1999;84:3490–7.

[51] Veldhuis JD, Patrie JT, Frick K, et al. Sustained GH and IGF-I responses to prolonged high-dose twice-daily GHRH stimulation in middle-aged and older men. J Clin Endocrinol Metab 2004;89:6325–30.

[52] Bowers CY, Granda R, Mohan S, et al. Sustained elevation of pulsatile growth hormone (GH) secretion and insulin-like growth factor I (IGF-I), IGF-binding protein-3 (IGFBP-3), and IGFBP-5 concentrations during 30-day continuous subcutaneous infusion of GH-releasing peptide-2 in older men and women. J Clin Endocrinol Metab 2004;89:2290–300.

[53] Arvat E, Ceda GP, Di Vito L, et al. Age-related variations in the neuroendocrine control, more than impaired receptor sensitivity, cause the reduction in the GH-releasing activity of GHRP's in human aging. Pituitary 1998;1:51–8.

[54] Jorgensen JO, Pedersen SA, Thuesen L, et al. Beneficial effects of growth hormone treatment in GH-deficient adults. Lancet 1989;1:1221–5.

[55] Salomon F, Cuneo RC, Hesp R, et al. The effects of treatment with recombinant human growth hormone on body composition and metabolism in adults with growth hormone deficiency. N Engl J Med 1989;321:1797–803.

[56] Bengtsson BA, Eden S, Lonn L, et al. Treatment of adults with growth hormone (GH) deficiency with recombinant human GH. J Clin Endocrinol Metab 1993;76:309–17.

[57] Hartman ML, Pezzoli SS, Hellmann PJ, et al. Pulsatile growth hormone secretion in older persons is enhanced by fasting without relationship to sleep stages. J Clin Endocrinol Metab 1996;81:2694–701.

[58] Reutens AT, Veldhuis JD, Hoffman DM, et al. A highly sensitive growth hormone (GH) ELISA uncovers increased contribution of a tonic mode of GH secretion in adults with organic GH deficiency. J Clin Endocrinol Metab 1996;81:1591–7.

[59] Greenwood FC, Landon J, Stamp TCB. The plasma sugar, free fatty acid, cortisol, and growth hormone response to insulin. I in control subjects. J Clin Invest 1966;45:429–36.

ELSEVIER
SAUNDERS

Endocrinol Metab Clin N Am
34 (2005) 865–876

ENDOCRINOLOGY
AND METABOLISM
CLINICS
OF NORTH AMERICA

Aging Somatotropic Axis: Mechanisms and Implications of Insulin-Like Growth Factor–Related Binding Protein Adaptation

Jan Frystyk, MD, PhD, DMSc*

Medical Research Laboratories, Aarhus University Hospital, Aarhus, Denmark

The insulin-like growth factor (IGF) system is considered to be the primary regulator of normal body growth and regeneration, affecting cell proliferation, differentiation and apoptosis, tissue growth, and various organ-specific functions [1,2]. In addition, the IGF system appears to have positive effects on insulin sensitivity and long-term glucose metabolism [3]. Not all effects of the IGF system appear to be beneficial, however, and numerous epidemiologic, experimental, and clinical data indicate that the IGF system is involved in the development of several common cancers [2,4–6] and frequent diseases such as atherosclerosis [7] and type 2 diabetes mellitus (T2DM) [8–10].

The IGF system is composed of a family of closely related peptides, including the two growth-promoting peptides, IGF-I and IGF-II, six specific high-affinity IGF-binding proteins (IGFBP-1 to -6), a large non–IGF-binding glycoprotein, which in contrast to the other components is acid labile, hence its name acid labile subunit (ALS), and several low-affinity IGFBP-related proteins (IGFBP-rPs) [1,11,12]. IGF-I is considered to be the most important member of the IGF system, and it exerts is biologic effects through activation of the IGF-I receptor (IGF-IR), which belongs to a family of cell membrane-associated tyrosine kinase receptors [13]. The IGF-IR is expressed in virtually all cell types, and this may explain the multiple actions of the IGF system. The exact roles of IGF-II and its ubiquitously expressed receptor (the IGF-IIR, which also binds mannose-6-phosphate, albeit at another site) are much less

* Medical Research Laboratories, Aarhus University Hospital, Norrebrograde 44, 8000 Aarhus C, Denmark.
E-mail address: jan@frystyk.dk

0889-8529/05/$ - see front matter © 2005 Elsevier Inc. All rights reserved.
doi:10.1016/j.ecl.2005.07.001

understood. It generally is believed that IGF-II is involved in intrauterine growth, and in tumorigenesis in adults. The effects of IGF-II, however, appear to be mediated though cross-reaction with the IGF-IR or the type A isoform of the insulin receptor (IR), which both bind IGF-II with considerably affinity. No intracellular signal has been observed following activation of the IGF-IIR. On the other hand, through clearance of IGF-II, the IGF-IIR may serve as a tumor suppressor [2,14–16].

The liver is the primary source of the circulating IGF system, and the blood stream contains the highest concentrations of all of the members of the IGF system. Virtually all cell types, however, are capable to synthesize IGF-I and –II, and therefore it is debatable whether the IGF system exerts its biologic effects through endocrine or paracrine/autocrine mechanisms. Numerous human and experimental in vivo studies have shown that IGF-I is able to act through endocrine mechanisms [17]. Recent experimental studies in knock-out (KO) mice devoid of the hepatic production of IGF-I suggest that the IGF-I–dependent growth is maintained primarily through paracrine/autocrine mechanisms, however. This hypothesis has been supported by a case report describing an individual with genetic ALS-deficiency [18,19]. Because of ALS deficiency, the patient had very low levels of circulating IGF-I, and although he suffered from a delayed onset and progress of puberty, there was only minimal slowing of his linear growth [19]. Both KO mice and the patient who had ALS deficiency, however, showed increased serum growth hormone (GH) levels. This observation may be explained by a reduced feedback inhibition of the pituitary, caused by subnormal circulating IGF-I levels, and it is likely that this secondary hypersomatropinemia leads to a compensatory up-regulation of the paracrine/autocrine-dependent growth at the expense of endocrine-mediated effects, making an extrapolation of data to normal physiology difficult. On the other hand, there is little doubt that circulating IGF-I, and in particular free IGF-I, is an important regulator of pituitary GH secretion [20,21]. The problem of defining whether the IGF system mostly acts through endocrine or paracrine/autocrine pathways is complicated further by the presence of the high-affinity IGFBPs, which bind IGF-I and -II with an affinity equal to or above that of the IGF-IR. As for IGF-I and -II, most cell types are capable of synthesizing IGFBPs, and it is likely that IGFBPs produced at the local tissue level will affect the bioactivity of endocrine and paracrine/autocrine derived IGF-I and -II. This issue is unclarified, however.

In the blood stream, most IGF-I and -II circulates in ternary protein complexes with either IGFBP-3 or IGFBP-5 and ALS, which does not bind directly to the IGFs, but associates with IGFBP-3 or -5 complexed IGF. The size of the ternary complex is between 130 kd and 150 kd, depending on whether it includes IGFBP-3 or IGFBP-5, and this size is considered to limit the egress of any ternary bound IGF. The remaining pool of circulating IGF exists primarily as binary complexes, which are believed to have rather unhindered access to the extravascular compartment [11,12,22].

There is an approximately 50% molar excess of IGFBPs over IGF-I plus IGF-II in the circulation, and this combined with the high affinity of the IGFBPs may explain why only about 1% or less circulates as free IGF-I and -II [20,23]. Originally, the IGFBPs were thought to serve as IGF-carrier proteins, stabilizing plasma levels and controlling the egress of IGF from the circulation to the extravascular compartment. Furthermore, it was assumed that IGFBP-complexed IGF was biologically more or less inactive, being deprived of its ability to interact with the IGF-IR. It later appeared, however, that in some experimental settings the IGFBPs stimulated rather than inhibited IGF-I mediated actions, and accordingly, the IGFBPs now often are termed modulators of IGF-I bioactivity. In addition, most IGFBPs exert IGF-I- and IGF-IR-independent effects, possible involving interactions with (postulated) IGFBP receptors, or docking proteins located at the cell surface and intracellularly [12,24,25].

The IGFBPs are structurally related peptides, characterized by highly conserved C- and N-terminal domains rich in disulfide bonds, whereas the central domain of the peptides is specific for each of the binding proteins. The central domain is subject to extensive post-translational modification, including phosphorylation, glycosylation, and enzymatic cleavage. In vitro studies have shown that phosphorylation and enzymatic cleavage affects IGF-ligand affinity, whereas glycosylation affects the ability of the IGFBPs to interact with cell surfaces. The physiologic significance of the posttranslational modifications, however, remains uncertain. Finally, all IGFBPs but IGFBP-1 are able to bind to glycosaminoglycans (GAGs), which are an important part of the extracellular matrix (ECM). The authors have unpublished data showing that in vitro, GAGs dose-dependently increase serum levels of free and bioactive IGF-I by competitive binding, supporting the hypothesis that binding of IGF–IGFBP complexes to ECM-associated GAG may serve to concentrate IGF-I near the IGF-IR and in this way to increase IGF-I bioactivity [11,12,26].

Although the IGFBPs are truly multifactorial proteins, there is little doubt that one of their most important functions is to act in concert to regulate circulating levels of free IGF-I. This article reviews current knowledge on changes in the IGFBPs during aging and discusses how this affects levels of free IGF-I and -II and hence the bioactivity of the circulating IGF system.

Age-related changes in the insulin growth factor binding proteins

Insulin growth factor binding protein–1

IGFBP-1 constitutes only about 10% of the circulating pool of IGFBPs [23], but it has gained considerable interest because of its unique properties. IGFBP-1 is the only binding protein showing a marked diurnal variation [27]. The diurnal variation is explained by its tight relationship with insulin, which by far is the most important single regulator of the hepatic IGFBP-1 synthesis [28]. Within less than 2 hours after exposure to insulin, the hepatic IGFBP-1 gene transcription and mRNA levels are suppressed fully [29,30], and serum IGFBP-1 declines with a half-life of approximately 1 hour after administration of insulin [31,32]. In addition, data indicate that GH also may down-regulate IGFBP-1 independently of insulin. The suppressive effect of GH, however, only is unmasked in the presence of low insulin levels, suggesting that the effect of GH on IGFBP-1 is less important than that of insulin [33]. The intimate relationship between insulin and IGFBP-1 and the observation that IGFBP-1 usually inhibits IGF-I mediated actions in vivo and in vitro [20,28] strongly indicate that insulin controls IGF-I bioactivity indirectly by means of IGFBP-1. Supportive of this idea, an inverse relationship between IGFBP-1 and free IGF-I has been observed in various physiologic and pathophysiologic conditions [20,34]. For instance, in chronic catabolic diseases such as type 1 diabetic mellitus (T1DM) and chronic renal failure (CRF), serum levels of IGFBP-1 are elevated highly, whereas levels of free IGF-I are down-regulated, and this observation likely explains the reduced linear growth observed in children suffering from these conditions [20].

The relationship between IGFBP-1 and free IGF-II is less settled. During an oral glucose tolerance test (OGTT), levels of IGFBP-1 correlated inversely with free IGF-I, whereas no such correlation was observed for free IGF-II and IGFBP-1 [35]. During 3 days of fasting, however, the reduction in free IGF-II was tightly inversely associated with the increase in IGFBP-1 [36]. Previous studies have indicated that highly phosphorylated IGFBP-1, which is the major isoform of IGFBP-1 in nonpregnant subjects, binds IGF-I with a 10-fold higher affinity than IGF–II [37]. Thus, IGFBP-1 appears to affect free IGF-II only when levels increase to very high values.

Overnight fasting levels of IGFBP-1 increase in elderly subjects [38–40]. When comparing IGFBP-1 levels in subjects aged 20 to 30 years versus 60 to 90 years, fasting IGFBP-1 levels are approximately threefold higher in aged subjects [38,39], and accordingly, age and IGFBP-1 levels are associated positively [41,42]. Notably, the inverse relationship between IGFBP-1 and insulin, which has been observed in numerous studies in young adults, seems to be preserved in elderly healthy subjects, despite the concomitant increase in both peptides [39]. It has been speculated that the age-related increase in IGFBP-1 levels is caused by the progressive decline in GH secretion [33,39]. This hypothesis needs further investigation. On the other hand, a recent Swedish study has reported that insulin, body mass index, and carbohydrate intake explain about 40% of the variability of serum IGFBP-1 in men aged 42 to 54 years, but only about 6% of the variability in serum IGFBP-1 in men aged 65 years or more [41]. Thus, there is some evidence suggesting that with age, factors other than insulin become increasingly important regulators of IGFBP-1. Levels of IGFBP-1 also are affected by insulin sensitivity and beta-cell function, which both become increasingly abnormal in aged subjects [43]. Nondiabetic subjects with insulin resistance are able to maintain euglycemia, but only at the expense of an increased insulin secretion, and in these subjects, hyperinsulinemia leads to low plasma IGFBP-1 levels. When the beta-cell function starts to deteriorate, however, plasma IGFBP-1 increases toward normal values [20,44]. Thus, a normal level of IGFBP-1 does not necessarily indicate a normal glucose homeostasis.

Sex steroids, in particular estrogens, also may affect IGFBP-1 levels in aged subjects. Estrogen replacement therapy increases levels of IGFBP-1 in women, whereas testosterone administration has no effects on IGFBP-1 in men [45]. On the other hand, irrespective of hormone replacement therapy, there does not appear to be any clear difference between IGFBP-1 levels in aged men and women [40,42].

It has been hypothesized that the age-related increase in IGFBP-1 through inhibition of free IGF-I may lead to a further decrease in IGF-I bioactivity than accounted for by the reduction in serum total IGF-I [42]. Although this hypothesis seems attractive, it needs confirmation. So far, one study in aged subjects (55 to 80 years of age) found an age-related increase in free IGF-I, despite reductions in serum total IGF-I and increases in IGFBP-1 [40]. Unchanged [46] and reduced levels of free IGF-I also have been reported in elderly subjects [47,48].

Insulin-like growth factor binding protein–2

The knowledge on IGFBP-2 regulation is incomplete. In vitro studies show that insulin down-regulates the hepatic IGFBP-2 synthesis [29,49], but in contrast to IGFBP-1, serum IGFBP-2 does not show any rapid changes in response to insulin, either during acute exposure to or following acute withdrawal of insulin [50,51]. IGFBP-2 has preference for IGF-II, and accordingly, there exists an inverse relationship between free IGF-II and IGFBP-2. Furthermore, both peptides appear to be influenced by nutritional factors (in a broad sense). Conditions with an increased nutritional intake such as obesity (with or without type 2 diabetes) are characterized by increased levels of free and total IGF-II and reduced serum IGFBP-2, whereas catabolic conditions such as type 1 diabetes and anorexia nervosa are characterized by suppressed free and total IGF-II levels and elevated serum IGFBP-2 [20]. IGFBP-1 and -2 are positively associated with homeostasis model assessment (HOMA) estimates of insulin sensitivity (ie, the lower insulin sensitivity, the lower levels of IGFBP-1 and -2). Whereas serum IGFBP-1 starts do increase toward normal values with decreasing beta-cell function and the development of type 2 diabetes, serum IGFBP-2 remains suppressed [20].

IGFBP-2 levels increase in senescence in some studies [52], in particular in subjects above 65 years of age [53,54]. The physiologic significance of this finding and its impact on the overall activity of the IGF system remain to be clarified, however. Elevated serum levels of IGFBP-2 have been linked to the development of several cancers, including malignancies of the lung, colon, adrenal glands, prostate, and central nervous system (CNS). Elevated serum IGFBP-2 levels also have been noted in patients suffering from Wilms' tumor and nonislet cell tumor hypoglycemia. The predictive value of IGFBP-2 for tumor risk, however, has not been determined [55]. Furthermore, having the carcinogenic potential of IGF-I and -II in mind [2], it remains a puzzle that IGFBP-2, which predominantly inhibits IGF-mediated actions, is increased rather than decreased in subjects suffering from neoplasias [55].

Insulin-like growth factor binding protein–3 and –5

IGFBP-3 is the most abundant IGF-binding protein, accounting for as much as 75% or more of the circulating IGF-binding capacity in healthy subjects [12,23]. IGFBP-3 shares functional properties with IGFBP-5 in that both peptides are able to form ternary complexes with ALS and either IGF-I or -II [56]. IGFBP-5, however, circulates in much lower concentrations than IGFBP-3, and in healthy subjects, the ternary complexes carry as much as 90% of IGFBP-3 but only about 50% of IGFBP-5 [22].

The turnover of the ternary complexes is very slow, and therefore, it originally was believed that IGFBP-3 (and IGFBP-5) primarily stabilized plasma IGF-I and -II and prolonged their half-life. Within the last decade, however, a paradigm shift in IGFBP-3 physiology has occurred. It has become increasingly evident that IGFBP-3, independent of IGF-I, induces apoptosis, and today IGFBP-3 is considered by some to serve as an anticancer molecule, apparently protecting against several common cancers [57]. IGFBP-5 appears to be involved in apoptosis of the mammary gland during involution [58], suggesting a link between breast cancer and IGFBP-5. Besides their role in apoptosis, IGFBP-3 and -5 have also attained attention because of their ability to stimulate bone formation [59].

ALS and IGFBP-3 and -5 are primarily GH-dependent; therefore, it is not surprising that all three peptides decline gradually after the pubertal growth spurt [60–66]. So far, there are only sparse data on IGFBP-5 and its relationship with other components of the IGF system in elderly subjects. In contrast, there are several studies on IGFBP-3. In men and women, the age-related decline in IGF-I is more pronounced than that in IGFBP-3, resulting in a reduction in the molar ratio of IGF-I to IGFBP-3 [39,67,68]. Furthermore, men appear to have lower levels of IGFBP-3 than women [40,69,70], whereas most studies have failed to show any major gender-related differences in IGF-I levels [10]. Because the ratio IGF-I and IGFBP-3 is reduced in patients who have GH deficiency and increased in acromegaly, the altered ratio in elderly men and women has been suggested to reflect the declining GH secretion and an altered GH sensitivity of the two peptides [39].

Serum levels of free IGF-I correlate positively with total IGF-I levels, which in healthy subjects are highly dependent on IGFBP-3 and to some extent IGFBP-5. Thus, IGFBP-3 correlated positively with free IGF-I in normal subjects and in many pathophysiologic conditions. The same appears to be true for IGFBP-5. Generally, however, the correlation between IGFBP-3 or IGFBP-5 and free IGF-I is statistically weaker than that between free and total IGF-I [20].

The ratio of IGF-I to IGFBP-3 often has been used as an estimate of levels of free and bioavailable IGF-I, and accordingly, it has been deduced that in elderly subjects IGF-I bioavailability is reduced further than what is indicated from measurement of IGF-I. However, there has been no clear relationship between the age-related levels of free IGF-I and the ratio between IGF-I and IGFBP-3. In the author's view, the IGF-I to IGFBP-3 ratio should be used with great caution for two reasons. First, the ratio does not take into account IGF-II. In elderly subjects, circulating IGF-II appears to remain more or less constant up to 65 years of age [54]. An age-related decline has been observed when subjects up to 90 years of age have been included [70,71], but overall there is little doubt that the age-related decline is less pronounced for IGF-II than IGF-I. Thus, it is plausible that the ratio between the sum of IGF-I plus IGF-II to IGFBP-3 may be more or less constant even in elderly subjects, and if this is the case, then the ratio between IGF-I and IGFBP-3 simply illustrates an altered relationship between IGF-I and -II concentrations. It is acknowledged, however, that further studies are required to test this hypothesis. The second reservation concerns the impact of IGFBP-1, IGFBP-2, and IGFBP-3 proteolysis on levels of free IGF-I. In metabolic abnormal conditions such as T1DM, T2DM, anorexia nervosa, fasting, obesity, and insulin resistance, levels of IGFBP-1 and -2 are highly abnormal. In pregnancy, virtually all IGFBP-3 is degraded enzymatically, and this is reported to lower IGF-I affinity. In CRF, a considerable fraction of serum IGFBP-3 immunoreactivity arises from IGFBP-3 split products that show markedly reduced IGF-binding capacity. Thus, in these conditions, the ratio of IGF-I to IGFBP-3 is likely to be misleading [20].

Insulin-like growth factor binding protein–4 and –6

IGFBP-4 circulates in concentrations similar to those of IGFBP-5, making these the second most abundant IGFBPs. Still, together IGFBP-4 and -5 constitute only about one third of the concentration of IGFBP-3 [23]. The knowledge on the regulation of IGFBP-4 is insufficient; so far it appears that neither GH, glucocorticosteroids, nor thyroid hormones have any major effect on serum IGFBP-4 levels [72]. In vitro, however, parathyroid hormone (PTH) and vitamin D_3 stimulate the synthesis of IGFBP-4 in cultured cells [73,74]. In vivo, IGFBP-4 levels have been shown to increase following treatment with vitamin D_3 [73], and a positive correlation between serum IGFBP-4 and serum PTH has been observed in one study [74], whereas two other studies have failed to confirm such a relationship [72,75]. IGFBP-4 is primarily an inhibitor of IGF-mediated actions, and increased serum levels have been observed in patients with previous osteoporotic fractures [76]. In constitutionally tall girls, treatment with high doses of estradiol increased serum IGFBP-4 levels approximately twofold [77]. The apparent association between PTH, vitamin D_3, estradiol, and IGFBP-4 indicates that gonads and bone are the primary target organs for IGFBP-4 [78].

The age relationship of serum IGFBP-4 is not fully clarified. One study observed an increasing tendency in subjects (n = 102) aged 20 to 80 years [74], whereas another study in a much larger cohort (n = 804) failed to show any significant changes with age [72]. Further, serum levels of IGFBP-4 correlate positively with IGF-II, whereas the relationship with IGF-I (free and total) is more questionable [72,76]. This observation is in agreement with the relative modest effect of age on serum IGF-II.

IGFBP-6 resembles IGFBP-4 in that the knowledge on its function and regulation is sparse. Furthermore, both proteins have preference for IGF-II. So far, IGFBP-6 has been shown to inhibit cell proliferation and tumor-igenic potency and to increase apoptosis in various cell lines. Further, IGFBP-6 appears in large quantities in the CNS). Transgenic mice with a CNS-targeted overexpression of IGFBP-6 show a reduced CNS growth and differentiation and marked alterations in their reproductive physiology [79,80].

In people, serum IGFBP-6 increases with increasing age [54,81], but the physiologic importance of this finding remains unclear. As for IGFBP-4, serum IGFBP-6 is unaffected by GH status and administration of glucocorticosteroids and estradiol [77,81], whereas increased levels have been observed in patients suffering from osteoporotic fractures [76].

Summary

Most of the IGFBPs undergo marked changes during aging: IGFBP-3 and -5 change more or less in parallel with levels of IGF-I, whereas IGFBP-1, -2, and -6 show an increasing tendency. Only IGFBP-4 appears to be relatively stable during senescence. After more than 30 years of research, knowledge on the IGFBPs remains incomplete and in some aspects, it is virtually absent. There is little doubt, however, that the IGFBPs are regulated by different hormone systems, and it seems plausible that these hormone systems use the IGFBPs to integrate and concert the overall activity of the IGF system. To understand this complex signaling cascade, one needs to understand the regulatory mechanisms of the IGFBPs and how this affect levels of free IGF-I.

References

[1] LeRoith D, Bondy C, Yakar S, et al. The somatomedin hypothesis: 2001. Endocr Rev 2001; 22(1):53–74.
[2] Pollak MN, Schernhammer ES, Hankinson SE. Insulin-like growth factors and neoplasia. Nat Rev Cancer 2004;4(7):505–18.
[3] Yuen K, Frystyk J, Umpleby M, et al. Changes in free rather than total insulin-like growth factor-I enhance insulin sensitivity and suppress endogenous peak growth hormone (GH)

release following short-term low-dose GH administration in young healthy adults. J Clin Endocrinol Metab 2004;89(8):3956–64.

[4] Khandwala HM, McCutcheon IE, Flyvbjerg A, et al. The effects of insulin-like growth factors on tumorigenesis and neoplastic growth. Endocr Rev 2000;21(3):215–44.

[5] Renehan AG, Zwahlen M, Minder PC, et al. Insulin-like growth factor (IGF)-I, IGF binding protein-3, and cancer risk: systematic review and meta-regression analysis. Lancet 2004; 363(9418):1346–53.

[6] Ibrahim YH, Yee D. Insulin-like growth factor-I and cancer risk. Growth Horm IGF Res 2004;14(4):261–9.

[7] Juul A, Scheike T, Davidsen M, et al. Low serum insulin-like growth factor I is associated with increased risk of ischemic heart disease: a population-based case-control study. Circulation 2002;106(8):939–44.

[8] Sandhu MS, Heald AH, Gibson JM, et al. Circulating concentrations of insulin-like growth factor-I and development of glucose intolerance: a prospective observational study. Lancet 2002;359(9319):1740–5.

[9] Vaessen N, Heutink P, Janssen JA, et al. A polymorphism in the gene for IGF-I: functional properties and risk for type 2 diabetes and myocardial infarction. Diabetes 2001;50(3): 637–42.

[10] Juul A. Serum levels of insulin-like growth factor I and its binding proteins in health and disease. Growth Horm IGF Res 2003;13(4):113–70.

[11] Hwa V, Oh Y, Rosenfeld RG. The insulin-like growth factor-binding protein (IGFBP) superfamily. Endocr Rev 1999;20(6):761–87.

[12] Firth SM, Baxter RC. Cellular actions of the insulin-like growth factor binding proteins. Endocr Rev 2002;23(6):824–54.

[13] De Meyts P, Whittaker J. Structural biology of insulin and IGF1 receptors: implications for drug design. Nat Rev Drug Discov 2002;1(10):769–83.

[14] Hawkes C, Kar S. The insulin-like growth factor-II/mannose-6-phosphate receptor: structure, distribution and function in the central nervous system. Brain Res Brain Res Rev 2004;44(2–3):117–40.

[15] Fowden AL. The insulin-like growth factors and feto-placental growth. Placenta 2003; 24(8–9):803–12.

[16] Scott CD, Firth SM. The role of the M6P/IGF-II receptor in cancer: tumor suppression or garbage disposal? Horm Metab Res 2004;36(5):261–71.

[17] Savage MO, Camacho-Hubner C, Dunger DB. Therapeutic applications of the insulin-like growth factors. Growth Horm IGF Res 2004;14(4):301–8.

[18] Yakar S, Liu JL, Stannard B, et al. Normal growth and development in the absence of hepatic insulin-like growth factor I. Proc Natl Acad Sci U S A 1999;96(13):7324–9.

[19] Domene HM, Bengolea SV, Martinez AS, et al. Deficiency of the circulating insulin-like growth factor system associated with inactivation of the acid-labile subunit gene. N Engl J Med 2004;350(6):570–7.

[20] Frystyk J. Free insulin-like growth factors—measurements and relationships to growth hormone secretion and glucose homeostasis. Growth Horm IGF Res 2004;14(5):337–75.

[21] Chen JW, Højlund K, Beck-Nielsen H, et al. Free rather than total circulating IGF-I determines the feedback on GH release in normal subjects. J Clin Endocrinol Metab 2005;90(1): 366–71.

[22] Baxter RC, Meka S, Firth SM. Molecular distribution of IGF binding protein-5 in human serum. J Clin Endocrinol Metab 2002;87(1):271–6.

[23] Rajaram S, Baylink DJ, Mohan S. Insulin-like growth factor-binding proteins in serum and other biological fluids: regulation and functions. Endocr Rev 1997;18(6):801–31.

[24] Ricort JM. Insulin-like growth factor binding protein (IGFBP) signaling. Growth Horm IGF Res 2004;14(4):277–86.

[25] Jones JI, Clemmons DR. Insulin-like growth factors and their binding proteins: biological actions. Endocr Rev 1995;16:3–34.

[26] Clemmons DR. Use of mutagenesis to probe IGF-binding protein structure/function relationships. Endocr Rev 2001;22(6):800–17.

[27] Frystyk J, Nyholm B, Skjærbæk C, et al. The circulating IGF-system and its relationship with 24-hour glucose regulation and insulin sensitivity in healthy subjects. Clin Endocrinol (Oxf) 2003;58:777–84.

[28] Lee PD, Giudice LC, Conover CA, et al. Insulin-like growth factor binding protein-1: recent findings and new directions. Proc Soc Exp Biol Med 1997;216(3):319–57.

[29] Ooi GT, Tseng LY, Rechler MM. Post-transcriptional regulation of insulin-like growth factor binding protein-2 mRNA in diabetic rat liver. Biochem Biophys Res Commun 1992;189: 1031–7.

[30] Pao CI, Farmer PK, Begovic S, et al. Regulation of insulin-like growth factor-I (IGF-I) and IGF-binding protein 1 gene transcription by hormones and provision of amino acids in rat hepatocytes. Mol Endocrinol 1993;7:1561–8.

[31] Conover CA, Lee PD, Kanaley JA, et al. Insulin regulation of insulin-like growth factor binding protein-1 in obese and nonobese humans. J Clin Endocrinol Metab 1992;74: 1355–60.

[32] Brismar K, Fernqvist Forbes E, et al. Effect of insulin on the hepatic production of insulin-like growth factor-binding protein-1 (IGFBP-1), IGFBP-3, and IGF-I in insulin-dependent diabetes. J Clin Endocrinol Metab 1994;79:872–8.

[33] Nørrelund H, Fisker S, Vahl N, et al. Evidence supporting a direct suppressive effect of growth hormone on serum IGFBP-1 levels. Experimental studies in normal, obese and GH- deficient adults. Growth Horm IGF Res 1999;9(1):52–60.

[34] Lang CH, Vary TC, Frost RA. Acute in vivo elevation of insulin-like growth factor (IGF) binding protein-1 decreases plasma free IGF-I and muscle protein synthesis. Endocrinology 2003;144(9):3922–33.

[35] Frystyk J, Grøfte T, Skjærbæk C, et al. The effect of oral glucose on serum free insulin-like growth factor-I and -II in healthy adults. J Clin Endocrinol Metab 1997;82(9): 3124–7.

[36] Frystyk J, Højlund K, Rasmussen KN, et al. Development and clinical evaluation of a novel immunoassay for the binary complex of insulin-like growth factor-I (IGF-I) and IGF-binding protein-1 in human serum. J Clin Endocrinol Metab 2002;87:260–6.

[37] Westwood M, Gibson JM, White A. Purification and characterization of the insulin-like growth factor binding protein-1 isoform found in normal plasma. Endocrinology 1997; 138(3):1130–6.

[38] Rutanen EM, Karkkainen T, Stenman UH, et al. Aging is associated with decreased suppression of insulin-like growth factor binding protein-1 by insulin. J Clin Endocrinol Metab 1993;77(5):1152–5.

[39] Benbassat CA, Maki KC, Unterman TG. Circulating levels of insulin-like growth factor (IGF) binding protein-1 and -3 in aging men: relationships to insulin, glucose, IGF, and dehydroepiandrosterone sulfate levels and anthropometric measures. J Clin Endocrinol Metab 1997;82(5):1484–91.

[40] Janssen JA, Stolk RP, Pols HA, et al. Serum free IGF-I, total IGF-I, IGFBP-1 and IGFBP-3 levels in an elderly population: relation to age and sex steroid levels. Clin Endocrinol (Oxf) 1998;48(4):471–8.

[41] Wolk K, Larsson SC, Vessby B, et al. Metabolic, anthropometric, and nutritional factors as predictors of circulating insulin-like growth factor binding protein-1 levels in middle-aged and elderly men. J Clin Endocrinol Metab 2004;89(4):1879–84.

[42] Nyström FH, Öhman PK, Ekman BA, et al. Population-based reference values for IGF-I and IGF-binding protein-1: relations with metabolic and anthropometric variables. Eur J Endocrinol 1997;136(2):165–72.

[43] Møller N, Gormsen L, Fuglsang J, et al. Effects of ageing on insulin secretion and action. Horm Res 2003;60(Suppl 1):102–4.

[44] Heald AH, Cruickshank JK, Riste LK, et al. Close relation of fasting insulin-like growth factor binding protein-1 (IGFBP-1) with glucose tolerance and cardiovascular risk in two populations. Diabetologia 2001;44(3):333–9.

[45] Gentili A, Mulligan T, Godschalk M, et al. Unequal impact of short-term testosterone repletion on the somatotropic axis of young and older men. J Clin Endocrinol Metab 2002;87(2): 825–34.

[46] Juul A, Holm K, Kastrup KW, et al. Free insulin-like growth factor I serum levels in 1430 healthy children and adults, and its diagnostic value in patients suspected of growth hormone deficiency. J Clin Endocrinol Metab 1997;82(8):2497–502.

[47] Frystyk J, Vestbo E, Skjærbæk C, et al. Free insulin-like growth factors in human obesity. Metabolism 1995;44:37–44.

[48] Gomez JM, Maravall FJ, Gomez N, et al. The IGF-I system component concentrations that decrease with ageing are lower in obesity in relationship to body mass index and body fat. Growth Horm IGF Res 2004;14(2):91–6.

[49] Boni-Schnetzler M, Schmid C, Mary JL, et al. Insulin regulates the expression of the insulin-like growth factor binding protein 2 mRNA in rat hepatocytes. Mol Endocrinol 1990;4(9): 1320–6.

[50] Attia N, Caprio S, Jones TW, et al. Changes in free insulin-like growth factor-1 and leptin concentrations during acute metabolic decompensation in insulin withdrawn patients with type 1 diabetes. J Clin Endocrinol Metab 1999;84(7):2324–8.

[51] Clemmons DR, Snyder DK, Busby WHJ. Variables controlling the secretion of insulin-like growth factor binding protein-2 in normal human subjects. J Clin Endocrinol Metab 1991; 73:727–33.

[52] Amin S, Riggs BL, Atkinson EJ, et al. A potentially deleterious role of IGFBP-2 on bone density in aging men and women. J Bone Miner Res 2004;19(7):1075–83.

[53] van den Beld AW, Blum WF, Pols HA, et al. Serum insulin-like growth factor binding protein-2 levels as an indicator of functional ability in elderly men. Eur J Endocrinol 2003; 148(6):627–34.

[54] Yu H, Mistry J, Nicar MJ, et al. Insulin-like growth factors (IGF-I, free IGF-I and IGF-II) and insulin-like growth factor binding proteins (IGFBP-2, IGFBP-3, IGFBP-6, and ALS) in blood circulation. J Clin Lab Anal 1999;13(4):166–72.

[55] Hoeflich A, Reisinger R, Lahm H, et al. Insulin-like growth factor-binding protein 2 in tumorigenesis: protector or promoter? Cancer Res 2001;61(24):8601–10.

[56] Twigg SM, Baxter RC. Insulin-like growth factor (IGF)-binding protein 5 forms an alternative ternary complex with IGFs and the acid-labile subunit. J Biol Chem 1998;273(11):6074–9.

[57] Ali O, Cohen P, Lee KW. Epidemiology and biology of insulin-like growth factor binding protein-3 (IGFBP-3) as an anti-cancer molecule. Horm Metab Res 2003;35(11–12):726–33.

[58] Collett-Solberg PF, Cohen P. Genetics, chemistry, and function of the IGF/IGFBP system. Endocrine 2000;12(2):121–36.

[59] Govoni KE, Baylink DJ, Mohan S. The multi-functional role of insulin-like growth factor binding proteins in bone. Pediatr Nephrol 2005;20(3):261–8.

[60] Blum WF, Albertsson-Wikland K, Rosberg S, et al. Serum levels of insulin-like growth factor I (IGF-I) and IGF binding protein 3 reflect spontaneous growth hormone secretion. J Clin Endocrinol Metab 1993;76(6):1610–6.

[61] Baxter RC. Circulating levels and molecular distribution of the acid-labile (alpha) subunit of the high molecular weight insulin-like growth factor-binding protein complex. J Clin Endocrinol Metab 1990;70:1347–53.

[62] Boisclair YR, Rhoads RP, Ueki I, et al. The acid-labile subunit (ALS) of the 150 kDa IGF-binding protein complex: an important but forgotten component of the circulating IGF system. J Endocrinol 2001;170(1):63–70.

[63] Juul A, Møller S, Mosfeldt-Laursen E, et al. The acid-labile subunit of human ternary insulin-like growth factor binding protein complex in serum: hepatosplanchnic release, diurnal

variation, circulating concentrations in healthy subjects, and diagnostic use in patients with growth hormone deficiency. J Clin Endocrinol Metab 1998;83(12):4408–15.

[64] Bowers CY, Granda R, Mohan S, et al. Sustained elevation of pulsatile growth hormone (GH) secretion and insulin-like growth factor I (IGF-I), IGF-binding protein-3 (IGFBP-3), and IGFBP-5 concentrations during 30-day continuous subcutaneous infusion of GH-releasing peptide-2 in older men and women. J Clin Endocrinol Metab 2004;89(5):2290–300.

[65] Baxter RC, Martin JL. Radioimmunoassay of growth hormone-dependent insulin-like growth factor binding protein in human plasma. J Clin Invest 1986;78:1504–12.

[66] Mohan S, Libanati C, Dony C, et al. Development, validation, and application of a radioimmunoassay for insulin-like growth factor binding protein-5 in human serum and other biological fluids. J Clin Endocrinol Metab 1995;80(9):2638–45.

[67] Gambera A, Scagliola P, Falsetti L, et al. Androgens, insulin-like growth factor-I (IGF-I), and carrier proteins (SHBG, IGFBP-3) in postmenopause. Menopause 2004;11(2):159–66.

[68] Juul A, Main K, Blum WF, et al. The ratio between serum levels of insulin-like growth factor (IGF)-I and the IGF binding proteins (IGFBP-1, 2 and 3) decreases with age in healthy adults and is increased in acromegalic patients. Clin Endocrinol (Oxf) 1994;41:85–93.

[69] Ceda GP, Dall'Aglio E, Magnacavallo A, et al. The insulin-like growth factor axis and plasma lipid levels in the elderly. J Clin Endocrinol Metab 1998;83(2):499–502.

[70] Pfeilschifter J, Scheidt-Nave C, Leidig-Bruckner G, et al. Relationship between circulating insulin-like growth factor components and sex hormones in a population-based sample of 50- to 80-year-old men and women. J Clin Endocrinol Metab 1996;81(7):2534–40.

[71] Raynaud-Simon A. Levels of plasma insulin-like growth factor I (IGF I), IGF II, IGF binding proteins, type 1 IGF receptor and growth hormone binding protein in community-dwelling elderly subjects with no malnutrition and no inflammation. J Nutr Health Aging 2003; 7(4):267–73.

[72] Van Doorn J, Cornelissen AJ, Buul-Offers SC. Plasma levels of insulin-like growth factor binding protein-4 (IGFBP-4) under normal and pathological conditions. Clin Endocrinol (Oxf) 2001;54(5):655–64.

[73] Scharla SH, Strong DD, Rosen C, et al. 1,25-Dihydroxyvitamin D3 increases secretion of insulin-like growth factor binding protein-4 (IGFBP-4) by human osteoblast-like cells in vitro and elevates IGFBP-4 serum levels in vivo. J Clin Endocrinol Metab 1993;77(5):1190–7.

[74] Honda Y, Landale EC, Strong DD, et al. Recombinant synthesis of insulin-like growth factor-binding protein-4 (IGFBP-4): development, validation, and application of a radioimmunoassay for IGFBP-4 in human serum and other biological fluids. J Clin Endocrinol Metab 1996;81(4):1389–96.

[75] Jehle PM, Ostertag A, Schulten K, et al. Insulin-like growth factor system components in hyperparathyroidism and renal osteodystrophy. Kidney Int 2000;57(2):423–36.

[76] Jehle PM, Schulten K, Schulz W, et al. Serum levels of insulin-like growth factor (IGF)-I and IGF binding protein (IGFBP)-1 to -6 and their relationship to bone metabolism in osteoporosis patients. Eur J Intern Med 2003;14(1):32–8.

[77] Rooman RP, De Beeck LO, Martin M, et al. IGF-I, IGF-II, free IGF-I and IGF-binding proteins-2 to -6 during high-dose oestrogen treatment in constitutionally tall girls. Eur J Endocrinol 2002;146(6):823–9.

[78] Mazerbourg S, Callebaut I, Zapf J, et al. Update on IGFBP-4: regulation of IGFBP-4 levels and functions, in vitro and in vivo. Growth Horm IGF Res 2004;14(2):71–84.

[79] Bach LA. Insulin-like growth factor binding protein-6: the forgotten binding protein? Horm Metab Res 1999;31(2–3):226–34.

[80] Bienvenu G, Seurin D, Grellier P, et al. Insulin-like growth factor binding protein-6 transgenic mice: postnatal growth, brain development, and reproduction abnormalities. Endocrinology 2004;145(5):2412–20.

[81] Van Doorn J, Ringeling AM, Shmueli SS, et al. Circulating levels of human insulin-like growth factor binding protein-6 (IGFBP-6) in health and disease as determined by radioimmunoassay. Clin Endocrinol (Oxf) 1999;50(5):601–9.

ELSEVIER
SAUNDERS

Endocrinol Metab Clin N Am
34 (2005) 877–893

ENDOCRINOLOGY
AND METABOLISM
CLINICS
OF NORTH AMERICA

Sex-Steroid Control of the Aging Somatotropic Axis

Johannes D. Veldhuis, MD[a],*, Dana Erickson, MD[a],
Ali Iranmanesh, MD[b,c], John M. Miles, MD[a],
Cyril Y. Bowers, MD[d]

[a]Endocrine Research Unit, Department of Internal Medicine,
Mayo School of Graduate Medical Education, General Clinical Research Center,
Mayo Clinic, Rochester, MN, USA
[b]Endocrine Service, Medical Section Salem, Veterans Affairs Medical Center,
Salem, VA, USA
[c]University of Virginia School of Medicine, Charlottesville, VA, USA
[d]Division of Endocrinology and Metabolism, Department of Internal Medicine,
Tulane University Medical Center, New Orleans, LA, USA

Growth hormone (GH) concentrations decline progressively with increasing age beginning in young adulthood (Fig. 1) [1–8]. In contrast, the maximal pituitary secretory capacity, plasma elimination kinetics, and hepatic actions of GH are preserved in older people [9–12]. Reduced availability of GH and thereby insulin-like growth factor (IGF-I) in the elderly adult has significant implications [13]. In particular, epidemiologic investigations correlate hyposomatotropism with reduced insulin sensitivity, dyslipidemia, increased cardiovascular mortality, intra-abdominal adiposity, sarcopenia, osteopenia, and diminished quality of life [14–18]. Obesity, especially excessive visceral fat mass, forecasts decreased GH secretion in the adult (see Fig. 1) [4,5,7,19,20]. In addition, sex steroid depletion at any age after adolescence predicts relative GH deficiency (see Fig. 1,) [3,4,6,21–23]. Conversely, supplementation with estradiol (E_2) or an aromatizable androgen, such as testosterone (Te), will stimulate GH production in aging and

The authors acknowledge support from the National Center for Research Resources (Rockville, MD) to the General Clinical Research Center (M01 RR00585, Mayo Clinic) and Grants R01-NIA AG 14,799 and R01-NIA AG 19,695 from the National Institutes of Health (Bethesda, MD) in the writing of this paper.

* Corresponding author. Endocrine Research Unit, Department of Internal Medicine, Mayo School of Graduate Medical Education, General Clinical Research Center, Mayo Clinic, 200 First Street Southwest, Rochester, MN 55905.

E-mail address: veldhuis.johannes@mayo.edu (J.D. Veldhuis).

0889-8529/05/$ - see front matter © 2005 Elsevier Inc. All rights reserved.
doi:10.1016/j.ecl.2005.07.006   *endo.theclinics.com*

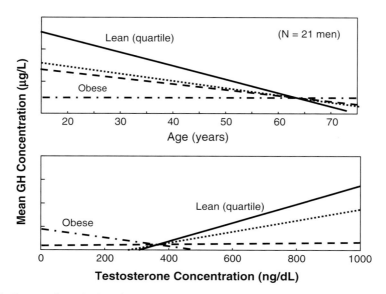

Fig. 1. Impact of age (*top*) and testosterone (Te) concentrations (*bottom*) on mean (24-hour) GH concentrations in 21 healthy men. Regression lines in each panel are stratified by quartiles of percentage body fat, thereby highlighting how relative adiposity interacts with age and androgen concentrations in determining GH secretion. The negative impact of age and the positive impact of Te are most evident in subjects who are lean (*uppermost continuous line*) and least evident in individuals who are obese (*lower broken lines*). The other two interrupted lines represent intermediate degrees of adiposity. (*Data from* Iranmanesh A, South S, Liem AY, et al. Unequal impact of age, percentage body fat, and serum testosterone concentrations on the somatotrophic, IGF-I, and IGF-binding protein responses to a three-day intravenous growth hormone-releasing hormone pulsatile infusion in men. Eur J Endocrinol 1998;139:59–71.)

hypogonadal adults [21,22,24]. Estrogens are primary agonists. Recent developments in this arena allow new clinical perspectives in aging, which are highlighted in this article.

Significance of growth hormone outflow to target tissues

GH, IGF-I (the tissue product of GH action), E_2, and Te collaborate in a tetrapartite interaction in puberty to promote statural and organ growth, modify body composition, ensure sexual maturation, facilitate psychosocial adaptation, and endow peak physical performance [23]. Table 1 highlights some of the mechanisms by which sex steroids collaborate with GH and IGF-I in mediating tissue-specific anabolism. The types of synergistic mechanisms engaged in puberty are relevant for the most part in aging. Therefore, the combined impoverishment of somatotropic and gonadal sex steroid hormones in older men and women signifies significant withdrawal of anabolic support.

Table 1
Illustrative mechanisms mediating anabolic synergy between sex steroids and growth hormone on insulin-like growth factor–I

Mechanisms	Anatomic site
Estradiol and testosterone increase GH secretion	Hypothalamic–pituitary unit
Estradiol increases IGF-I receptor	Brain
Testosterone increases IGF-I peptide	Muscle
Testosterone decreases IGFBP-4 protein	Muscle
Testosterone increases GH-stimulated IGF-I synthesis	Bone
Estradiol increases GH receptor	Liver (alternative transcript, GHR1)
IGF-I increases estradiol action	Neurons

Laboratory experiments indicate that GH governs gene expression in part by inducing in situ IGF-I production and modifying local availability of IGF-binding proteins (IGFBPs) [10,28]. In addition, GH can stimulate lipolysis, prechondrocyte proliferation, growth of erythroid precursors, hepatic synthesis of the low-density lipoprotein (LDL) receptor, and selected metabolic enzymes directly [29–33]. In certain organs, such as the liver and kidneys, GH promotes organotypic and systemic production of IGF-I and certain IGFBPs [29]. Accordingly, the contributions of blood-borne IGF-I (somatomedin hypothesis) to peripheral tissues and local IGF-I production are complementary rather than mutually exclusive. In fact, marked (greater than 70%) depletion of systemic IGF-I concentrations achieved transgenically in mice does not restrict somatic growth after birth, but impairs insulin-dependent fat and carbohydrate balance and reduces bone density in the adult animal [29].

E_2 and Te modulate the actions of GH, IGF-I, and IGFBPs in diverse target tissues [34,35]. For example, E_2 directs IGF-I production, turnover, and signaling in the brain, thereby putatively enhancing neurogenesis, synaptic differentiation, and possibly memory [36]. Joint actions of E_2 and GH in bone promote net calcium accretion [23]. Analogously, combined effects of Te and GH in muscle induce in situ IGF-I synthesis, stimulate protein anabolism, and increase lean body mass [23].

Mechanisms of estrogen-driven growth hormone secretion in postmenopausal women

Quantitation of dynamic control is challenging, because GH secretion proceeds in discrete bursts (pulses), nycthemeral (24-hour rhythmic) variations, and feedback-sensitive (entropic) patterns (Fig. 2). Aging alters each of these regulated attributes [10,13]. To understand the underlying causes, recent clinical investigative strategies included the implementation of specific high-sensitivity GH assays, frequent blood sampling, infusion of biosynthetic secretagogues, validated analytical methods, and model-assisted formulations. Collective observations established that low mean GH concentrations

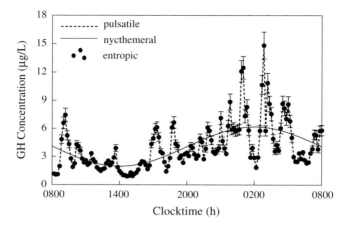

Fig. 2. Dynamic modes of regulated GH secretion: pulsatile (burst-like), nycthemeral (24-hour rhythmic), and entropic (feedback-sensitive pattern regularity).

in aging individuals reflect a reduction in the amount of GH secreted per burst (defined as μg GH released per unit distribution volume per event) [5,7,19,21,22]. This adaptation is specific, because there is minimal or no change in the basal release, pulse frequency, or plasma half-life of GH [4,7,19,21,22]. The insight that aging impoverishes GH secretory burst mass is crucial by way of focusing studies on the mechanisms that normally sustain high-amplitude GH pulses [10,13].

An emerging concept is that coordinated interactions among systemic, hypothalamic, and pituitary peptides; and nonpeptidyl effectors, such as sex steroids and glucocorticoids, govern the amount of GH secreted per burst [10,37–40]. By way of caveat, the species selectivity of certain mechanisms of sex steroid action makes inferences gained in the rat, mouse, pig, and sheep illustrative of, rather than definitive to, people. For example, estrogens repress and nonaromatizable androgens increase GH pulse height in the rat, but exert opposite effects in people [10,21,25–27,41,42]. Thus, further discussion will focus on clinical physiology and pathophysiology.

Estrogenic stimulation of growth hormone release

GH concentrations and pulsatile secretion double in the preovulatory phase of the menstrual cycle, when E_2 secretion rises [43–45]. Increased estrogen concentrations also predict higher GH concentrations and larger GH pulses in pre- and postmenopausal women than comparably aged men [3,6,46,47]. Additionally, estrogen supplementation in girls with Turner syndrome, postmenopausal women, male-to-female transsexual men, and patients with prostatic cancer elevates GH concentrations by 1.8 to 3.3-fold (Fig. 3) [16,17,21,26,27,48,49]. The stimulatory effect of estrogen depends upon the concentration achieved rather than the route of delivery, in that

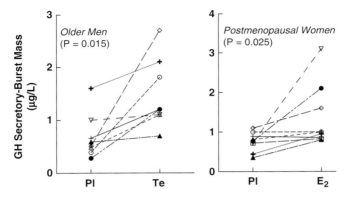

Fig. 3. Supplementation with testosterone (Te) or estradiol (E$_2$) versus placebo (Pl) amplifies the amount of GH secreted per burst (GH secretory-burst mass). Data are from healthy older (older than 60 years of age) men and women. (*Data from* Shah N, Evans WS, Veldhuis JD. Actions of estrogen on the pulsatile, nyctohemeral, and entropic modes of growth hormone secretion. Am J Physiol 1999;276:R1351–R1358; and Gentili A, Mulligan T, Godschalk M, et al. Unequal impact of short-term testosterone repletion on the somatotropic axis of young and older men. J Clin Endocrinol Metab 2002;87:825–34.)

intravenous, intramuscular, oral, intravaginal, intranasal and transdermal administration can stimulate GH secretion and either lower or not affect total IGF-I concentrations [8,17,21,27,48,50]. When assessed analytically, the mechanisms of sex steroid action entail amplification of GH secretory burst mass (see Fig. 3) [22,23,47]. Understanding how E$_2$ stimulates GH secretion is important in aging individuals, in part to foster alternative strategies to obviate hyposomatotropism. Nonsteroidal avenues become especially relevant to men with prostatic disease and women at increased risk of E$_2$-related neoplastic, cerebro- and cardiovascular, thrombophlebitic or cholestatic adverse effects.

Concept of ensemble control

Estrogen's capability to augment pulsatile GH secretion selectively is significant, because aging and hypogonadism primarily reduce pulsatile GH production; burst-like GH secretion constitutes most (85%) of total daily GH output [4,5,7,19,21,22,46,47,51], and GH secretory burst mass is determined by a well-articulated set of key peptidyl signals: GH-releasing hormone (GHRH), somatostatin (SS), ghrelin/GHRP, GH, and IGF-I (Fig. 4) [10,52–61]. Because of such complexity, a growing clinical challenge is intuitively visualizing how time-delimited, reciprocal, concentration-dependent nonlinear interactions among the primary signals serve to control GH output [10,23]. This issue has fostered the recent development of simplified biomathematical models that incorporate the principal connections recognized among the five major peptides (see Fig. 4) [37–40]. Analytical

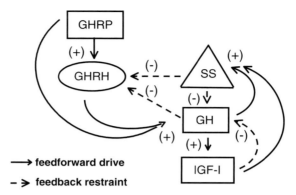

Fig. 4. Simplified ensemble of principal regulatory peptides that direct pulsatile GH secretion. GHRP denotes the GH-releasing peptide, ghrelin; GHRH, GH-releasing hormone; and SS, somatostatin, an inhibitory peptide. GHRH stimulates (*continuous arrow* [+]) the synthesis and secretion of GH. GHRP (ghrelin) induces hypothalamic GHRH and pituitary GH secretion directly. SS represses neuronal GHRH outflow and inhibits somatotrope GH release (*interrupted arrow* [−]) without blocking GH synthesis. GH and its tissue product, IGF-I, feed back negatively on GH secretion by driving SS and suppressing GHRH output. IGF-I also may directly pituitary GH synthesis and secretion inhibit. Aging appears to reduce feedforward by GHRH and GHRP and augment feedback by SS. E2 and Te exert distinct actions on each signaling pathway.

simulations demonstrate that consensus linkages among GHRH, SS, ghrelin, and GH/IGF-I are sufficient to confer self-renewing, high-amplitude GH secretory bursts with gender-specific pulse patterns.

Multi-site actions of estradiol

Recent clinical experiments have unveiled novel mechanisms by which E_2 amplifies GH secretion. Specifically, E_2 supplementation in postmenopausal women:

- Enhances submaximal stimulation by pulses of recombinant human (rh) GHRH-1,44-amide (increases secretagogue potency)
- Attenuates submaximal inhibition by infused SS (blunts inhibitory sensitivity)
- Potentiates dose-dependent stimulation by synthetic GHRP
- Mutes negative feedback by a pulse of rh GH
- Amplifies the rebound-like release of GH after SS withdrawal
- Paradoxically accentuates inhibition of fasting GH secretion by IGF-I (Fig. 5) [54–57,60,62–68]

Thus, E_2 regulates multiple interactions among GHRH, SS, ghrelin, GH, and IGF-I. The overall outcome is to enhance the size (mass and amplitude) of GH pulses and quench a given pulse by IGF-I negative feedback.

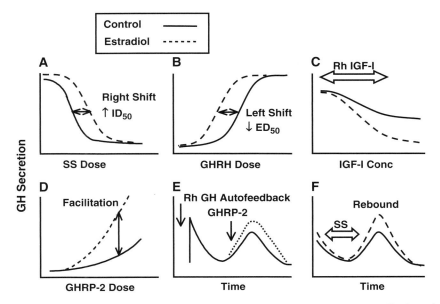

Fig. 5. Estradiol (E_2) modulates multiple mechanisms that control the size (amplitude and mass) of GH pulses. (*A*) E_2 reduces the inhibitory potency of infused SS (increases the one-half maximally suppressive dose of SS); (*B*) enhances the stimulatory potency of GHRH; (*C*) accentuates negative feedback by systemic IGF-I, thus quenching a GH pulse to allow renewal of the next burst; (*D*) potentiates feedforward by the ghrelin analog, GHRP-2; (*E*) mutes negative feedback by a single pulse of rh GH; and (*F*) augments rebound-like GH release induced by sequential exposure to and withdrawal of SS.

Investigation of ensemble mechanisms in aging

A consequence of interactive control is that modulation of any given regulatory locus will perforce alter the output of all interconnected sites [10,13,23]. For example, the observation that E_2 amplifies GH secretory burst mass following a submaximal GHRH stimulus [56] could signify that estrogen:

- Upregulates somatotrope GHRH receptors
- Reduces negative feedback by systemic GH or IGF-I
- Attenuates inhibition by SS
- Augments GHRH-releasable GH stores
- Potentiates ghrelin/GHRP action, which itself stimulates GH secretion and synergizes with GHRH [10,13,58,69]

A corollary clinical finding is that oral supplementation with E_2 lowers total IGF-I and elevates IGFBP-1 concentrations, which predictively would reduce free (unbound) IGF-I concentrations, restrict negative feedback, and thereby disinhibit GH secretion (Fig. 6).

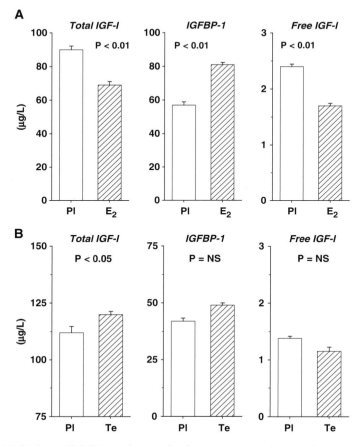

Fig. 6. (*A*) Oral estradiol (E_2) supplementation in postmenopausal women lowers total IGF-I and elevates IGFBP-1 concentrations, thereby putatively reducing free (unbound) IGF-I availability. Lower free IGF-I concentrations would be expected to disinhibit negative feedback, and thus further augment pulsatile GH secretion. (*B*) Intramuscular testosterone (Te) administration in healthy older men significantly increases total IGF-I but not IGFBP-1 concentrations, thereby preserving free IGF-I availability to a greater extent than E_2. (*Data from* Gentili A, Mulligan T, Godschalk M, et al. Unequal impact of short-term testosterone repletion on the somatotropic axis of young and older men. J Clin Endocrinol Metab 2002;87:825–34.)

Given the ensemble nature of GH control, determining precisely how E_2 directs multi-peptide regulation from any single intervention becomes difficult. For this reason, several recent clinical studies have used simultaneous infusion of two or more secretagogues to unravel interactive mechanisms [13,65,67,70,71]. Even then, the capability to interpret complex physiologic adaptations in GH secretion in aging depends in part upon the availability, practicability, reliability, and incisiveness of clinical experiments and analytical tools. The reader is referred to examples of enhanced analytical methodologies available to clinical investigators [28,39,40,72–74].

Mechanisms of testosterone-stimulated growth hormone secretion in older men

Comparisons by gender indicate that within the premenopausal age range, the rate (slope) of decline in GH production with age is 50% greater in men than women [6]. Extrapolation from cross-sectional data in healthy men further suggests that beginning in young adulthood 24-hour GH secretion falls by approximately 50% every 7 to 12 years (see Fig. 1) [4,5,7,19]. Accordingly, compared with 18- to 21 year-old men, middle-aged and older individuals exhibit an 80% or greater reduction in 24-hour integrated GH concentrations. From a regulatory perspective, attenuated GH secretion in later adulthood may arise (nonexclusively) from decreased stimulation by endogenous GHRH or ghrelin and increased inhibition by SS, GH, or IGF-I [10,75].

To test the role of relative GHRH deficiency, two clinical studies administered low doses of GHRH for up to 21 days in aging men [10]. Neither paradigm achieved a sustained elevation of both GH and IGF-I concentrations into the young adult range. In an investigation of 4 months duration in older men and women, once-daily injection of GHRH stimulated GH secretion for several hours after each injection without increasing morning IGF-I concentrations [76]. A recent analysis showed, however, that administration of a high dose of rh GHRH twice daily in older men will elevate GH and IGF-I concentrations throughout a 3-month intervention [77].

Te stimulates production of GH and IGF-I but not IGFBP-1 in hypoandrogenemic men and boys and genotypic females undergoing gender reassignment [10,22,42,48,78]. The increase in IGF-I concentrations induced by Te is not mimicked by estrogen administration, unless a synthetic progestin is added (Table 2) [13,21]. In fact, at higher concentrations, E_2 inhibits GH receptor-mediated hepatic signaling of IGF-I synthesis [79]. Because Te does not increase hepatic IGF-I synthesis directly [10,25], Te-induced GH secretion seems to be the proximate basis for increased IGF-I production [25–27,41]. In this regard, high interpulse nadir GH concentrations particularly induce hepatic IGF-I synthesis [80].

Classical principles of negative feedback predict that the Te-induced rise in GH and IGF-I concentrations should inhibit GH secretion. For example, infusion of rh GH or rh IGF-I in older adults to mimic midpubertal concentrations rapidly suppresses burst-like GH secretion [10,57,61,68]. Conversely, partial (34%) reduction of systemic IGF-I concentrations by administration of a selective GH-receptor antagonist doubles pulsatile GH secretion in young adults [60]. Recent studies may explain this paradox, in as much as supplementation with Te relieves GH and IGF-I-dependent negative feedback in healthy older men [81,82]. On the other hand, E_2 appears to

Table 2
Sex steroid actions in humans

Outcome	E_2[a]	Te[a]
Total daily GH secretion	↑	↑
GH secretory burst mass	↑	↑
Irregularity (ApEn[b])	↑	↑
Basal GH secretion	↔	↑
IGF-I	↓	↑
IGFBP-1	↑	↔
IGFBP-3	↔	↔
GH negative feedback	↓	↓
IGH-I feedback	↑	↓

Disorderliness increases (ApEn decreases) when feedback is muted and/or augmented, as in puberty. The actions of E_2 and Te differ in that Te elevates IGF-I concentrations, stimulates basal (nonpulsatile) GH secretion, and mutes negative feedback by IGF-I, whereas E_2 elevates IGFBP-1 concentrations, lowers IGF-1 concentrations, and accentuates negative feedback by rhIGF-1.

[a] Regulate specific attributes of GH secretion, concentrations of IGF-I, IGFBP-1, IGFBP-3, and feedback by GH and IGF-I.

[b] Denotes approximate entropy, a measure of the regularity of subpatterns.

potentiate autoinhibition by IGF-I in postmenopausal women [68]. The basis for this apparent dichotomy of sex steroid regulation is not known (see Table 2).

The endogenous GHRP, ghrelin, is unique by way of inducing somatotrope GH secretion directly, stimulating central nervous system (CNS) release of GHRH, synergizing with available GHRH, and antagonizing the hypothalamic and pituitary actions of SS (see Fig. 4). Aging decreases the maximal individual and combined stimulatory effects of GHRH and GHRP [10,83]. Impaired GH secretion is relieved when both peptides are infused after L-arginine injection, which putatively reduces hypothalamic SS release [9,10,84]. Such clinical observations and laboratory experiments suggest that elevated or unvarying SS release in older individuals attenuates the amplitude of GH pulses [10]. This point is important, in as much as E_2 supplementation mutes SS inhibition [55]. Whether Te exerts this effect remains unknown.

The cause of inferably increased SS restraint in older adults has not been established. In as much as age and GH deficiency both enhance hepatic sensitivity to GH [11,12,85], a plausible notion is that aging increases CNS sensitivity to GH feedback-induced SS release [10,83]. Although this hypothesis has not been tested, aging decreases the expression of GH receptor gene transcripts in the brain [86].

Gender contrasts in growth hormone axis regulation in aging adults

Aging impairs hypothalamo–pituitary responses to most clinically used individual GH secretagogues, except insulin-induced hypoglycemia (Fig. 7)

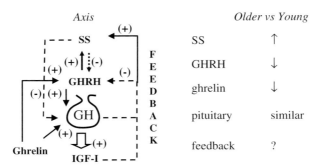

Fig. 7. Postulated mechanisms that contribute to reduced GH secretion and thereby decreased IGF-I production in healthy older adults. Aging augments (*up arrow*) inhibitory outflow of somatostatin (SS) and attenuates stimulatory drive by GHRH and ghrelin (GHRP, *down arrows*). Maximal pituitary secretory capacity is preserved in elderly subjects. The impact of age itself upon GH and IGF-I–dependent negative feedback is not known. Inhibition is shown by interrupted lines (−) and stimulation by continuous lines (+).

[10]. For example, compared with young subjects, older adults have diminished responses to L-arginine, aerobic exercise, GHRH, GHRP-2, and somatostatin withdrawal-induced rebound GH release [10,75]. More recent studies indicate that age, gender, and sex-steroid concentrations jointly determine the maximally stimulatory effects of distinct GH secretagogues [22,54,56,66–68,70,81]. For example, spontaneous GH secretion is greater in women than comparably aged men [46,47,84]. In contrast, somatostatin-induced rebound GH release is several-fold greater in older men than women [70]. From a mechanistic vantage, withdrawal of SS triggers rebound-like secretion of a burst of hypothalamic GHRH and thereby GH [10,67,75]. Estrogen supplementation in ovariprival women enhances rebound GH secretion, possibly because E_2 increases GHRH potency [56,67]. The fact that older men respond more to this intervention than E_2-withdrawn women could indicate that systemic Te in men provides effectual substrate for in situ E_2 synthesis.

Partial molecular silencing of the neuronal ghrelin/GHRP receptor in transgenic mice reduces GH pulse amplitude and IGF-I concentrations in the adult female but not male animal [52]. In consonance with this gender difference, E_2 but not Te potentiates GHRP stimulation in older adults [54,57,81]. E_2 and Te, however, both potentiate GHRP stimulation in children [49]. The latter contrast points to unexplained developmental factors, which might modulate the capability of E_2 to induce transcription of the human GHRP-receptor gene and thus augment GHRP drive [87].

In consonance with the facilitative role of E_2, continuous subcutaneous infusion of GHRP-2 for 30 days amplifies burst-like GH secretion twofold more in postmenopausal estrogen-replaced women than comparably aged men [84]. In addition, constant intravenous infusion of GHRP-2 stimulates pulsatile GH production more in female than male patients with protracted critical illness [88]. In both of these contexts, greater GHRP action correlates with higher estrogen availability.

Summary

Fourfold depletion of GH, IGF-I, Te, and E_2 in healthy aging adults is accompanied by an increased prevalence of clinical, hormonal, biochemical, and structural features of frailty, disability, and reduced quality of life. In principle, the consequences of diminished GH availability could be overcome by supplementation with rh GH [89–92]. There are no definitive safety data that justify long-term GH administration in healthy older individuals, however. Safety issues are paramount, in as much as injection of high doses of rh GH in certain clinical settings (such as protracted critical illness) exacerbates mortality and in GH-deficient adults may elicit mild acromegalic features [93,94]. Mechanistic understanding of normal GH secretion may allow near-physiologic repletion of GH in selected subgroups of older adults at increased catabolic risk. In consideration of this eventual expectation, Fig. 7 summarizes current understanding of mechanistic deficits in aging individuals. The salient distinctions inferred between aging and young adults are a decrease in feedforward by GHRH and GHRP/ghrelin and an increase in feedback by SS.

Te and E_2 both augment GH secretion in older individuals. Recent clinical studies have unveiled that Te and E_2 exert a complex cascade of specific effects on signaling by GHRH and ghrelin/GHRP (stimulatory), somatostatin (inhibitory), and GH and IGF-I (feedback) (see Table 2). The conjoined outcome is amplification of pulsatile GH secretion. Further clinical studies are needed to determine how Te and E_2 drive multi-signal–dependent GH production and modulate organ-specific actions of GH, IGF-I, and IGFBPs in aging individuals.

Acknowledgments

The authors thank Kris Nunez for excellent support of manuscript preparation, Kandace Bradford for assistance in analyses and graphical work, the General Clinical Research Center (GCRC) for conducting research protocols.

References

[1] Finkelstein JW, Roffwarg HP, Boyar RM, et al. Age-related change in the twenty-four-hour spontaneous secretion of growth hormone. J Clin Endocrinol Metab 1972;35:665–70.
[2] Zadik Z, Chalew SA, McCarter RJ Jr, et al. The influence of age on the 24-hour integrated concentration of growth hormone in normal individuals. J Clin Endocrinol Metab 1985;60:513–6.

[3] Ho KKY, Evans WS, Blizzard RM, et al. Effects of sex and age on the 24-hour profile of growth hormone secretion in man: importance of endogenous estradiol concentrations. J Clin Endocrinol Metab 1987;64:51–8.

[4] Iranmanesh A, Lizarralde G, Veldhuis JD. Age and relative adiposity are specific negative determinants of the frequency and amplitude of growth hormone (GH) secretory bursts and the half-life of endogenous GH in healthy men. J Clin Endocrinol Metab 1991;73: 1081–8.

[5] Iranmanesh A, Grisso B, Veldhuis JD. Low basal and persistent pulsatile growth hormone secretions are revealed in normal and hyposomatotropic men studied with a new ultrasensitive chemiluminescence assay. J Clin Endocrinol Metab 1994;78:526–35.

[6] Weltman A, Weltman JY, Hartman ML, et al. Relationship between age, percentage body fat, fitness, and 24-hour growth hormone release in healthy young adults: effects of gender. J Clin Endocrinol Metab 1994;78:543–8.

[7] Iranmanesh A, South S, Liem AY, et al. Unequal impact of age, percentage body fat, and serum testosterone concentrations on the somatotrophic, IGF-I, and IGF-binding protein responses to a three-day intravenous growth hormone-releasing hormone pulsatile infusion in men. Eur J Endocrinol 1998;139:59–71.

[8] Lieman HJ, Adel TE, Forst C, et al. Effects of aging and estradiol supplementation on GH axis dynamics in women. J Clin Endocrinol Metab 2001;86:3918–23.

[9] Arvat E, Ceda GP, Di Vito L, et al. Age-related variations in the neuroendocrine control, more than impaired receptor sensitivity, cause the reduction in the GH-releasing activity of GHRPs in human aging. Pituitary 1998;1:51–8.

[10] Giustina A, Veldhuis JD. Pathophysiology of the neuroregulation of growth hormone secretion in experimental animals and the human. Endocr Rev 1998;19:717–97.

[11] Lissett CA, Shalet SM. The insulin-like growth factor-I generation test: peripheral responsiveness to growth hormone is not decreased with ageing. Clin Endocrinol (Oxf) 2003;58: 238–45.

[12] Arvat E, Ceda G, Ramunni J, et al. The IGF-I response to very low rhGH doses is preserved in human ageing. Clin Endocrinol (Oxf) 1998;49:757–63.

[13] Veldhuis JD, Bowers CY. Sex steroid modulation of growth hormone (GH) secretory control: tripeptidyl ensemble regulation under dual feedback restraint by GH and IGF-I. Endocrine 2003;22:25–40.

[14] Juul A, Scheike T, Davidsen M, et al. Low serum insulin-like growth factor I is associated with increased risk of ischemic heart disease: a population-based case-control study. Circulation 2002;106:939–44.

[15] Laughlin GA, Barrett-Connor E, Criqui MH, et al. The prospective association of serum insulin-like growth factor I (IGF-I) and IGF-binding protein-1 levels with all cause and cardiovascular disease mortality in older adults: the Rancho Bernardo study. J Clin Endocrinol Metab 2004;89:114–20.

[16] Frantz AG, Rabkin MT. Effects of estrogen and sex difference on secretion of human growth hormone. J Clin Endocrinol Metab 1965;25:1470–80.

[17] Wiedemann E, Schwartz E, Frantz AG. Acute and chronic estrogen effects upon serum somatomedin activity, growth hormone, and prolactin in man. J Clin Endocrinol Metab 1976; 42:942–52.

[18] Rosilio M, Blum WF, Edwards DJ, et al. Long-term improvement of quality of life during growth hormone (GH) replacement therapy in adults with GH Deficiency, as measured by Questions on Life Satisfaction-Hypopituitarism (QLS-H). J Clin Endocrinol Metab 2004; 89:1684–93.

[19] Veldhuis JD, Liem AY, South S, et al. Differential impact of age, sex-steroid hormones, and obesity on basal versus pulsatile growth hormone secretion in men as assessed in an ultrasensitive chemiluminescence assay. J Clin Endocrinol Metab 1995;80:3209–22.

[20] Pijl H, Langendonk JG, Burggraaf J, et al. Altered neuroregulation of GH secretion in viscerally obese premenopausal women. J Clin Endocrinol Metab 2001;86:5509–15.

[21] Shah N, Evans WS, Veldhuis JD. Actions of estrogen on the pulsatile, nyctohemeral, and entropic modes of growth hormone secretion. Am J Physiol 1999;276:R1351–8.

[22] Gentili A, Mulligan T, Godschalk M, et al. Unequal impact of short-term testosterone repletion on the somatotropic axis of young and older men. J Clin Endocrinol Metab 2002;87:825–34.

[23] Veldhuis JD, Roemmich JN, Richmond EJ, et al. Endocrine control of body composition in infancy, childhood and puberty. Endocr Rev 2005;26(1):114–46.

[24] Veldhuis JD, Evans WS, Bowers CY, et al. Interactive regulation of postmenopausal growth hormone insulin-like growth factor axis by estrogen and growth hormone-releasing peptide-2. Endocrine 2001;14:45–62.

[25] Weissberger AJ, Ho KKY. Activation of the somatotropic axis by testosterone in adult males: evidence for the role of aromatization. J Clin Endocrinol Metab 1993;1407:1412.

[26] Devesa J, Lois N, Arce V, et al. The role of sexual steroids in the modulation of growth hormone (GH) secretion in humans. J Steroid Biochem Mol Biol 1991;40:165–73.

[27] Veldhuis JD, Metzger DL, Martha PM Jr, et al. Estrogen and testosterone, but not a non-aromatizable androgen, direct network integration of the hypothalamo-somatotrope (growth hormone)-insulin-like growth factor I axis in the human: evidence from pubertal pathophysiology and sex steroid hormone replacement. J Clin Endocrinol Metab 1997;82:3414–20.

[28] Keenan DM, Roelfsema F, Biermasz N, et al. Physiological control of pituitary hormone secretory-burst mass, frequency and waveform: a statistical formulation and analysis. Am J Physiol 2003;285:R664–73.

[29] Le Roith D, Bondy C, Yakar S, et al. The somatomedin hypothesis: 2001. Endocr Rev 2001; 22:53–74.

[30] Achermann JC, Brook CG, Robinson IC, et al. Peak and trough growth hormone (GH) concentrations influence growth and serum insulin like growth factor-1 (IGF-1) concentrations in short children. Clin Endocrinol (Oxf) 1999;50:301–8.

[31] Jaffe CA, Turgeon DK, Lown K, et al. Growth hormone secretion pattern is an independent regulator of growth hormone actions in humans. Am J Physiol Endocrinol Metab 2002;283: E1008–15.

[32] Lindahl A, Isgaard J, Carlsson L, et al. Differential effects of growth hormone and insulin-like growth factor I on colony formation of epiphyseal chondrocytes in suspension culture in rats of different ages. Endocrinology 1987;121:1061–9.

[33] Mauras N, O'Brien KO, Welch S, et al. Insulin-like growth factor I and growth hormone (GH) treatment in GH-deficient humans: differential effects on protein, glucose, lipid, and calcium metabolism. J Clin Endocrinol Metab 2000;85:1686–94.

[34] Johannsson G, Bjarnason R, Bramnert M, et al. The individual responsiveness to growth hormone (GH) treatment in GH-deficient adults is dependent on the level of GH-binding protein, body mass index, age, and gender. J Clin Endocrinol Metab 1996;81:1575–81.

[35] Duenas M, Torres-Aleman I, Naftolin F, et al. Interaction of insulin-like growth factor-I and estradiol signaling pathways on hypothalamic neuronal differentiation. Neuroscience 1996; 74:531–9.

[36] Lichtenwalner RJ, Forbes ME, Bennett SA, et al. Intracerebroventricular infusion of insulin-like growth factor-I ameliorates the age-related decline in hippocampal neurogenesis. Neuroscience 2001;107:603–13.

[37] Farhy LS, Straume M, Johnson ML, et al. A construct of interactive feedback control of the GH axis in the male. Am J Physiol 2001;281:R38–51.

[38] Farhy LS, Straume M, Johnson ML, et al. Unequal autonegative feedback by GH models the sexual dimorphism in GH secretory dynamics. Am J Physiol 2002;282:R753–64.

[39] Farhy LS, Veldhuis JD. Joint pituitary hypothalamic and intrahypothalamic autofeedback construct of pulsatile growth hormone secretion. Am J Physiol Regul Integr Comp Physiol 2003;285:R1240–9.

[40] Farhy LS, Veldhuis JD. Putative GH pulse renewal: periventricular somatostatinergic control of an arcuate-nuclear somatostatin and GH-releasing hormone oscillator. Am J Physiol 2004;286:R1030–42.

[41] Metzger DL, Kerrigan JR. Estrogen receptor blockade with tamoxifen diminishes growth hormone secretion in boys: evidence for a stimulatory role of endogenous estrogens during male adolescence. J Clin Endocrinol Metab 1994;79:513–8.

[42] Fryburg DA, Weltman A, Jahn LA, et al. Short-term modulation of the androgen milieu alters pulsatile but not exercise or GHRH-stimulated GH secretion in healthy men. J Clin Endocrinol Metab 1997;82:3710–9.

[43] Yen SSC, Vela P, Rankin J, et al. Hormonal relationships during the menstrual cycle. JAMA 1970;211:1513–7.

[44] Faria ACS, Bekenstein LW, Booth RA Jr, et al. Pulsatile growth hormone release in normal women during the menstrual cycle. Clin Endocrinol (Oxf) 1992;36:591–6.

[45] Ovesen P, Vahl N, Fisker S, et al. Increased pulsatile, but not basal, growth hormone secretion rates and plasma insulin-like growth factor I levels during the preovulatory interval in normal women. J Clin Endocrinol Metab 1998;83:1662–7.

[46] van den Berg G, Veldhuis JD, Frolich M, et al. An amplitude-specific divergence in the pulsatile mode of GH secretion underlies the gender difference in mean GH concentrations in men and premenopausal women. J Clin Endocrinol Metab 1996;81:2460–6.

[47] Veldhuis JD, Roemmich JN, Rogol AD. Gender and sexual maturation-dependent contrasts in the neuroregulation of growth hormone secretion in prepubertal and late adolescent males and females—a general clinical research center-based study. J Clin Endocrinol Metab 2000; 85:2385–94.

[48] van Kesteren P, Lips P, Deville W, et al. The effect of one-year cross-sex hormonal treatment on bone metabolism and serum insulin-like growth factor-1 in transsexuals. J Clin Endocrinol Metab 1996;81:2227–32.

[49] Loche S, Colao A, Cappa M, et al. The growth hormone response to hexarelin in children: reproducibility and effect of sex steroids. J Clin Endocrinol Metab 1997;82:861–4.

[50] Lissett CA, Shalet SM. The impact of dose and route of estrogen administration on the somatotropic axis in normal women. J Clin Endocrinol Metab 2003;88:4668–72.

[51] Hartman ML, Faria AC, Vance ML, et al. Temporal structure of in vivo growth hormone secretory events in man. Am J Physiol 1991;260:E101–10.

[52] Shuto Y, Shibasaki T, Otagiri A, et al. Hypothalamic growth hormone secretagogue receptor regulates growth hormone secretion, feeding, and adiposity. J Clin Invest 2002;109:1429–36.

[53] Low MJ, Otero-Corchon V, Parlow AF, et al. Somatostatin is required for masculinization of growth hormone-regulated hepatic gene expression but not of somatic growth. J Clin Invest 2001;107:1571–80.

[54] Anderson SM, Shah N, Evans WS, et al. Short-term estradiol supplementation augments growth hormone (GH) secretory responsiveness to dose-varying GH-releasing peptide infusions in healthy postmenopausal women. J Clin Endocrinol Metab 2001;86:551–60.

[55] Bray MJ, Vick TM, Shah N, et al. Short-term estradiol replacement in postmenopausal women selectively mutes somatostatin's dose-dependent inhibition of fasting growth hormone secretion. J Clin Endocrinol Metab 2001;86:3143–9.

[56] Veldhuis JD, Evans WS, Bowers CY. Estradiol supplementation enhances submaximal feed-forward drive of growth hormone (GH) secretion by recombinant human GH-releasing hormone-1,44-amide in a putatively somatostatin-withdrawn milieu. J Clin Endocrinol Metab 2003;88:5484–9.

[57] Anderson SM, Wideman L, Patrie JT, et al. Estradiol supplementation selectively relieves GH's autonegative feedback on GH-releasing peptide-2-stimulated GH secretion. J Clin Endocrinol Metab 2001;86:5904–11.

[58] Hataya Y, Akamizu T, Takaya K, et al. A low dose of ghrelin stimulates growth hormone (GH) release synergistically with GH-releasing hormone in humans. J Clin Endocrinol Metab 2001;86:4552.

[59] Di Vito L, Broglio F, Benso A, et al. The GH-releasing effect of ghrelin, a natural GH secretagogue, is only blunted by the infusion of exogenous somatostatin in humans. Clin Endocrinol (Oxf) 2002;56:643–8.

[60] Veldhuis JD, Bidlingmaier M, Anderson SM, et al. Lowering total plasma insulin-like growth factor I concentrations by way of a novel, potent, and selective growth hormone (GH) receptor antagonist, pegvisomant (B2036-peg), augments the amplitude of GH secretory bursts and elevates basal/nonpulsatile GH release in healthy women and men. J Clin Endocrinol Metab 2001;86:3304–10.

[61] Camacho-Hubner C, Woods KA, Miraki-Moud F, et al. Effects of recombinant human insulin-like growth factor I (IGF-I) therapy on the growth hormone-IGF system of a patient with a partial IGF-I gene deletion. J Clin Endocrinol Metab 1999;84:1611–6.

[62] Shah N, Evans WS, Bowers CY, et al. Tripartite neuroendocrine activation of the human growth-hormone (GH) axis in women by continuous 24-hour GH-releasing peptide (GHRP-2) infusion: pulsatile, entropic, and nyctohemeral mechanisms. J Clin Endocrinol Metab 1999;84:2140–50.

[63] Shah N, Evans WS, Bowers CY, et al. Oral estradiol administration modulates continuous intravenous growth hormone (GH)-releasing peptide-2 driven GH secretion in postmenopausal women. J Clin Endocrinol Metab 2000;85:2649–59.

[64] Evans WS, Anderson SM, Hull LT, et al. Continuous 24-hour intravenous infusion of recombinant human growth hormone (GH)-releasing hormone-(1, 44)-amide augments pulsatile, entropic, and daily rhythmic GH secretion in postmenopausal women equally in the estrogen-withdrawn and estrogen-supplemented states. J Clin Endocrinol Metab 2001;86: 700–12.

[65] Veldhuis JD, Evans WS, Bowers CY. Impact of estradiol supplementation on dual peptidyl drive of growth hormone secretion in postmenopausal women. J Clin Endocrinol Metab 2002;87:859–66.

[66] Veldhuis JD, Patrie J, Wideman L, et al. Contrasting negative-feedback control of endogenously driven and exercise-stimulated pulsatile growth hormone secretion in women and men. J Clin Endocrinol Metab 2004;89:840–6.

[67] Veldhuis JD, Anderson SM, Patrie JT, et al. Estradiol supplementation in postmenopausal women doubles rebound-like release of growth hormone (GH) triggered by sequential infusion and withdrawal of somatostatin: evidence that estrogen facilitates endogenous GH-releasing hormone drive. J Clin Endocrinol Metab 2004;89:121–7.

[68] Veldhuis JD, Anderson SM, Kok P, et al. Estradiol supplementation modulates growth hormone (GH) secretory-burst waveform and recombinant human insulin-like growth factor-I-enforced suppression of endogenously driven GH release in postmenopausal women. J Clin Endocrinol Metab 2004;89:1312–8.

[69] Bowers CY. New insight into the control of growth hormone secretion. In: Kleinberg DL, Clemmons DR, editors. Central and peripheral mechanisms in pituitary disease. Bristol (UK): BioScientifica Ltd; 2002. p. 163–75.

[70] Veldhuis JD, Patrie JT, Brill KT, et al. Contributions of gender and systemic estradiol and testosterone concentrations to maximal secretagogue drive of burst-like GH secretion in healthy middle-aged and older adults. J Clin Endocrinol Metab 2004;89(12): 6291–6.

[71] Erickson D, Keenan DM, Mielke K, et al. Dual secretagogue drive of burst-like growth hormone secretion in postmenopausal compared with premenopausal women studied under an experimental estradiol clamp. J Clin Endocrinol Metab 2004;89:4746–54.

[72] Pincus SM, Mulligan T, Iranmanesh A, et al. Older males secrete luteinizing hormone and testosterone more irregularly, and jointly more asynchronously, than younger males. Proc Natl Acad Sci U S A 1996;93:14100–5.

[73] Keenan DM, Licinio J, Veldhuis JD. A feedback-controlled ensemble model of the stress-responsive hypothalamo-pituitary-adrenal axis. Proc Natl Acad Sci U S A 2001;98: 4028–33.

[74] Keenan DM, Alexander SL, Irvine CHG, et al. Reconstruction of in vivo time-evolving neuroendocrine dose-response properties unveils admixed deterministic and stochastic elements in interglandular signaling. Proc Natl Acad Sci U S A 2004;101:6740–5.

[75] degli Uberti EC, Ambrosio MR, Cella SG, et al. Defective hypothalamic growth hormone (GH)-releasing hormone activity may contribute to declining GH secretion with age in man. J Clin Endocrinol Metab 1997;82:2885–8.

[76] Khorram O, Laughlin GA, Yen SSC. Endocrine and metabolic effects of long-term administration of [Nle^{27}]growth hormone-releasing hormone-(1–29)-NH$_2$ in age-advanced men and women. J Clin Endocrinol Metab 1997;82:1472–9.

[77] Veldhuis JD, Patrie JT, Frick K, et al. Sustained GH and IGF-I responses to prolonged high-dose twice-daily GHRH stimulation in middle-aged and older men. J Clin Endocrinol Metab 2004;89:6325–30.

[78] Giustina A, Scalvini T, Tassi C, et al. Maturation of the regulation of growth hormone secretion in young males with hypogonadotropic hypogonadism pharmacologically exposed to progressive increments in serum testosterone. J Clin Endocrinol Metab 1997;82:1210–9.

[79] Span JP, Pieters GF, Sweep CG, et al. Gender difference in insulin-like growth factor I response to growth hormone (GH) treatment in GH-deficient adults: role of sex hormone replacement. J Clin Endocrinol Metab 2000;85:1121–5.

[80] Hartman ML, Pincus SM, Johnson ML, et al. Enhanced basal and disorderly growth hormone secretion distinguish acromegalic from normal pulsatile growth hormone release. J Clin Invest 1994;94:1277–88.

[81] Veldhuis JD, Evans WS, Iranmanesh A, et al. Short-term testosterone supplementation relieves growth hormone autonegative feedback in men. J Clin Endocrinol Metab 2004;89:1285–90.

[82] Veldhuis JD, Anderson SM, Iranmanesh A, et al. Testosterone blunts feedback inhibition of GH secretion by experimentally elevated IGF-I concentrations. J Clin Endocrinol Metab 2005;90(3):1613–7.

[83] Mueller EE, Locatelli V, Cocchi D. Neuroendocrine control of growth hormone secretion. Physiol Rev 1999;79:511–607.

[84] Bowers CY, Granda R, Mohan S, et al. Sustained elevation of pulsatile growth hormone (GH) secretion and insulin-like growth factor I (IGF-I), IGF-binding protein-3 (IGFBP-3), and IGFBP-5 concentrations during 30-day continuous subcutaneous infusion of GH-releasing peptide-2 in older men and women. J Clin Endocrinol Metab 2004;89:2290–300.

[85] Aimaretti G, Fanciulli G, Bellone S, et al. Enhancement of the peripheral sensitivity to growth hormone in adults with GH deficiency. Eur J Endocrinol 2001;145:267–72.

[86] Nyberg F. Aging effects on growth hormone receptor binding in the brain. Exp Gerontol 1997;32:521–8.

[87] Petersenn S, Rasch AC, Penshorn M, et al. Genomic structure and transcriptional regulation of the human growth hormone secretagogue receptor. Endocrinology 2001;142:2649–59.

[88] Van den Berghe G, Baxter RC, Weekers F, et al. A paradoxical gender dissociation within the growth hormone/insulin-like growth factor I axis during protracted critical illness. J Clin Endocrinol Metab 2000;85:183–92.

[89] Johannsson G, Grimby G, Sunnerhagen KS, et al. Two years of growth hormone (GH) treatment increase isometric and isokinetic muscle strength in GH-deficient adults. J Clin Endocrinol Metab 1997;82:2877–84.

[90] Cuneo RC, Salomon F, Watts GF, et al. Growth hormone treatment improves serum lipids and lipoproteins in adults with growth hormone deficiency. Metabolism 1993;42:1519–23.

[91] Johannsson G, Marin P, Lonn L, et al. Growth hormone treatment of abdominally obese men reduces abdominal fat mass, improves glucose and lipoprotein metabolism, and reduces diastolic blood pressure. J Clin Endocrinol Metab 1997;82:727–34.

[92] Johannsson G, Bengtsson BA. Growth hormone and the acquisition of bone mass. Horm Res 1997;48(Suppl 5):72–7.

[93] Bengtsson BA. Rethink about growth hormone therapy for critically ill patients. Lancet 1999;354:1403–4.

[94] Carvalho LR, de Faria ME, Osorio MG, et al. Acromegalic features in growth hormone (GH)-deficient patients after long-term GH therapy. Clin Endocrinol (Oxf) 2003;59:788–92.

ELSEVIER
SAUNDERS

Endocrinol Metab Clin N Am
34 (2005) 895–906

ENDOCRINOLOGY
AND METABOLISM
CLINICS
OF NORTH AMERICA

Testing Pituitary Function in Aging Individuals

Roberta Giordano, MD[a],
Gianluca Aimaretti, MD, PhD[a],
Fabio Lanfranco, MD[a], Mario Bo, MD[b],
Matteo Baldi, MD[a], Fabio Broglio, MD, PhD[a],
Roberto Baldelli, MD[a], Silvia Grottoli, MD[a],
Ezio Ghigo, MD[a], Emanuela Arvat, MD[a],*

[a]Division of Endocrinology and Metabolism, Department of Internal Medicine,
University of Turin, Turin, Italy
[b]Section of Geriatrics, Department of Medical and Surgical Disciplines,
University of Turin, Turin, Italy

Changes in endocrine function in aging individuals often reflect age-related impairment in animal and human neuroendocrine regulation of pituitary function. Growth hormone/insulin-like growth factor (GH/IGF)-I hypofunction in the elderly is a clear example of decreased activity as a function of age-related changes in the neural control of somatotroph cells [1–4]. GH secretion undergoes clear variations during an individual's lifespan: its secretion is maximal at birth, strongly increased during puberty, and progressively decreased thereafter showing very low secretion in the aged [5]. Mechanisms underlying the age-related changes of GH secretion involve peripheral influences (ie, gonadal steroids and adiposity), but age-related changes in hypothalamic neuropeptide and neurotransmitter release, mainly GHRH and somatostatin (SS), play a major role. GHRH and SS are likely to reflect age-dependent changes in suprahypothalamic functions [1–4]. Animal and human studies indicate that age-related changes in neurotransmitter regulation leading to GHRH

This article is based on the personal studies of the authors supported by the Ministero Istruzione Università e Ricerca (MIUR, Rome, Italy) and the University of Turin and SMEM Foundation of Turin (Turin, Italy).
  * Corresponding author. Division of Endocrinology and Metabolism, Department of Internal Medicine, University of Turin, Corso Dogliotti 14, 10126 Turin, Italy.
  E-mail address: emanuela.arvat@unito.it (E. Arvat).

hypoactivity and absolute or relative SS hyperactivity mainly account for the reduction of spontaneous and stimulated GH secretion in the elderly [1–4].

Cholinergic impairment in the aging brain involves hypothalamic pathways and contributes to the disrupted GHRH/SS interplay that underlies GH/IGF-I hyposecretion [6]. Also, age-related variations in the ghrelin system (ghrelin being a gastric hormone discovered as a natural GH secretagogue [GHS] acting within the central nervous system [CNS] and the hypothalamus) could play a role in the decreased GH secretion that connotes aging [7–9].

From a clinical point of view, aging is associated with changes in body composition, metabolism, and structural functions and results in reduced lean mass, increased adiposity, decreased bone mass, and protein synthesis [1,10]. These alterations are similar to those in young adults with GH deficiency (GHD) [11,12], and this evidence, together with demonstrated age-related declining activity of the GH/IGF-I axis, has led to the neologism *somatopause*, which indicates the potential link between age-related decline in GH and IGF-I levels and frailty in the aging [13].

Taking into account the clinical and hormonal features of somatopause, diagnosis of GHD in the aging is the subject of much controversy. GHD must be carefully distinguished from the reduction in GH secretion that accompanies normal aging and obesity. To avoid overtreatment, GH replacement is warranted only for severe GHD [14]. There is consensus that very low IGF-I levels may be representative of adult GHD, although normal IGF-I levels do not rule out the presence of severe GHD [15–18]. As total IGF-I levels are often within the normal age-related limits, subjects suspected of having adult GHD often undergo provocative testing of GH secretion, which determines whether somatotroph function is impaired or normal [14,18,19]. The importance of accurate diagnosis of GHD in the elderly is based on evidence that elderly patients who have GHD do benefit from replacement treatment with recombinant human GH (rhGH), while the efficacy of rejuvenating the GH/IGF-I axis in somatopause has not been proven.

Provocative tests for somatotroph release as a function of age

Insulin-induced hypoglycemia: insulin tolerance test

The insulin tolerance test (ITT) is considered the gold standard test to investigate somatotroph function. Hypoglycemia stimulates GH secretion by means of multifactorial central mechanisms representing the hypothalamic neuroendocrine response to a stressful condition and includes activation of the hypothalamus-pituitary-adrenal axis. An increase in endogenous GHRH activity with a concomitant decrease in hypothalamic SS release, and an increase in catecholamine release with α-adrenergic activation seem to be the most significant mechanisms that lead to an increase in GH. GH response to ITT (0.05 to 0.15 IU regular insulin intravenously) undergoes age-related variations, increasing from childhood to adulthood without significant change in the aging. GH response to ITT does not appear to be affected by sex, but is reduced in obesity, where it shows poor intraindividual reproducibility, implying low specificity. It is generally contraindicated and risky when CNS or cardiovascular diseases are present or suspected [19–26].

Arginine and ornithine

The mechanisms of action of arginine are not unlike those of ornithine, an arginine metabolite, but other amino acids (eg, methyonine) act by means of other unknown mechanisms. Arginine likely acts primarily by means of negative modulation of hypothalamic SS release, although this assumption is based on indirect evidence only [8]. The arginine-induced GH response (0.5 g/kg infused for 30 minutes intravenously) is independent of age, but not sex (more prevalent in women than in men as a function of the positive influence of estrogens), and reduced in obesity. Poor intraindividual reproducibility of GH response to this test has been demonstrated, which implies low specificity. It is generally well-tolerated, although vomiting can occur as function of overdose or rapid infusion [24–29].

Glucagon

Intramuscular or subcutaneous, but not intravenous, administration of glucagon is followed by a marked increase in GH and corticotropin (ACTH)/cortisol. Thus, glucagon is not a true stimulus of somatotroph secretion. The mechanisms of action are likely related to products of its degradation. There is no confirmed data about GH response to intramuscular glucagon (1.0 mg) as a function of age and sex, although glucagon's stimulatory effect is reduced obesity. Poor intraindividual reproducibility of GH response to this test has been demonstrated, which implies low specificity. It is generally well-tolerated, although vomiting can occur as a function of overdose or rapid infusion [19,26,30–32].

Levodopa

Levodopa, another one of the oldest provocative tests, stimulates GH by means of dopaminergic activation, which, in turn, likely inhibits hypothalamic SS release or stimulates endogenous GHRH activity. There is no confirmed data about GH response to levodopa as a function of age, sex, and body weight. Levodopa (125, 250, and 500 mg by mouth for a body weight less than 15 kg, between 15 and 30 kg, and more than 30 kg, respectively) is a stimulus weaker than ITT, arginine, and intramuscular glucagon. Very poor intraindividual reproducibility of the response to this test has been demonstrated, implying low specificity. Levodopa administration often induces nausea and vomiting [25,26,33].

Clonidine

Clonidine, an α2-adrenergic agonist, displays the GH-releasing effect in agreement with the positive influence of α-adrenergic receptors on somatotroph function. The stimulatory effect of clonidine comprises concomitant stimulation of GHRH–secreting neurons and inhibition of SS-secreting neurons. There is no definitive data supporting the GH-releasing effect of clonidine as a function of age and sex, although its effect is reduced obesity. It is assumed that clonidine represents a stimulus weaker than ITT, arginine, and intramuscular glucagons. An assumption based on low oral doses (0.15 mg/m^2) which are usually administered to avoid more marked vascular adverse effects observed after intravenous administration. Very poor intraindividual reproducibility of the response to this test has been demonstrated, implying low specificity [26,33,34].

Other neuroactive substances used as stimuli of growth hormone secretion

In agreement with the evidence that acetylcholine plays a major role in the neural regulation of GH secretion, through the negative modulation of hypothalamic SS release, cholinergic agonists such as pyridostigmine stimulate GH secretion. Although several cholinergic agonists have been shown to significantly increase GH secretion, pyridostigmine has been the most studied in people. The GH response to pyridostigmine in children and adults is similar, although it is reduced in elderly subjects. It seems independent of sex but influenced by body weight, being decreased in obesity. Pyridostigmine (60 mg by mouth in children and 120 mg by mouth in adults) elicits a GH response lower than that recorded after ITT, arginine, and glucagon. Cholinergic adverse effects (fasciculations, abdominal pain) often are observed after drug administration [24,29,33,35].

Galanin

Galanin is a neuropeptide that stimulates GH secretion by means of concomitant GHRH increase and SS inhibition. Its effect depends on age (less marked in the aging) and sex (more marked in women) and decreased obesity. Galanin (80 pmol/kg/min intravenously) has been investigated as a potentially new provocative test for GH secretion, but it represents a stimulus weaker than ITT, arginine, and glucagon and cannot be used in current clinical practice [33].

Steroids

Glucocorticoids play a dual role in GH secretion. Besides long-term inhibition following overexposure to natural and synthetic glucocorticoids, acute administrations of synthetic glucocorticoids stimulate GH secretion, probably by inhibiting hypothalamic SS release. Synthetic glucocorticoids have been proposed as new provocative test, but their advantage over other classical provocative tests has not yet been demonstrated [36].

Although gonadal steroids are devoid of a direct stimulatory effect on GH secretion, they have been often used to sensitize GH response to classical provocative stimuli in children. In fact, pretreatment with androgens and estrogens has been shown to increase GH responsiveness to stimulatory agents in boys and girls. This procedure was popular in past years, but never validated, and there is no consensus about usefulness of priming with sex steroids before provocative tests. Gonadal steroids also enhance spontaneous and stimulated GH secretion in the aging. Somatotroph pulsatility is, in fact, amplified by both estrogens and androgens in elderly women and men, respectively. Moreover, estrogen pretreatment significantly increased GHRH-induced GH release in postmenopausal women. Priming with gonadal steroids, however, has never been proposed in clinical practice for evaluating somatotrope function in aging [5,37,38].

Growth hormone-releasing hormone

By activating pituitary GHRH receptors, GHRH is a neurohormone that specifically stimulates somatotroph cell proliferation, GH synthesis, and release. Its tight interaction with SS is needed to generate GH pulsatility. Although originally considered a more useful stimulus for GH secretion in the diagnosis of childhood and adult GHD in comparison with classical tests, GHRH has poor reproducibility and reliability as a provocative test. This variability likely reflects variations in endogenous somatostatinergic tone and makes it difficult to define reliable normative limits for this test, the specificity of which is very low. It remains debatable whether GH response to GHRH (1 µg/kg intravenously) is sex-dependent (having been reported to be higher in women and enhanced by exposure to estrogens). GH response to GHRH is influenced by body weight and less effective obesity. It has been demonstrated that the GH-releasing effect of GHRH changes during an individual's lifespan. It is at its peak in newborns, similar in children and young adults, slightly higher than that seen after ITT, and markedly decreased in the elderly, likely a consequence of hypothalamic SS hyperactivity. In about 30% of elderly subjects, however, a normal GH response to GHRH can be detected, which is in agreement with evidence in animals showing that pituitary somatotroph capacity is preserved with advancing age. As a consequence of the age-related decline in the GH-releasing activity of GHRH, testing with GHRH is not useful in the diagnosis of GHD in elderly people, unless combined with other neuroactive substances that inhibit SS release. GHRH administration does not induce significant adverse effects, except for mild and transient facial flushing [19,24–26,33].

Natural and synthetic growth hormone secretagogues

Synthetic GHS and the natural ligand of GHS receptors (ie, ghrelin) strongly stimulate GH secretion by directly stimulating the pituitary gland and primarily activating GHRH-secreting neurons in the hypothalamus. Their action as functional antagonists of somatostatin also has demonstrated [9].

The GH response to both ghrelin and synthetic GHS (1 or 2 µg/kg intravenously) is independent of sex, although it is decreased in ratio of increasing body weight. The GH-releasing activity of ghrelin and synthetic GHS undergoes marked age-related variations, different from those recorded after GHRH. In fact, as opposed to GHRH, GH response to GHS is low at birth, significantly increased during puberty, and progressively decreased with advancing age, likely a consequence of age-dependent changes in the hypothalamic neuroendocrine regulation of somatotroph function (ie, GHRH hypoactivity and SS hyperactivity). Even in the elderly, however, ghrelin and GHS are more potent than GHRH in stimulating GH secretion. Good intraindividual reproducibility of the GH response to GHS has been demonstrated, but normative limits, which should be age-related, have not been defined. The administration of ghrelin and GHS does not induce relevant adverse effects, except for mild, transient facial flushing and hunger [7–9,39].

Growth hormone-releasing hormone in combination with arginine, pyridostigmine, or growth hormone secretagogues

GHRH has been shown to be one of the most powerful and reproducible stimuli of GH secretion when given in combination with substances with the capacity to increase its GH-releasing activity by counteracting the SS tone (Figs. 1 and 2). Several neuroactive substances are able to strengthen GH

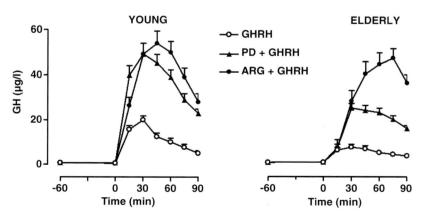

Fig. 1. GH responses (mean ± SEM) to GHRH (1 µg/kg as intravenous bolus at 0 min), pyridostigmine (PD, 120 mg orally at −60 min) + GHRH or arginine (ARG, 0.5 g/kg intravenously over 30 minutes from 0 to +30 min) + GHRH in young and elderly subjects.

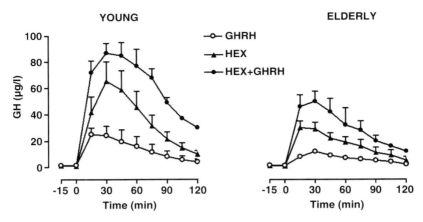

Fig. 2. GH responses (mean ± SEM) to GHRH (1 µg/kg as intravenous bolus at 0 min), hexarelin (HEX, 2 µg/kg as intravenous bolus at 0 min) or HEX + GHRH in young and elderly subjects.

response to GHRH: propranolol, pyridostigmine, arginine, galanin, ghrelin, and synthetic GHS. By inhibiting SS release or antagonizing its inhibitory activity on somatotroph cells, these molecules allow GHRH to fully express its GH-releasing action and assess the maximal releasable pool of GH. This, in turn, reflects the appropriate function of hypothalamic mechanisms regulating GH synthesis and secretion. Particularly, GHRH + pyridostigmine, GHRH + arginine, and GHRH + GHRP-6 or hexarelin, two synthetic GHS, have been proposed as provocative tests for diagnosing GHD. GH response to these tests does not seem to be dependent on sex, although it is inversely associated with body mass.

As far as the utility of these provocative stimulations in the elderly is concerned, the GH-releasing effect of GHRH combined with pyridostigmine or GHS is strongly age-dependent, showing reduced activity with advancing age. This likely reflects age-related changes in the primary regulation of GH secretion, involving impairment of cholinergic activity and SS hypertone. Thus, they are not as reliable in the aged as in young subjects to distinguish normal from GHD-aged subjects. Conversely, GHRH when combined with arginine, does not show age-related GH responses, demonstrating a similar GH response during an individual's life span. This evidence implies at least two major considerations:

1. The maximal somatotroph capacity is preserved in human aging, in agreement with animal studies, indicating that the age-related GH decline mostly reflects central variations in neuroendocrine control of pituitary function.
2. The normal cut-off limit of the GH response to this test can be assumed to be the same in all ages, making this a good provocative test for diagnosing GHD through the life span.

Very good diagnostic reliability of GHRH + arginine test has been shown in the period from childhood to the elderly years. Thus, this testing procedure is considered as an alternative provocative test for diagnosing adult GHD when ITT is contraindicated. This procedure is brief (30, 45, and 60 minutes), which reduces testing time and costs. The adverse effects recorded during this test are negligible, and similar to those reported after GHRH or arginine alone [24,26,39–44].

Diagnosis of growth hormone deficiency in the aging individual

Following the Consensus Guidelines of the Growth Hormone Research Society, it is recommended that the diagnosis of GHD in adulthood be established biochemically by provocative testing of GH secretion [14]. An evaluation for GHD should be considered only in patients for whom there is high suspicion for acquired hypothalamic-pituitary disease or in patients with childhood-onset GHD [14,24,45].

That the diagnosis of adult GHD requires a clear failure to respond to provocative testing is based on evidence that such tests (eg, insulin-induced hypoglycemia, but not GH surrogates such as IGF-I and IGFBP-3) can distinguish between normal and GHD subjects [21]. In fact, IGF-I levels are often overlapping in normal adults and patients who have GHD, and this is even more evident in aging individuals, based on age-related IGF-I decline [4,16–18].

GH secretion undergoes age-related variations that are generally mirrored by IGF-I levels (the best marker of GH status) in both animals and humans; the notable exception being at birth [1–4]. A progressive fall in 24-hour GH secretory rates occurs during the aging process (~14% per decade) [46,47]. The distinction between normal and GHD subjects based on the amount of spontaneous GH concentration is difficult to determine even in adulthood based on remarkable overlap between normal and GHD subjects on the individual basis and compounded in the elderly [11,19]. Accordingly, although IGF-I levels generally reflect the GH status in aging and in adulthood, IGF-I levels in normal and GHD subjects show remarkable overlap that reduces the diagnostic value of total IGF-I measurement for diagnosing severe GHD. In the absence of nutritional impairment, however, low IGF-I levels strongly point toward possible severe GHD [16–19].

Thus, in aging and in adulthood, the diagnosis of severe GHD must be shown biochemically by single provocative testing, provided that a reproducible test with clear normative limits is available [14,21]. It has been demonstrated that at least some provocative tests distinguish GHD from normal.

As anticipated, ITT is considered the test of choice, and severe GHD, requiring treatment with rhGH, was defined arbitrarily as a GH response below 3 μg/L [14,21]. Based on the ITT contraindications (ischemic heart disease, seizure disorders, and aging), however, this test is unlikely to be that of choice to test elderly subjects suspected for GHD [23]. Alternative provocative tests with appropriate cut-off limits have been validated. Among classical tests, it has been reported that glucagon is reliable to distinguish normal from GHD subjects, even in aging [19].

GHRH + arginine has been shown to be a reliable means of diagnosing severe GHD, also in the aging individual by distinguishing GHD from normal elderly subjects, while assuming a cut-off point of 9 µg/L GH peak. This reliability reflects the age-independent GH-releasing action of the GHRH and arginine combination [42].

On the other hand, the GHRH, synthetic GHS, and arginine combination represents another potent and reproducible provocative test, which has been shown to distinguish GHD from normal subjects even in the elderly. The cut-off point, below which severe GHD is demonstrated by this test, has been defined as 10 µg/L GH peak. The GH-releasing action has been reported to independent of age [40–42]. The GH response to GHRH in combination with arginine or GHS is likely to depend negatively on BMI; therefore, lower cut-off points should be considered in the presence of obesity [42].

Summary

GH provocative tests remain the only hormonal investigation that provides data on somatotroph function during an individual's lifespan. Diagnosis of GHD in the elderly is difficult because of age-related GH secretory decline or somatopause. In aging and adulthood, the evaluation of spontaneous GH secretion and IGF-I levels does not provide grounds for distinguishing GHD subjects from normal subjects. Thus, severe GHD must be biochemically demonstrated by provocative testing. Among classical tests, ITT is considered the gold standard, while arginine and glucagon are considered reliable alternatives. ITT, however, has contraindications that are particularly relevant to elderly subjects. GHRH in combination with arginine or synthetic GHS has become the most potent and reproducible stimulus of GH secretion because it explores the maximal secretory capacity of somatotroph cells and is independent of aging. This approach to somatotroph test function shows high specificity and very good sensitivity as it can distinguish between normal and GHD subjects even in the elderly. GHRH in combination with arginine or GHS is safe and has no known contraindications. This profile is therefore relevant in term of availability of a good provocative test for GH secretion in aging individuals. In fact, even in this period of life, diagnosis of GHD may be crucial, based on the evidence that treating GHD patients with rhGH replacement therapy counteracts several clinical symptoms that are more likely associated with GHD than aging.

Acknowledgments

The authors wish to thank Prof. Camanni for his support and suggestions.

References

[1] Corpas E, Harman SM, Blackman MR. Human growth hormone and human aging. Endocr Rev 1993;14:20–39.

[2] Muller EE, Cella SG, Parenti M, et al. Somatotropic dysregulation in old mammals. Horm Res 1995;43:39–45.

[3] Ghigo E, Arvat E, Gianotti L, et al. Human aging and the GH-IGF-I axis. J Pediatr Endocrinol Metab 1996;9:271–8.

[4] Arvat E, Giordano R, Gianotti L, et al. Neuroendocrinology of the human growth-hormone-insulin-like growth factor I axis during aging. Growth Horm IGF Res 1999;9(Suppl A):111–5.

[5] Giustina A, Veldhuis JD. Pathophysiology of the neuroregulation of growth hormone secretion in experimental animals and the human. Endocr Rev 1998;19:717–97.

[6] White P, Hiley CR, Goodhardt MJ, et al. Neocortical cholinergic neurons in elderly people. Lancet 1977;1(8013):668–71.

[7] Kojima M, Hosoda H, Date Y, et al. Ghrelin is a growth-hormone-releasing acylated peptide from stomach. Nature 1999;402:656–60.

[8] Ghigo E, Arvat E, Giordano R, et al. Biologic activities of growth hormone secretagogues in humans. Endocrine 2001;14:87–93.

[9] van der Lely AJ, Tschop M, Heiman ML, et al. Biological, physiological, pathophysiological, and pharmacological aspects of ghrelin. Endocr Rev 2004;25:426–57.

[10] Rudman D, Feller AG, Nagraj HS, et al. Effects of human growth hormone in men over 60 years old. N Engl J Med 1990;323:1–6.

[11] de Boer H, Blok GJ, Van der Veen EA. Clinical aspects of growth hormone deficiency in adults. Endocr Rev 1995;16:63–86.

[12] Toogod AA, Shalet SM. Ageing and growth hormone status. Baillieres Clin Endocrinol Metab 1998;12:281–96.

[13] Toogood AA, O'Neill PA, Shalet SM. Beyond the somatopause: growth hormone deficiency in adults over the age of 60 years. J Clin Endocrinol Metab 1996;81:460–5.

[14] Growth Hormone Research Society (GRS). Consensus guidelines for the diagnosis and treatment of adults with GH deficiency. Statement of the GRS Workshop on Adult GHD. J Clin Endocrinol Metab 1998;83:379–81.

[15] Hartman ML, Crowe BJ, Biller BM, et al. Which patients do not require a GH stimulation test for the diagnosis of adult GH deficiency? J Clin Endocrinol Metab 2002;87:477–85.

[16] Aimaretti G, Corneli G, Razzore P, et al. Usefulness of IGF-I assay for the diagnosis of GH deficiency in adults. J Endocrinol Invest 1998;21:506–11.

[17] Aimaretti G, Corneli G, Baldelli R, et al. Diagnostic reliability of a single IGF-I measurement in 237 adults with total anterior hypopituitarism and severe GH deficiency. Clin Endocrinol (Oxf) 2003;59:56–61.

[18] Aimaretti G, Corneli G, Rovere S, et al. Insulin-like growth factor I levels and the diagnosis of adult growth hormone deficiency. Horm Res 2004;62(Suppl 1):26–33.

[19] Shalet SM, Toogood A, Rahim A, et al. The diagnosis of growth hormone deficiency in children and adults. Endocr Rev 1998;19:203–23.

[20] Fish HR, Chernow B, O'Brian JT. Endocrine and neurophysiologic response of the pituitary to insulin-induced hypoglycaemia: a review. Metabolism 1986;35:763–80.

[21] Hoffman DM, O Sullivan AJ, Baxter RC, et al. Diagnosis of growth-hormone deficiency in adults. Lancet 1994;343(8905):1064–8.

[22] Hoeck HC, Vestergaard P, Jakobsen E, et al. Test of growth hormone secretion in adults: poor reproducibility of the insulin tolerance test. Eur J Endocrinol 1995;133:305–12.

[23] Thorner MO, Bengtsson BA, Ho KY, et al. Diagnosis of growth hormone deficiency in adults. J Clin Endocrinol Metab 1995;80:3097–8.

[24] Ghigo E, Aimaretti G, Gianotti L, et al. New approach to the diagnosis of growth hormone deficiency in adults. Eur J Endocrinol 1996;134:352–6.

[25] Biller BMK, Samuels MH, Zagar A, et al. Sensitivity and specificity of six tests for the diagnosis of adult GH deficiency. J Clin Endocrinol Metab 2002;87:2067–79.

[26] Aimaretti G, Bellone S, Baldelli R, et al. Growth Hormone stimulation tests in pediatrics. Endocrinologist 2004;14:216–21.

[27] AlbaRoth J, Albrecht Muller O, Schophl J, et al. Arginine stimulates GH secretion by suppressing endogenous somatostatin secretion. J Clin Endocrinol Metab 1988;67:1186–92.

[28] Ghigo E, Goffi S, Nicolosi M, et al. GH responsiveness to combined administration of arginine and GHRH does not vary with age in man. J Clin Endocrinol Metab 1990;71: 1481–5.

[29] Procopio M, Maccario M, Savio P, et al. GH response to GHRH combined with pyridostigmine or arginine in different conditions of low somatotrope secretion in adulthood: obesity and Cushing's syndrome in comparison with hypopituitarism. Panminerva Med 1998;40: 13–7.

[30] Ghigo E, Bartolotta E, Imperiale E, et al. Glucagon stimulates GH secretion after intramuscular administration but not intravenous administration. Evidence against the assumption that glucagon per se has a GH-releasing activity. J Endocrinol Invest 1994;17:849–54.

[31] Arvat E, Maccagno B, Ramunni J, et al. Glucagon is an ACTH secretagogue as effective as hCRH after intramuscular administration while it is ineffective when given intravenously in normal subjects. Pituitary 2000;3:169–73.

[32] Tassone F, Grottoli S, Rossetto R, et al. Glucagon administration elicits blunted GH but exaggerated ACTH response in obesity. J Endocrinol Invest 2002;25:551–6.

[33] Aimaretti G, Baffoni C, DiVito L, et al. Comparisons among old and new provocative tests of GH secretion in 178 normal adults. Eur J Endocrinol 2000;142:347–52.

[34] Gil-Ad I, Gurewitz R, Marcovici O, et al. Effects of aging on human plasma growth hormone response to clonidine. Mech Ageing Dev 1984;27:97–100.

[35] Ghigo E, Goffi S, Arvat E, et al. Pyridostigmine partially restores the GH responsiveness to GHRH in normal aging. Acta Endocrinol (Copenh) 1990;123:169–74.

[36] Dieguez C, Mallo F, Senaris R, et al. Role of glucocorticoids in the neuroregulation of growth hormone secretion. J Pediatr Endocrinol Metab 1996;9:255–60.

[37] Kerrigan J, Rogol AD. The impact of gonadal steroid hormone action on growth hormone secretion during childhood and adolescence. Endocr Rev 1992;13:281–98.

[38] Wehrenberg WB, Giustina A. Mechanisms and pathways of gonadal steroids modulation of growth hormone secretion. Endocr Rev 1992;13:299–308.

[39] Ghigo E, Arvat E, Aimaretti G, et al. Diagnostic and therapeutic uses of growth hormone-releasing substances in adult and elderly subjects. Baillieres Clin Endocrinol Metab 1998;12: 341–58.

[40] Popovic V, Leal A, Micic D, et al. GH-releasing hormone and GH-releasing peptide-6 for diagnostic testing in GH-deficient adults. Lancet 2000;356:1137–42.

[41] Popovic V, Pekic S, Doknic M, et al. The effectiveness of arginine + GHRH test compared with GHRH + GHRP-6 test in diagnosing growth hormone deficiency in adults. Clin Endocrinol (Oxf) 2003;59:251–7.

[42] Ghigo E, Aimaretti G, Arvat E, et al. Growth hormone-releasing hormone combined with arginine or growth hormone secretagogues for the diagnosis of growth hormone deficiency in adults. Endocrine 2001;15:29–38.

[43] Aimaretti G, Corneli G, Razzore P, et al. Comparison between insulin-induced hypoglycemia and growth hormone (GH)-releasing hormone + arginine as provocative tests for the diagnosis of GH deficiency in adults. J Clin Endocrinol Metab 1998;83:1615–8.

[44] Arvat E, Gianotti L, Grottoli S, et al. Arginine and growth hormone-releasing hormone restore the blunted growth hormone-releasing activity of hexarelin in elderly subjects. J Clin Endocrinol Metab 1994;79:1440–3.

[45] Gharib H, Cook DM, Saenger PH, et al. American Association of Clinical Endocrinologists medical guidelines for clinical practice for growth hormone use in adults and children—2003 update. Endocr Pract 2003;9(1):64–76.

[46] Zadik Z, Chalew SA, McCarter RJ Jr, et al. The influence of age on the 24-hour integrated concentration of growth hormone in normal individuals. J Clin Endocrinol Metab 1985;60: 513–6.

[47] Ho KY, Evans WS, Blizzard RM, et al. Effects of sex and age on the 24-hour profile of growth hormone secretion in man: importance of endogenous estradiol concentrations. J Clin Endocrinol Metab 1987;64:51–8.

ELSEVIER
SAUNDERS

Endocrinol Metab Clin N Am
34 (2005) 907–922

ENDOCRINOLOGY
AND METABOLISM
CLINICS
OF NORTH AMERICA

Perimenopausal Reproductive Endocrinology

Georgina E. Hale, MD[a],*, Henry G. Burger, MD[b]

[a]Department of Obstetrics and Gynaecology, University of Sydney, Sydney, NSW, Australia
[b]Prince Henry's Institute of Medical Research, Monash Medical Centre,
Clayton, VIC, Australia

Major reproductive endocrine changes affect the hypothalamo-pituitary-ovarian axis at several times during the life of the normal female, including the neonatal period, puberty, and in the transition to menopause. These changes affect the gonadotropins, sex steroids, and inhibins. Changes also occur in circulating preandrogens and androgens, but such changes are primarily age related rather than reproductive aging related and are beyond the scope of this article. For most women, the transition to menopause is symptomatic, and the range of experiences is a reflection of the complexity of the underlying endocrinologic processes.

The menopause transition, or perimenopause, was first officially referred to by the World Health Organization (WHO) in 1996 as, "that period of time immediately before menopause when the endocrinological, biological and clinical features of approaching menopause commence" [1]. The WHO discouraged the use of the term "climacteric" and encouraged the use of the terms "menopause transition" and "perimenopause." There was a need for further clarification given that the clinical features of the menopause transition remained undefined at this time. In the meantime, investigators often proposed their own guidelines to determine entry into the menopause transition [2–4]. In the prospective Massachusetts' Women's Health Study, a self-report of between 3 and 12 months of amenorrhea was used for entry into perimenopause [2]. Similar criteria were used for entry into the late menopause transition in the Seattle Midlife Women's Health Project [3]. A self-report of a change in menstrual flow, menstrual flow duration, or cycle length was used for entry into the early menopause

* Corresponding author. Department of Obstetrics and Gynaecology, University of Sydney, Queen Elizabeth II Building (DO2), 2006 Sydney, NSW, Australia.
E-mail address: ghale@med.usyd.edu.au (G.E. Hale).

0889-8529/05/$ - see front matter © 2005 Elsevier Inc. All rights reserved.
doi:10.1016/j.ecl.2005.07.013   *endo.theclinics.com*

transition, and new-onset variability in cycle length (two or more consecutive cycles that differ in length by at least 7 days) was used as entry into the midperimenopause [3]. In a major longitudinal study of the experiences of menopause, Dennerstein and colleagues [4] also used self-reported new-onset menstrual cycle irregularity as the marker of entry into the early transition and absence of menses for between 3 and 11 months for entry into the late transition.

The rationale underlying any staging system in reproductive ageing should be to indicate what a normal pattern of progression to menopause would look like and to give an approximation of proximity to the final menstrual period. An intermenstrual interval of 60 days has often been used as a criterion for entry into the late menopause transition and has been shown to be associated with ovulatory failure [5]. It also predicts the final menstrual period more consistently than any other menstrual criteria during the menopause transition [6]. In women over the age of 45, a 60-day intermenstrual interval has been shown to have the best balance of sensitivity (94%) and specificity (91%) in predicting the final menstrual period within 2 years [7]. The range of cycle length has also been shown to be predictive of the final menstrual period. As demonstrated in the Melbourne Midlife Health Project, a mean running range of 42 days (the difference between the length of the longest and shortest cycles) predicts the final menstrual period within 2 years and is more reliable than a self-report of irregular menstrual cycles [8].

The first standardized classification guidelines for perimenopause were proposed in 2001 at The Stages of Reproductive Aging Workshop (STRAW) [9]. These criteria were proposed "to develop a relevant and useful staging system, to revise the nomenclature and to identify gaps in knowledge that should be addressed by the research community" (Fig. 1). The stages were nominated using the final menstrual period as a reference point and were based on changes in menstrual cycle patterns and follicle-stimulating hormone (FSH) levels. Subjective data, such as menstrual flow changes or vasomotor symptoms, were thought to be too variable or too unreliably recorded to be used in the criteria. The criteria were recommended only for use in women who are nonsmokers, have a body mass index between 18 and 30, do not participate in intense regular exercise, do not have chronic menstrual irregularities, and who have no history of hysterectomy or abnormal reproductive anatomy.

The STRAW criteria for entry into the early menopause transition (stage 2) are somewhat ambiguous, with the menstrual cycle criteria being stated in Fig. 1 as when menstrual cycles become "of variable length or more than 7 days different from normal" but in the text as "when the menstrual cycles remain 'regular', but where the cycle length changes by 7 days or more." There is no indication in the criteria as to what is considered to be a normal cycle length. This would be useful given a normal cycle length may still be evident despite changes in length of 7 or more days. It may be more

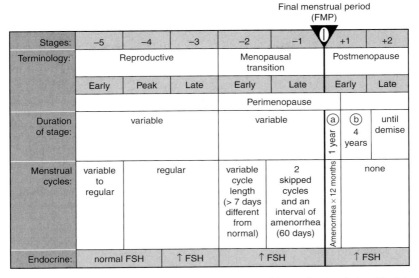

Fig. 1. Staging system recommended at the 2001 Stages of Reproductive Aging Workshop. FSH, follicle stimulating hormone; ↑, elevated. (*Adapted from* Soules MR, Sherman S, Parrott E, et al. Executive summary: Stages of Reproductive Aging Workshop (STRAW). Climacteric 2001;4(4):267–71; with permission.)

appropriate to use criteria that take into account normal cycle length and irregularity, as some investigators have done. For example, on the basis of the work by Taffe and colleagues [8], Burger and colleagues [10] suggested that the early menopause transition begins on "the date of the first of more than two cycles in any consecutive series of 10 cycles, the length of which lies outside the normal reproductive range of 23–35 days." Even with use of this latter criterion, prior knowledge of cycle length is important when assigning stage of transition because some women may have had cycle lengths outside this normal range for most of their reproductive life.

The hormonal characteristics of the normal menstrual cycle

The endocrine changes that occur with reproductive aging and the menopause transition involve changes in the normally highly coordinated relationship between the hypothalamus, pituitary, and ovary, a unit referred to as the hypothalamo-pituitary-ovarian axis. Communication between the pituitary and the hypothalamus involves transfer of hypothalamus-derived neurotransmitters to the anterior pituitary. Cells within the median eminence of the hypothalamus secrete gonadotropin-releasing hormone (GnRH) in a pulsatile manner within a critical range of frequency and amplitude to successfully stimulate anterior pituitary gonadotropin release. The cyclical balance between GnRH, the gonadotropins, and ovarian sex steroids underlies the normal menstrual cycle. In the first half of the menstrual cycle, when estrogen levels are low, synthesis, secretion, and storage levels of FSH and luteinizing hormone (LH) are low. As the follicular phase progresses, selection of a dominant follicle occurs under the influence of specific concentrations of estradiol and FSH. This is followed by a sharp increase in estradiol and inhibin A secretion by the dominant follicle. Rising follicular phase levels of estradiol increase the synthesis and storage of LH but at the same time inhibit its secretion [11]. This results in a buildup of stored LH in preparation for the midcycle surge. The GnRH also primes the pituitary by increasing the concentration of its own receptors on the pituitary gonadotrope, a process that requires the presence of estrogen and progesterone [11,12]. The brief rise in progesterone before the LH surge is also important in augmenting the LH surge [13] and, together with LH, suppresses estrogen secretion, causing the pre-LH peak fall in estrogen levels. The preovulatory rise in progesterone also contributes to the midcycle FSH peak, which assists in the maturation of the dominant follicle and plays a critical role in ensuring an adequate amount of functional LH receptors on the dominant follicle granulosa cells and complete luteinization after ovulation [14]. Inhibin A levels also fall transiently at the time of ovulation then rise and remain elevated for the remainder of the luteal phase (Fig. 2A). Inhibin B levels normally rise from the beginning of the cycle to the midfollicular phase and then fall from this point onward and remain low for the remainder of the luteal phase [15].

After ovulation, full luteinization of the dominant follicle occurs, resulting in a marked increase in progesterone secretion (Fig. 2B). During the ensuing luteal phase, estrogen and progesterone have an inhibitory effect on gonadotropin secretion. Progesterone inhibits GnRH at the level of the hypothalamus [16] and blocks estrogen responses to GnRH in the pituitary [17]. Progesterone levels reach a peak after about 7 to 8 days, after which time the corpus luteum rapidly declines and continues to regress unless rescued by human chorionic gonadotropin in pregnancy [18]. After a 13- to 14-day luteal phase and in the absence of pregnancy, progesterone and estradiol levels decline and precipitate a menstrual bleed [19,20]. The factors influencing the lifespan and functional capacity of the corpus luteum are not fully understood, but lower-than-normal levels of follicular phase FSH and lower luteal phase levels of LH are associated with luteal insufficiency [21,22]. The role of luteal phase estradiol in limiting the lifespan of the corpus luteum is unclear, but high levels are thought to be luteolytic [21] despite the absence of estrogen receptors in luteal tissue [23]. During the late luteal phase and about 4 days before a menstrual bleed, FSH levels begin to rise in response to falling levels of estrogen, progesterone, and inhibin A (Fig. 2C). Toward the end of the cycle, these rising levels of FSH stimulate antral follicular development, and activity is indicated by increasing secretion of estradiol and inhibin B from the antral follicles (Fig. 2B). Inhibin B secretion occurs

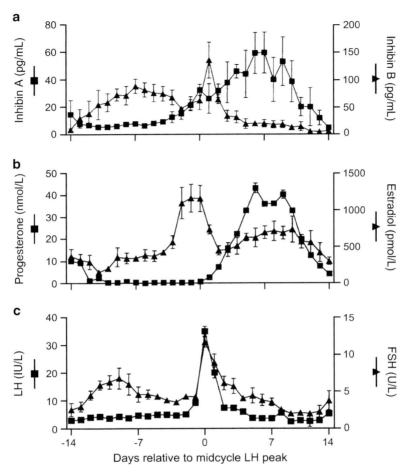

Fig. 2. Hormonal series from pooled midreproductive age data illustrating cyclical changes in inhibin A and inhibin B (*A*), estradiol and progesterone (*B*), and LH and FSH (*C*). (*From* Groome NP, Illingworth PJ, O'Brien M, et al. Measurement of dimeric inhibin B throughout the human menstrual cycle. J Clin Endocrinol Metab 1996;81:1403; with permission.)

secondary to the FSH-stimulated antral follicle development and granulose cell proliferation. By the midproliferative phase, the rise in inhibin B levels leads a fall in FSH secretion (Fig. 2C) [24].

Gonadotropin release during the menstrual cycle is closely regulated by inhibin A and inhibin B, which are dimeric glycoproteins consisting of two subunits (alpha and βA or βB). Bioactive inhibin A is a dimer of an α and a βA subunit, and bioactive inhibin B is a dimer of an α and a βB sub-unit. The main action of inhibin A and B is to inhibit synthesis and secretion of FSH. Inhibin A is primarily a product of the dominant follicle and corpus luteum, and its secretion pattern is similar to estradiol, rising slowly during the early follicular phase and reaching a peak with maturation of the dominant follicle in the late follicular phase [25]. It falls transiently at the time of ovulation then rises and remains elevated for the remainder of the luteal phase, contributing to FSH suppression and prevention of follicle development during the luteal phase (Fig. 2A). As well as being regulated by FSH, inhibin A is also likely to be regulated by LH, especially during the luteal phase [26]. Inhibin B is a product of the preantral and antral follicles, and levels rise from the beginning of the cycle to the midfollicular phase and start to fall in the late follicular phase (Fig. 2A) [27]. After a brief peak around the time of ovulation, levels fall and remain low for the remainder of the luteal phase [15]. Both inhibin A and B are stimulated by FSH in the follicular phase in a dose-dependent manner, but inhibin B seems to be the more important regulator of FSH during the follicular phase [28].

The endocrinology of late reproductive aging

The STRAW definition for late reproductive age (Stage -3) is an elevated early-cycle FSH in the setting of regular menstrual cycles [9]. An elevated early follicular phase FSH level has become recognized as a hallmark of reproductive aging [29–34] and precedes the onset of irregular cycles and the menopause transition by 3 to 10 years [31,35–39]. This rise in early follicular phase FSH levels has been shown to be associated with a decrease in follicular phase length and menstrual cycle length. In women of late reproductive age, the length of time from the beginning of the cycle to the rise in estradiol from dominant follicle selection (ie, estrogen take off) has been shown to be inversely correlated to the early follicular phase rise in FSH [40]. Klein and colleagues [41] have shown that this correlation is most likely caused by the increased FSH levels triggering an earlier rather than an accelerated follicle development and dominant follicle selection. The rise in early follicular phase FSH levels has been observed to begin as early as 30 years of age in infertility clinic patients [42] and by 40 years of age in randomly selected healthy women [36,43]. The FSH rise, however, does not occur in all women at these ages [43] and is not consistent between cycles from the same women [44]. In addition, although FSH levels are correlated with age between the ages of 20 and 50, follicular phase levels of FSH are only higher than the normal range in a minority of women 35 to 40 years of age [45].

In view of the inconsistency of FSH levels between women and from cycle to cycle, single-time FSH measurements have a limited capacity to reliably predict reproductive status [46]. In regular cycles where there are high follicular levels of FSH, levels of LH are minimally increased [31,32,47] or unchanged [29,34,35,48–51], although increases in LH pulse frequency and amplitude have been noted [39] along with a reduced pituitary LH sensitivity to GnRH stimulation [50]. In general, the rise in LH levels occurs later than FSH, becoming most pronounced after the onset of the menopause transition [42].

The rise in FSH in advancing reproductive age was initially thought to be secondary to a fall in estradiol levels. Many subsequent studies, however, have revealed that the rise in FSH is associated with normal or higher than normal estradiol levels [30–33,36,46,52–55]. Significantly elevated mean cycle levels of estradiol have been observed in regularly cycling women, even up to 55 years of age [56]. Several other studies in women of late reproductive age have revealed nonsignificant elevations in mean cycle [38,49] or mean follicular phase levels estradiol [31,39,56] compared with midreproductive control subjects. Lee and colleagues [31] sampled 94 healthy regularly cycling women aged between 24 and 50 years of age and found increased follicular phase estradiol and FSH in the subjects aged 39 to 44 [31]. Elevated mean cycle and luteal phase estrogen excretion levels have also been found in regularly cycling women of late reproductive aged compared with control subjects [57].

The observation of high levels of estradiol in association with high levels of FSH suggests that, in at least some menstrual cycles, the ovary responds to the increased FSH levels by increasing estrogen secretion. It is unclear whether this response is attributable to increased estrogen secretion from the developing antral follicles or the dominant follicle or why FSH levels are not always associated with increased levels of estradiol. It is also unclear why high FSH levels are not always associated with increased levels of estradiol. Further studies are needed to determine whether there are specific menstrual cycle patterns or within-cycle hormone secretion patterns that are associated with an increase in estrogen secretion. It is also important to determine if changes in estrogen secretion are linked to changes in luteal phase function because some studies suggest that advanced reproductive age is associated with lower luteal phase progesterone levels [30,48] or lower luteal phase urinary excretion of pregnanediol 3-glucuronide (PdG) [57], although this has not been found in all studies [29,31,32,44].

Elevated levels of follicular phase FSH in late reproductive age have been found to be associated with decreased levels of inhibin B [33,58–62], with numerous studies reporting higher FSH and lower inhibin B levels in women of advanced reproductive aged compared with younger women [33,59,63–67]. Follicular phase inhibin B levels have been found to be inversely correlated with, and to be significant independent predictors of, follicular phase levels of FSH [43]. Decreased levels of inhibin B may occur only during cycles with elevated levels of FSH and, like FSH levels, vary from cycle to cycle [59,64,65]. Given the variability in inhibin B and FSH levels from cycle to cycle, it follows that the stimulus for inhibin B secretion also changes from cycle to cycle. It has been shown that inhibin B levels are correlated with the number of developing antral follicles seen on ultrasonography during the early follicular phase [68] and that levels fall in parallel with number of antral follicles in the ovary [64]. Part of the reason inhibin B secretion varies from cycle to cycle may lie in the variable number of antral follicles that are recruited during each menstrual cycle, which is likely to be influenced by the size of the remaining pool of primordial follicles.

Inhibin A is a product of the dominant follicle and, in contrast to inhibin B, does not seem to change in late reproductive age [33,58,59,69]. Klein and colleagues [33] found no difference in early follicular phase levels of inhibin A between women 45 to 47 years of age and women 20 to 25 years of age [33]. Although Welt and colleagues [59] found similar mean follicular and luteal phase inhibin A levels in regularly cycling women 20 to 34 years of age and women 35 to 47 years of age, lower peak levels of inhibin A were found on the day after the LH peak in the older subjects despite normal follicular phase levels of FSH and lower mean cycle levels of inhibin B [59]. Lower peak levels of inhibin A during the follicular phase and luteal phase have been found in another study of 16 women 40 to 50 years of age with increased cycle-day 3 FSH levels (> 8 mIU/mL) [65]. Lower mean luteal phase inhibin A levels in late reproductive age have been found [66], but this was not associated with any change in inhibin A levels in the dominant follicle fluid [33,70].

The endocrinology of the menopause transition

Irregular cycles herald the onset of the menopause transition and precede the final menstrual period by 4 to 5 years [71]. The main contributing factor to the onset of cycle irregularity seems to be the diminishing pool of ovarian follicles. The numbers of primordial follicles and the number of developing antral follicles decrease with increasing reproductive age [72,73], and, by the time of onset of irregular cycles, there are only between 100 and 1000 primordial follicles [74]. The fall in primordial follicle numbers and the resultant decrease in the number of antral follicles developing during each menstrual cycle influence the balance of hormonal communication between the ovary and hypothalamo-pituitary unit. The most common endocrinologic manifestations of this fall in follicle numbers are ovulatory failure, an increase in FSH levels, and a decrease in inhibin B levels. The rise in FSH becomes more pronounced and more variable from cycle to cycle compared with late reproductive age [29,75,76], whereas luteinizing hormone levels become more consistently elevated [31,35,47,75,77–79].

The changes in estrogen secretion across the transition have been of interest to a number of investigators, with a number of studies observing elevated estradiol levels during the early menopause transition [30,39,45,48] and others observing no change [44,79] or decreased levels [45,75]. Lower-than-normal levels of estradiol have been observed in late menopause transition, primarily in studies of menstrual cycles in which the ovulatory status is unknown [37]. When analyses of estradiol data are performed according to ovulatory status, the fall in estradiol levels is seen to be largely confined to anovulatory cycles [80]. In a recent detailed longitudinal study of 13 women by Landgren and colleagues [44], there were no changes in ovulatory cycle estradiol or progesterone levels during the 4- to 9-year period before the final menstrual. There were significantly decreased levels of these hormones during anovulatory cycles or cycles in which ovulation may have occurred outside the 30-day period of blood sampling.

Few other studies have sampled serum estradiol levels in comparable numbers of women classified as early or late perimenopause, but there have been numerous studies on urinary estrogen excretion during the menopause transition. Two large studies, the British FREEDOM study (Fertility Recognition and Enabling Early Detection of Menopause) and the North American Study of Women's Health Across the Nation (SWAN), have recently been reported. In the Freedom study, daily urine samples were collected from 37 women over a mean of 11 cycles during the menopause transition. Low levels of estrogen excretion were found to be associated with prolonged ovulatory cycles during the lag period between the menstrual phase and the onset of the follicular phase [81]. This lag period was associated with marked elevations in FSH and moderate elevations in LH excretion, a finding consistent with limited data from smaller studies [1,52,75,82]. In contrast to the inverse correlation between the length of this lag period and follicular phase FSH seen in late reproductive age, in the menopause transition during elongated cycles, this correlation was shown to be positive [81]. When the follicular phase commenced in the elongated ovulatory cycles, estrogen excretion was significantly higher than normal, with a positive correlation between the amount of estrogen excreted during the luteal phase and the length of the lag period [81]. The amount of estrogen excretion was correlated to follicular phase LH levels rather than FSH levels [81]. Although a rise in estrogen excretion during ovulatory cycles has been found during the menopause transition in a number of small studies [47,52,57,78,83], mean ovulatory cycle estrone excretion was found to be unchanged in the large SWAN cohort with 833 irregularly cycling peri-menopausal women [84]. It is possible that in previous studies that found falls in estradiol levels or estrogen excretion across the menopause transition [45,79,85,86], hormonal data from normal ovulatory cycles was pooled with data from elongated ovulatory cycles or anovulatory cycles. The latter two types of cycles in particular become more common with the progression of menopause and would contribute to a lower group mean estradiol level.

Few studies have measured serum progesterone during irregular ovulatory cycles in peri-menopausal women [29,59]. In one study of daily blood samples taken during three menstrual cycles in three subjects, there was a decrease in luteal phase progesterone secretion in the three subjects being studied over time with the development of irregular cycles [59]. In another study, prolonged ovulatory cycles were associated with abnormally low progesterone levels [29]. Studies exploring the excretion of progesterone's major urinary metabolite, PdG, have been more numerous and have consistently shown a decrease in PdG excretion with the onset of irregular cycles [5,29,35,52,57,85,87]. In one of these studies, ovulatory cycles from women with a history of intermenstrual intervals of 60 days or more had significantly lower peak luteal phase PdG excretion [87]. PdG excretion during ovulatory cycles was also found to be lower than midreproductive levels in the SWAN and FREEDOM studies, with PdG excretion being inversely correlated with the length of the lag phase and with luteal phase LH excretion [40].

Increased follicular [29,34,37,52,57,76,83] and luteal phase [40,52,57, 84,88] levels of FSH have been reported widely during the menopause transition, especially during long intermenstrual intervals or anovulatory cycles when estradiol levels are low [40]. As indicated in a recent report of detailed endocrine data, FSH and estradiol levels may be relatively unchanged during normal-length ovulatory cycles during the 4- to 9-year period before the final menstrual period [44]. This report and other data illustrating the variability of FSH levels suggest that single measurements of FSH levels during the menopause transition are highly dependent on cycle length and ovulatory status of the cycle being sampled and are thus unreliable predictors of reproductive stage. In addition, recent data on cycle-day 2 to 4 FSH levels in women of late reproductive age revealed that FSH was less able to predict the onset of the menopause transition (irregular cycles) than anti-mullerian hormone or inhibin B [89].

Given the variability in FSH and estradiol secretion and the increased incidence of anovulatory cycles in the menopause transition, it seems that as ovarian follicles decline in number, there is increased ovarian refractoriness to gonadotropin stimulation. Given that inhibin B is a marker of ovarian reserve, it is likely that ovarian refractoriness is reflected by low levels of inhibin B [68]. There are minimal changes in inhibin A or inhibin B during ovulatory cycles of normal length in peri-menopausal subjects, but during prolonged ovulatory cycles or anovulatory cycles, there is a significant decrease in inhibin B levels along with lower levels of estradiol [44]. More studies are needed to explore within-cycle temporal relationships between the gonadotropins and inhibins during irregular cycles and the activities of these hormones underlying the variability in ovarian responses during different phases of the cycle.

Consequences of the changes in reproductive hormone secretion

There are few recognized symptoms associated with the subtle hormonal changes in late reproductive age, but with the onset of irregular cycles in the menopause transition, hormonal changes become more marked, and experiences such as breast tenderness, menorrhagia, vasomotor symptoms, sleep difficulties, and labile mood become common [90–93]. Breast tenderness is associated with the early menopause transition [92] and has been thought to be caused by an increase in estradiol levels, although no studies on simultaneously measured hormones and symptoms have been performed. Subjective menorrhagia during ovulatory cycles has been shown to be associated with increased estradiol levels during the follicular [94,95] and luteal phases

[48]. When the increase in estrogen secretion is accompanied by a decrease in progesterone secretion, there may be an increased incidence of endometrial hyperplasia [94] and a hypothetical increased risk of endometrial cancer [96].

Vasomotor symptoms are normally associated with low levels of estrogen and have been shown to be most common in the late menopause transition and menopause [92]. They can also occur during ovulatory cycles in the menopause transition [97], perhaps as a result of an increase in estrogen level fluctuations. Other experiences that are commonly reported by midlife and peri-menopausal women include poor concentration, memory disturbances, and labile mood [98], but the hormonal dynamics underlying these experiences have not been investigated. There is an improbable association between the menopause transition and depression, and no clear relationship has been found between the incidence and severity of depression and estrogen levels [99]. Given the complexity of changes occurring during the transition, further investigation of peri-menopausal experiences would be best studied by measuring day-to-day and cycle-to-cycle hormone levels while simultaneously recording experiences.

Summary

Hormonal changes in reproductive aging reflect a marked decline in ovarian follicle numbers, decreasing inhibin B secretion and consequent increases in FSH levels. During late reproductive age and the menopause transition, the ovary demonstrates a progressive decrease in the capacity to respond to increasing levels of FSH. In late reproductive age, ovarian responsiveness seems to be relatively well preserved, with minimal changes occurring in cycle length and ovulation. In the early menopause transition, before significant elongation of the menstrual cycle occurs, ovarian responsiveness becomes less consistent and results in noticeable changes in cycle length and discernible experiences that include menstrual flow changes. By the late menopause transition, the attainment of a critical number of ovarian follicles leads to significant ovarian refractoriness to FSH, and the primary manifestation of this is prolonged ovulatory cycles, resulting from delayed estradiol secretion response and an increased incidence of anovulatory cycles. In the prolonged ovulatory cycles, dominant follicle development may lead to higher-than-normal levels of estradiol but lower luteal phase levels of progesterone. Further studies on whether the increased estradiol secretion relative to progesterone is associated with an increased risk of endometrial hyperplasia and endometrial cancer precursor development are warranted.

References

[1] WHO Scientific Group. Research on the menopause in the 1990's: a report of the WHO Scientific Group. World Health Organisation 1996;866:1–79.

[2] Brambilla DJ, McKinlay SM, Johannes CB. Defining the perimenopause for application in epidemiologic investigations. Am J Epidemiol 1994;140:1091–5.

[3] Mitchell ES, Woods NF, Mariella A. Three stages of the menopausal transition from the Seattle Midlife Women's Health Study: toward a more precise definition. Menopause 2000;7: 334–49.

[4] Dennerstein L. Well-being, symptoms and the menopausal transition. Maturitas 1996;23: 147–57.

[5] Metcalf MG. Incidence of ovulation from the menarche to the menopause: observations of 622 New Zealand women. N Z Med J 1983;96:645–8.

[6] Lisabeth LD, Harlow SD, Gillespie B, et al. Staging reproductive aging: a comparison of proposed bleeding criteria for the menopausal transition. Menopause 2004;11:186–97.

[7] Taylor SM, Kinney AM, Kline JK. Menopausal transition: predicting time to menopause for women 44 years or older from simple questions on menstrual variability [see comment]. Menopause 2004;11:40–8.

[8] Taffe JR, Dennerstein L. Menstrual patterns leading to the final menstrual period. Menopause 2002;9:32–40.

[9] Soules MR, Sherman S, Parrott E, et al. Stages of Reproductive Aging Workshop (STRAW). J Womens Health Gend Based Med 2001;10:843–8.

[10] Burger HG, Robertson D, Baksheev L, et al. The relationship between the endocrine characteristics and the regularity of menstrual cycles in the approach to menopause. Menopause 2005;12:267–74.

[11] Urban RJ, Veldhuis JD, Dufau ML. Estrogen regulates the gonadotropin-releasing hormone-stimulated secretion of biologically active luteinizing hormone. J Clin Endocrinol Metab 1991;72:660–8.

[12] Hoff JD, Lasley BL, Yen SS. The functional relationship between priming and releasing actions of luteinizing hormone-releasing hormone. J Clin Endocrinol Metab 1979;49:8–11.

[13] Couzinet B, Brailly S, Bouchard P, et al. Progesterone stimulates luteinizing hormone secretion by acting directly on the pituitary. J Clin Endocrinol Metab 1992;74:374–8.

[14] Smith SK, Lenton EA, Cooke ID. Plasma gonadotrophin and ovarian steroid concentrations in women with menstrual cycles with a short luteal phase. J Reprod Fertil 1985;75:363–8.

[15] Groome NP, Illingworth PJ, O'Brien M, et al. Measurement of dimeric inhibin B throughout the human menstrual cycle. J Clin Endocrinol Metab 1996;81:1401–5.

[16] Kasa-Vubu JZ, Dahl GE, Evans NP, et al. Progesterone blocks the estradiol-induced gonadotropin discharge in the ewe by inhibiting the surge of gonadotropin-releasing hormone. Endocrinology 1992;131:208–12.

[17] Araki S, Chikazawa K, Motoyama M, et al. Reduction in pituitary desensitization and prolongation of gonadotropin release by estrogen during continuous administration of gonadotropin-releasing hormone in women: its antagonism by progesterone. J Clin Endocrinol Metab 1985;60:590–8.

[18] Catt KJ, Dufau ML, Vaitukaitis JL. Appearance of hCG in pregnancy plasma following the initiation of implantation of the blastocyst. J Clin Endocrinol Metab 1975;40:537–40.

[19] McNeely MJ, Soules MR. The diagnosis of luteal phase deficiency: a critical review [see comments]. Fertil Steril 1988;50:1–15.

[20] Lenton EA, Landgren BM, Sexton L, et al. Normal variation in the length of the follicular phase of the menstrual cycle: effect of chronological age. Br J Obstet Gynaecol 1984;91: 681–4.

[21] Soules MR, Clifton DK, Steiner RA, et al. The corpus luteum: determinants of progesterone secretion in the normal menstrual cycle. Obstet Gynecol 1988;71:659–66.

[22] Soules MR, Steiner RA, Clifton DK, et al. Abnormal patterns of pulsatile luteinizing hormone in women with luteal phase deficiency. Obstet Gynecol 1984;63:626–9.

[23] Hild-Petito S, Stouffer RL, Brenner RM. Immunocytochemical localization of estradiol and progesterone receptors in the monkey ovary throughout the menstrual cycle. Endocrinology 1988;123:2896–905.

[24] Welt CK, Martin KA, Taylor AE, et al. Frequency modulation of follicle-stimulating hormone (FSH) during the luteal-follicular transition: evidence for FSH control of inhibin B in normal women. J Clin Endocrinol Metab 1997;82:2645–52.

[25] Groome NP, Illingworth PJ, O'Brien M, et al. Detection of dimeric inhibin throughout the human menstrual cycle by two-site enzyme immunoassay. Clin Endocrinol (Oxf) 1994;40: 717–23.

[26] Welt CK, Adams JM, Sluss PM, et al. Inhibin A and inhibin B responses to gonadotropin withdrawal depends on stage of follicle development. J Clin Endocrinol Metab 1999;84: 2163–9.

[27] Welt CK, Schneyer AL. Differential regulation of inhibin B and inhibin a by follicle-stimulating hormone and local growth factors in human granulosa cells from small antral follicles. J Clin Endocrinol Metab 2001;86(1):330–6.

[28] Burger HG, Groome NP, Robertson DM. Both inhibin A and B respond to exogenous follicle-stimulating hormone in the follicular phase of the human menstrual cycle. J Clin Endocrinol Metab 1998;83:4167–9.

[29] Sherman BM, West JH, Korenman SG. The menopausal transition: analysis of LH, FSH, estradiol, and progesterone concentrations during menstrual cycles of older women. J Clin Endocrinol Metab 1976;42:629–36.

[30] Reyes FI, Winter JS, Faiman C. Pituitary-ovarian relationships preceding the menopause: a cross-sectional study of serum follicle-stimulating hormone, luteinizing hormone, prolactin, estradiol, and progesterone levels. Am J Obstet Gynecol 1977;129:557–64.

[31] Lee SJ, Lenton EA, Sexton L, et al. The effect of age on the cyclical patterns of plasma LH, FSH, oestradiol and progesterone in women with regular menstrual cycles. Hum Reprod 1988;3:851–5.

[32] Fitzgerald CT, Seif MW, Killick SR, et al. Age related changes in the female reproductive cycle. Br J Obstet Gynaecol 1994;101:229–33 [erratum appears in Br J Obstet Gynaecol 1994;101:360].

[33] Klein NA, Illingworth PJ, Groome NP, et al. Decreased inhibin B secretion is associated with the monotropic FSH rise in older, ovulatory women: a study of serum and follicular fluid levels of dimeric inhibin A and B in spontaneous menstrual cycles. J Clin Endocrinol Metab 1996;81:2742–5.

[34] MacNaughton J, Banah M, McCloud P, et al. Age related changes in follicle stimulating hormone, luteinizing hormone, oestradiol and immunoreactive inhibin in women of reproductive age. Clin Endocrinol (Oxf) 1992;36:339–45.

[35] Metcalf MG, Donald RA, Livesey JH. Pituitary-ovarian function in normal women during the menopausal transition. Clin Endocrinol (Oxf) 1981;14:245–55.

[36] Lenton EA, Sexton L, Lee S, et al. Progressive changes in LH and FSH and LH: FSH ratio in women throughout reproductive life. Maturitas 1988;10:35–43.

[37] Burger HG, Dudley EC, Hopper JL, et al. The endocrinology of the menopausal transition: a cross-sectional study of a population-based sample. J Clin Endocrinol Metab 1995;80: 3537–45.

[38] Klein NA, Battaglia DE, Clifton DK, et al. The gonadotropin secretion pattern in normal women of advanced reproductive age in relation to the monotropic FSH rise. J Soc Gynecol Investig 1996;3:27–32.

[39] Reame NE, Kelche RP, Beitins IZ, et al. Age effects of follicle-stimulating hormone and pulsatile luteinizing hormone secretion across the menstrual cycle of premenopausal women. J Clin Endocrinol Metab 1996;81:1512–8.

[40] Miro F, Parker SW, Aspinall LJ, et al. Origins and consequences of the elongation of the human menstrual cycle during the menopause transition: the FREEDOM Study. J Clin Endocrinol Metab 2004;89:4910–5.

[41] Klein NA, Harper AJ, Houmard BS, et al. Is the short follicular phase in older women secondary to advanced or accelerated dominant follicle development? J Clin Endocrinol Metab 2002;87:5746–50.

[42] Ahmed Ebbiary NA, Lenton EA, Cooke ID. Hypothalamic-pituitary ageing: progressive increase in FSH and LH concentrations throughout the reproductive life in regularly menstruating women. Clin Endocrinol (Oxf) 1994;41:119–206.

[43] Burger HG, Dudley E, Mamers P, et al. Early follicular phase serum FSH as a function of age: the roles of inhibin B, inhibin A and estradiol. Climacteric 2000;3:17–24.

[44] Landgren BM, Collins A, Csemiczky G, et al. Menopause transition: annual changes in serum hormonal patterns over the menstrual cycle in women during a nine-year period prior to menopause. J Clin Endocrinol Metab 2004;89:2763–9.

[45] Burger HG, Dudley EC, Hopper JL, et al. Prospectively measured levels of serum follicle-stimulating hormone, estradiol, and the dimeric inhibins during the menopausal transition in a population-based cohort of women. J Clin Endocrinol Metab 1999;84: 4025–30.

[46] Burger HG. Diagnostic role of follicle-stimulating hormone (FSH) measurements during the menopausal transition: an analysis of FSH, oestradiol and inhibin. Eur J Endocrinol 1994; 130:38–42.

[47] Adamopoulos DA, Loraine JA, Dove GA. Endocrinological studies in women approaching the menopause. J Obstet Gynaecol Br Commonw 1971;78:62–79.

[48] Ballinger CB, Browning MC, Smith AH. Hormone profiles and psychological symptoms in peri-menopausal women. Maturitas 1987;9:235–51.

[49] Klein NA, Battaglia DE, Fujimoto VY, et al. Reproductive aging: accelerated ovarian follicular development associated with a monotropic follicle-stimulating hormone rise in normal older women. J Clin Endocrinol Metab 1996;81:1038–45.

[50] Fujimoto VY, Klein NA, Battaglia DE, et al. The anterior pituitary response to a gonadotropin-releasing hormone challenge test in normal older reproductive-age women. Fertil Steril 1996;65:539–44.

[51] Hall Moran V, Leathard HL, Coley J. Urinary hormone levels during the natural menstrual cycle: the effect of age. J Endocrinol 2001;170:157–64.

[52] Shideler SE, DeVane GW, Kalra PS, et al. Ovarian-pituitary hormone interactions during the perimenopause. Maturitas 1989;11:331–9.

[53] Burger HG, Dudley E, Mamers P, et al. The ageing female reproductive axis I. Novartis Found Symp 2002;242:161–7 [discussion: 167–71].

[54] Robertson DM, Burger HG. Reproductive hormones: ageing and the perimenopause. Acta Obstet Gynecol Scand 2002;81:612–6.

[55] Burger HG, Dudley EC, Robertson DM, et al. Hormonal changes in the menopause transition. Recent Prog Horm Res 2002;57:257–75.

[56] Klein NA, Houmard BS, Hansen KR, et al. Age-related analysis of inhibin A, inhibin B, and activin a relative to the intercycle monotropic follicle-stimulating hormone rise in normal ovulatory women. J Clin Endocrinol Metab 2004;89:2977–81.

[57] Santoro N, Brown JR, Adel T, et al. Characterization of reproductive hormonal dynamics in the perimenopause. J Clin Endocrinol Metab 1996;81:1495–501.

[58] Burger HG, Cahir N, Robertson DM, et al. Serum inhibins A and B fall differentially as FSH rises in perimenopausal women. Clin Endocrinol (Oxf) 1998;48:809–13 [erratum appears in Clin Endocrinol (Oxf) 1998;49:550].

[59] Welt CK, McNicholl DJ, Taylor AE, et al. Female reproductive aging is marked by decreased secretion of dimeric inhibin. J Clin Endocrinol Metab 1999;84:105–11.

[60] Welt CK, Pagan YL, Smith PC, et al. Control of follicle-stimulating hormone by estradiol and the inhibins: critical role of estradiol at the hypothalamus during the luteal-follicular transition. J Clin Endocrinol Metab 2003;88:1766–71.

[61] Findlay JK, Sai X, Shukovski L. Role of inhibin-related peptides as intragonadal regulators. Reprod Fertil Dev 1990;2:205–18.

[62] Hughes EG, Robertson DM, Handelsman DJ, et al. Inhibin and estradiol responses to ovarian hyperstimulation: effects of age and predictive value for in vitro fertilization outcome. J Clin Endocrinol Metab 1990;70:358–64.

[63] Soules MR, Battaglia DE, Klein NA. Inhibin and reproductive aging in women. Maturitas 1998;30:193–204.

[64] Danforth DR, Arbogast LK, Mroueh J, et al. Dimeric inhibin: a direct marker of ovarian aging. Fertil Steril 1998;70:119–23.

[65] Muttukrishna S, Child T, Lockwood GM, et al. Serum concentrations of dimeric inhibins, activin A, gonadotrophins and ovarian steroids during the menstrual cycle in older women. Hum Reprod 2000;15:549–56.

[66] Santoro N, Adel T, Skurnick JH. Decreased inhibin tone and increased activin A secretion characterize reproductive aging in women. Fertil Steril 1999;71:658–62.

[67] Reame NE, Wyman TL, Phillips DJ, et al. Net increase in stimulatory input resulting from a decrease in inhibin B and an increase in activin A may contribute in part to the rise in follicular phase follicle-stimulating hormone of aging cycling women. J Clin Endocrinol Metab 1998;83:3302–7.

[68] Tinkanen H, Blauer M, Laippala P, et al. Correlation between serum inhibin B and other indicators of the ovarian function. Eur J Obstet Gynecol Reprod Biol 2001;94:109–13.

[69] Reame NE, Sauder SE, Kelch RP, et al. Pulsatile gonadotropin secretion during the human menstrual cycle: evidence for altered secretion of gonadotropin-releasing hormone. J Clin Endocrinol Metab 1984;59:328–37.

[70] Klein NA, Battaglia DE, Miller PB, et al. Ovarian follicular development and the follicular fluid hormones and growth factors in normal women of advanced reproductive age. J Clin Endocrinol Metab 1996;81:1946–51.

[71] den Tonkelaar I, te Velde ER, Looman CW. Menstrual cycle length preceding menopause in relation to age at menopause. Maturitas 1998;29:115–23.

[72] Faddy MJ, Gosden RG. A model conforming the decline in follicle numbers to the age of menopause in women. Hum Reprod 1996;11:1484–6.

[73] Scheffer GJ, Broekmans FJ, Looman CW, et al. The number of antral follicles in normal women with proven fertility is the best reflection of reproductive age. Hum Reprod 2003; 18:700–6.

[74] Richardson SJ, Senikas V, Nelson JF. Follicular depletion during the menopausal transition: evidence for accelerated loss and ultimate exhaustion. J Clin Endocrinol Metab 1987;65: 1231–7.

[75] Sherman BM, Korenman SG. Hormonal characteristics of the human menstrual cycle throughout reproductive life. J Clin Invest 1975;55:699–706.

[76] Hee J, MacNaughton J, Bangah M, et al. Perimenopausal patterns of gonadotrophins, immunoreactive inhibin, oestradiol and progesterone. Maturitas 1993;18:9–20.

[77] Rannevik G, Jeppsson S, Johnell O, et al. A longitudinal study of the perimenopausal transition: altered profiles of steroid and pituitary hormones, SHBG and bone mineral density. Maturitas 1995;21:103–13.

[78] Papanicolaou AD, Loraine JA, Dove GA, et al. Hormone excretion patterns in perimenopausal women. J Obstet Gynaecol Br Commonw 1969;76:308–16.

[79] Abe T, Yamaya Y, Wada Y, et al. Pituitary-ovarian relationships in women approaching the menopause. Maturitas 1983;5:31–7.

[80] Prior JC. Perimenopause: the complex endocrinology of the menopausal transition. Endocr Rev 1998;19:397–428.

[81] Miro F, Parker SW, Aspinall LJ, et al. Relationship between follicle-stimulating hormone levels at the beginning of the human menstrual cycle, length of the follicular phase and excreted estrogens: the FREEDOM study. J Clin Endocrinol Metab 2004;89:3270–5.

[82] O'Connor KA, Holman DJ, Wood JW. Menstrual cycle variability and the perimenopause. Am J Human Biol 2001;13:465–78.

[83] van Look PF, Lothian H, Hunter WM, et al. Hypothalamic-pituitary-ovarian function in perimenopausal women. Clin Endocrinol (Oxf) 1977;7:13–31.

[84] Santoro N, Lasley B, McConnell D, et al. Body size and ethnicity are associated with menstrual cycle alterations in women in the early menopausal transition: The Study of Women's

Health across the Nation (SWAN) Daily Hormone Study. J Clin Endocrinol Metab 2004;89: 2622–31.

[85] Longcope C, Franz C, Morello C, et al. Steroid and gonadotropin levels in women during the peri-menopausal years. Maturitas 1986;8:189–96.

[86] Randolph JF Jr, Sowers M, Bondarenko IV, et al. Change in estradiol and follicle-stimulating hormone across the early menopausal transition: effects of ethnicity and age. J Clin Endocrinol Metab 2004;89:1555–61.

[87] Metcalf MG. Incidence of ovulatory cycles in women approaching the menopause. J Biosoc Sci 1979;11:39–48.

[88] Metcalf MG, Mackenzie JA. Menstrual cycle and exposure to oestrogens unopposed by progesterone: relevance to studies on breast cancer incidence. J Endocrinol 1985;104:137–41.

[89] van Rooij IAJ, den Tonkelaar I, Broekmans FJ, et al. Anti-mulluarian hormone is promising predictor for the occurrence of the menopausal transition. Menopause 2004;11:601–6.

[90] Mitchell ES, Woods NF. Symptom experiences of midlife women: observations from the Seattle Midlife Women's Health Study [see comments]. Maturitas 1996;25:1–10.

[91] Greene JG. A factor analytic study of climacteric symptoms. J Psychosom Res 1976;20: 425–30.

[92] Dennerstein L, Dudley EC, Hopper JL, et al. A prospective population-based study of menopausal symptoms. Obstet Gynecol 2000;96:351–8.

[93] McKinlay SM. The normal menopause transition: an overview. Maturitas 1996;23:137–45.

[94] van Look PF, Hunter WM, Michie EA, et al. Pituitary-ovarian function in perimenopausal women with dysfunctional uterine bleeding. J Endocrinol 1977;73:22P–3P.

[95] Brown JB, Matthew GD. The application of urinary estrogen measurements to problems in gynecology. Recent Prog Horm Res 1962;18:337.

[96] Hale GE, Hughes CL, Cline JM. Clinical review 139-Endometrial cancer: hormonal factors, the perimenopausal "window of risk, " and isoflavones [review]. J Clin Endocrinol Metab 2002;87:3–15.

[97] Hale GE, Hitchcock CL, Williams LA, et al. Cyclicity of breast tenderness and nighttime vasomotor symptoms in midlife women: information collected using the daily perimenopause diary. Climacteric 2003;6:128–39.

[98] Bromberger JT, Assmann SF, Avis NE, et al. Persistent mood symptoms in a multiethnic community cohort of pre- and perimenopausal women. Am J Epidemiol 2003;158:347–56.

[99] Freeman EW, Sammel MD, Liu L, et al. Hormones and menopausal status as predictors of depression in women in transition to menopause. Arch Gen Psychiatry 2004;61:62–70.

ELSEVIER
SAUNDERS

Endocrinol Metab Clin N Am
34 (2005) 923–933

ENDOCRINOLOGY
AND METABOLISM
CLINICS
OF NORTH AMERICA

Mechanisms of Premature Menopause

Robert W. Rebar, MD[a,b,*]

[a]*American Society for Reproductive Medicine, Birmingham, AL, USA*
[b]*Department of Obstetrics and Gynecology, University of Alabama, Birmingham,
Birmingham, AL, USA*

Normal menopause, defined as the permanent cessation of menses, generally occurs at about the age of 51 years. In contrast, menopause generally is regarded as premature when it begins before the age of 40. Premature menopause is known by several different names, including premature ovarian failure, primary hypogonadism, hypergonadotropic amenorrhea, hypergonadotropic hypogonadism, and ovarian insufficiency. Premature menopause generally describes a syndrome consisting of amenorrhea (of 3 or more months' duration) and elevated gonadotropin levels and decreased estrogen levels typical of those found in postmenopausal women [1]. Previously, follicle-stimulating hormone (FSH) levels in the menopausal range were regarded as prima facie evidence of depletion of ovarian follicles, resulting in irreversible and permanent cessation of ovarian function [2]. It is now clear, however, that approximately 50% of women with apparent premature menopause may have intermittent and unpredictable ovarian function; 25% may ovulate, and 6% to 8% may conceive after the diagnosis is made [3–6]. One of the women seen by the author even ovulated after 8 years of amenorrhea [3]. Thus, the term premature menopause is inappropriate, and it may be more correct to use a term such as primary hypogonadism or hypergonadotropic amenorrhea.

Similarities and differences compared with normal menopause

Individuals with premature menopause appear to have many similarities compared with normal postmenopausal women but they have distinct differences also. In one study, 85.6% (83 of 97) of women with secondary

---

* American Society for Reproductive Medicine, 1209 Montgomery Highway, Birmingham, AL 35216.
E-mail address: rrebar@asrm.org

0889-8529/05/$ - see front matter © 2005 Elsevier Inc. All rights reserved.
doi:10.1016/j.ecl.2005.07.002
endo.theclinics.com

amenorrhea and apparent premature menopause and 22.2% (4 of 18) of those with primary amenorrhea noted symptoms of estrogen deficiency [4]. These findings are similar to numerous reports documenting such symptoms in 75% to 85% of women during the menopausal transition [7,8]. Years after the onset of symptoms, ovulation and pregnancy may occur in women with presumptive premature menopause [3].

Ovarian biopsies [3] and serial ultrasound examinations [9] indicate that significant numbers of ovarian follicles exist in about half of women diagnosed with premature menopause. This is in distinct contrast to postmenopausal women, in whom isolated follicles are detected only rarely [10].

After menopause, FSH and luteinizing hormone (LH) levels are increased to more than 30 mIU/mL, and pulsatile secretion is apparent. Circulating levels of estradiol and estrone also are decreased markedly. During the years that comprise the transition to menopause, menstrual cycles may occur regularly up to the very last menstrual period. Alternatively, and much more frequently, variable cycles may occur, with some being ovulatory, and others being anovulatory [8,11–15]. Cycles may become shorter, because of a shortened follicular phase, or they become longer. FSH levels may be increased at times, particularly early in the follicular phase, and estradiol levels may be increased, decreased, or normal. Progesterone levels may be decreased or normal.

Women with premature menopause may have concentrations of gonadotropins and sex steroids that are identical to those of postmenopausal women, but they also may have gonadotropin levels indicative of follicular activity and ovulation [3]. Women with incipient premature menopause may have variable cycles, with some being short, some long, and some of normal length. Some cycles may be ovulatory and others anovulatory. Intermittent elevations in FSH may be present, and estradiol levels may be decreased, normal, or increased. Progesterone levels may be normal or decreased.

Thus, it is clear that individuals with premature menopause may have symptoms, follicle numbers, and hormonal profiles identical to those of women going through the normal menopausal transition and entering menopause. It is also apparent, however, that these parameters may be quite distinct in women with premature menopause. The age at which menses ceases in women with secondary amenorrhea and premature menopause comprises a bell-shaped curve with a mean of 28 years, quite separate from the bell-shaped curve surrounding the normal age at menopause [4]. Moreover, it is clear that those women with primary amenorrhea and hypergonadotropic hypogonadism form yet a third population.

Multiple etiologies

Given the many differences between women entering normal menopause and those with premature menopause, it is not surprising that investigators and clinicians have identified several apparent causes of premature menopause. Indeed, even de Moraes-Ruehsen and Jones [1] suggested three possible explanations for the disorder at a time when they presumed that no viable ovarian follicles remained in women identified as having premature menopause. These explanations were: a decreased germ cell endowment, accelerated loss of oocytes (ie, atresia), and postnatal germ cell destruction. Available data now indicate that this was a simplistic approach to classification. This section attempts to offer a classification, with the understanding that no categorization is perfect and that changes no doubt will occur as additional information about this enigmatic disorder is identified (Box 1). It is becoming clear that there is a genetic component to many, if not most, of the causes and apparent mechanisms for premature menopause. This is not surprising given data from mice indicating that the numbers of oocytes and rates of atresia vary widely among different strains [16].

Cytogenetic abnormalities involving the X chromosome

Individuals with the various forms of gonadal dysgenesis typically present with hypergonadotropic amenorrhea regardless of the extent of pubertal development and the absence or presence of associated anomalies. Studies of individuals with a 45,X karyotype indicate that two intact X chromosomes are necessary for maintaining oocytes, because the ovaries of 45,X fetuses contain a normal number of oocytes at 20 weeks' gestation, but the oocytes present undergo rapid atresia such that most are gone by birth [17]. Primary and secondary amenorrhea with elevated gonadotropin levels may occur in women with deletions in either the short or the long arm of the X chromosome, Xp and Xq, respectively. In fact, two independent loci on the X chromosome have been identified at Xq26–q28 (POF1) and Xq13.3–q22 (POF2). One gene in the POF2 region has homology to DIA allele, mutants of which in *Drosophila* cause male and female infertility [18]. Molecular defects in ovarian maintenance genes located in these loci could account for reports of familial aggregates of premature menopause in karyotypically normal women.

Fragile X premutations in the FMR1 gene, once thought to be an asymptomatic carrier state, can be associated with premature menopause or a neurodegenerative disorder characterized by tremor and ataxia [19–21]. Approximately 14% of women with familial premature menopause have a premutation in the FMR1 gene, compared with 2% of women with isolated premature menopause [22]. Women found to have a premutation in the FMR1 gene are at risk of having a child with mental retardation, should they be among the few women with premature menopause who conceive. Thus, individuals with a family history of fragile X syndrome, unexplained mental retardation, dementia, a child with developmental delay, or a tremor/ataxia syndrome should be tested for permutations of the FMR1 gene.

Box 1. Possible classification of premature menopause

Cytogenetic abnormalities involving the X chromosome
Structural alterations or absence of an X chromosome
Trisomy X with or without mosaicism
Association with fragile X premutations

Enzymatic defects
17α-Hydroxylase or 17,20-lyase deficiency
Aromatase deficiency
Galactosemia

Other genetic mutations
Forkhead transcription factor (FOXL2) gene (blepharophimosis)
E1F2B genes (leukodystrophy)
Inhibin alpha gene
Autoimmune regulator (AIRE) gene
Phosphomannomutase 2 (PMM2) gene
Bone morphogenetic protein-15 (BMP15) gene

Defective gonadotropin secretion or action
Mutations in FSH and LH receptors
Circulating FSH antagonists (low molecular weight)
Secretion of altered gonadotropins

Immune disturbances
Circulating antibodies to the FSH receptor
In association with other autoimmune disturbances
Isolated
In association with congenital thymic aplasia

Physical causes
Ionizing radiation
Chemotherapeutic agents
Viral infection
Surgical injury or extirpation

An excess of X chromosomes also may be associated with premature menopause [23,24]. In most of these individuals, normal ovarian function is present for several years before the onset of premature menopause. Yet even here a few individuals with sexual infantilism have been reported.

Enzymatic defects

Three separate enzymatic defects have been associated with premature menopause: 17α-hydroxylase or 17,20-lyase deficiency, aromatase deficiency, and galactose-1-phosphate uridyl transferase deficiency (ie, galactosemia).

Individuals with the rare disorder of 17α-hydroxylase deficiency are identified easily because of the characteristic constellation of findings including primary amenorrhea, sexual infantilism, hypergonadotropinism, hypertension, hypokalemic alkalosis, and increased circulating levels of deoxycorticosterone and progesterone [25–27]. Ovarian biopsies of a few affected individuals have shown the presence of numerous large cysts and follicular cysts, with complete absence of orderly follicular maturation [27].

Women with galactosemia, characterized by mental retardation, cataracts, hepatosplenomegaly, and renal tubular dysfunction when untreated, develop amenorrhea with elevated gonadotropin levels even when treatment with a galactose-restricted diet begins at an early age [28,29]. The precise etiology of the premature menopause in galactosemia is unknown.

Other genetic alterations

Increasing numbers of rare genetic mutations have been associated with premature menopause. One well-characterized association includes alterations in the forkhead transcription factor (FOXL2) gene at map locus 3p23, in which premature menopause is associated with a familial syndrome that includes the eyelid defects blepharophimosis, ptosis, and epicanthus inversus [30].

Mutations in three of the five E1F2B genes (2, 4, and 5) cause leukodystrophy syndrome with a clinical spectrum ranging from a severe, rapidly progressive congenital or early infantile encephalopathy to a slowly progressive motor deterioration that may be associated with premature menopause [31,32].

Mutations in a small number of other genes, including those encoding inhibin alpha [33,34], phosphomannomutase 2 (PMM2) [34,35], autoimmune regulator (AIRE) [34,35], and bone morphogenetic protein-15 (BMP15) [36], also have been reported.

Defective gonadotropin secretion or action

Defects in gonadotropin secretion or action likely are caused by genetic mutations; thus, it is not clear exactly where to place these defects in any classification scheme. In any case, FSH receptor mutations (gene map locus 2p21–p16) have been reported as an inherited cause of premature menopause in Finnish women. This appears to be an uncommon cause of premature menopause in North America, however [37,38]. Partial loss of the FSH receptor also has been associated with premature menopause; this has been documented by the finding of a woman with premature menopause who had compound heterozygotic mutations located in the extracellular domain and in the third loop of the FSH receptor, respectively [39]. Inactivating mutations of the LH receptor gene, although apparently even more rare than mutations involving the FSH receptor gene, also have been associated with premature menopause [40].

That gonadotropin action may be affected also is suggested by one study of 27 women with hypergonadotropic amenorrhea and evidence of intermittent ovarian function. Sera from two of the individuals had low molecular weight FSH receptor-binding activity, which was an antagonist of FSH action [41].

The possibility that defects in gonadotropin structure might result in premature menopause is only theoretical. Abnormal molecular forms of gonadotropin, especially FSH, might have reduced or absent biological activity and might lead to accelerated follicular atresia. Support for the need for normal levels of gonadotropins early in development is provided by the observation that fetal removal of the pituitary gland in rhesus monkeys leads to newborns having ovaries containing no oocytes [42]. Moreover, altered forms of immunoreactive LH and FSH have been noted in urinary extracts from women with premature menopause compared with those from oophorectomized and postmenopausal women [43], suggesting that metabolism or excretion of gonadotropins and possibly their subunits are altered in some cases of this disorder.

Immune disturbances

Although premature menopause has been observed in association with numerous autoimmune disorders [44], it is not clear if the incidence of autoimmune disorders is increased in women with this syndrome. Autoimmune thyroiditis is the most commonly associated syndrome, being found in more than 15% of women with premature menopause (Box 2). More worrisome are the 4% of women who have steroidogenic cell autoimmunity and are at risk of developing adrenal insufficiency [45]. When premature menopause and adrenal insufficiency occur together, the ovarian failure presents first in 9 of 10 cases.

A few women with premature menopause also have autoimmune polyendocrinopathy-candidiasis-ectodermal dystrophy (APECED) [34]. This is an autosomal recessive disorder caused by mutations to the autoimmune regulator (AIRE) gene mapped to chromosome 21q22.3 and characterized by variable autoimmune destruction of tissues, primarily endocrine glands; mucocutaneous candidiasis; and ectodermal dystrophy.

It is also conceivable that autoimmune oophoritis can occur alone in some women. Antibodies to any of several ovarian enzymes or tissue components might affect follicular development. Most convincing is a report of two women with ovarian failure who had circulating IgG that blocked binding of FSH to its receptor [46]. Alternatively, ovarian failure might result from cell-mediated autoimmunity, and autoantibodies to ovarian tissue may appear only because of resultant cell death.

Box 2. Most common autoimmune disorders associated with premature menopause

Thyroid disorders, including Graves' disease and thyroiditis
Hypoadrenalism (Addison's disease)
Diabetes mellitus
Alopecia
Mucocutaneous candidiasis
Hypoparathyroidism
Myasthenia gravis
Polyendocrinopathies (type I, type II, and unspecified)
Vitiligo
Rheumatoid arthritis
Systemic lupus erythematosus

Evidence also is accumulating to suggest that the presence of the thymus gland is necessary for normal gonadotropin secretion and to prevent accelerated follicular atresia in utero [47]. Congenitally athymic girls who die before puberty have ovaries devoid of oocytes on autopsy [48]. Moreover, fetal thymectomy in monkeys in utero results in markedly reduced numbers of oocytes at birth [49].

Physical causes

Destruction of oocytes by various environmental insults is one potential cause of ovarian failure [50]. Conditions that have been implicated include ionizing radiation, various chemotherapeutic (especially alkylating agents), certain viral infections, and cigarette smoking.

It is clear that 8 Gy to the ovaries over 3 days is generally sufficient to induce ovarian failure. Permanent ovarian failure has occurred in about 50% of women subjected to 4 to 5 Gy to the ovaries over 4 to 6 weeks during treatment for malignancies; in some of the others, only temporary ovarian failure has resulted [51].

Chemotherapeutic agents, especially alkylating agents such as cyclophosphamide, also may produce temporary or permanent ovarian failure [52–54]. In general, the younger the individual patient at the time of therapy, the more likely it is that ovarian function will not be compromised by the chemotherapeutic agents.

It has been difficult to document any effect of viruses on ovarian function. Three presumptive cases in which mumps oophoritis preceded premature menopause, including cases in a mother and her daughter in which the mother had documented mumps parotiditis and abdominal pain during pregnancy just before delivery of the daughter, provide reasonable evidence [55].

Finally, no discussion of environmental insults to the ovary would be complete without noting that menopause occurs earlier in cigarette smokers than nonsmokers, although it is advanced only by several months [56].

Final considerations

Although this article has focused on potential mechanisms for premature menopause, it seems appropriate to end with a few comments about diagnosis and treatment. It is important to identify those causes that have important health consequences for the patient or any children. Once hypergonadotropic amenorrhea is identified, it is important to communicate this information to the patient with sensitivity. Young women are unprepared emotionally for the diagnosis of premature menopause. Moreover, as has been noted, the ovarian failure is not always permanent, and it is not always possible to identify those who will ovulate or conceive in the future. Professional counseling may be necessary, as may referral to an organization such as the Premature Ovarian Failure Support Group (available at http://pofsupport.org). Because young women with premature menopause have pathologically low levels of serum estradiol at least some of the time, and commonly suffer from signs and symptoms of estrogen deficiency, it seems rational to replace ovarian steroid hormones even in the absence of randomized controlled trials proving safety. There are no controlled trials regarding the ideal hormone replacement strategy for women with premature menopause, however. Typically, young women require twice as much estrogen as women going through normal menopause for relief of menopausal symptoms. This makes sense given that circulating levels of estradiol through the menstrual cycle average about 100 pg. Combination oral contraceptives are not recommended as hormone replacement in women with premature menopause, because such preparations contain much more steroid hormone (two to four times) than is required for physiologic replacement. Moreover, for unknown reasons neither oral contraceptives nor hormone replacement prevent ovulation or pregnancy in women with premature menopause [4]. For women with this disorder who wish to have children, use of donor oocytes and adoptions are the most viable options.

References

[1] De Moraes-Ruehsen M, Jones GS. Premature ovarian failure. Fertil Steril 1967;18:440–61.
[2] Goldenberg RL, Grodin RL, Rodbard D, et al. Gonadotropins in women with amenorrhea. Am J Obstet Gynecol 1973;116:1003–9.
[3] Rebar RW, Erickson GF, Yen SSC. Idiopathic premature ovarian failure: clinical and endocrine characteristics. Fertil Steril 1982;37:35–41.
[4] Rebar RW, Connolly HV. Clinical features of young women with hypergonadotropic amenorrhea. Fertil Steril 1990;53:804–10.
[5] Aiman J, Smentek C. Premature ovarian failure. Obstet Gynecol 1985;66:9–14.

[6] Brown JR, Skurnick JH, Sharma N, et al. Frequent intermittent ovarian function in women with premature menopause: a longitudinal study. Endocr J 1993;1:467–74.

[7] Anderson E, Hamburger S, Liu JH, et al. Characteristics of menopausal women seeking assistance. Am J Obstet Gynecol 1987;156:428–33.

[8] McKinlay SM, Brambilla DJ, Posner JG. The normal menopause transition. Maturitas 1992;14:103–15.

[9] Nelson LM, Anasti JN, Kimzey LM, et al. Development of luteinized Graafian follicles in patients with karyotypically normal spontaneous premature ovarian failure. J Clin Endocrinol Metab 1994;79:1470–5.

[10] Richardson SJ, Senikas V, Nelson JF. Follicular depletion during the menopausal transition: evidence for accelerated loss and ultimate exhaustion. J Clin Endocrinol Metab 1987;65: 1231–7.

[11] Sherman BM, West JH, Korenman SG. The menopausal transition: analysis of LH, FSH, estradiol, and progesterone concentrations during menstrual cycles of older women. J Clin Endocrinol Metab 1976;42:629–36.

[12] Burger HG, Dudley EC, Hopper JL, et al. The endocrinology of the menopausal transition: a cross-sectional study of a population-based sample. J Clin Endocrinol Metab 1995;80: 3537–45.

[13] Santoro N, Brown JR, Adel T, Skurnick JH. Characterization of reproductive hormonal dynamics in the perimenopause. J Clin Endocrinol Metab 1996;81:1495–501.

[14] Prior JC. Perimenopause: the complex endocrinology of the menopausal transition. Endocr Rev 1998;19:397–428.

[15] Liu JH, Kao L, Rebar RW, Muse K. Urinary β-FSH subunit concentrations in perimenopausal and postmenopausal women: a biomarker for ovarian reserve. Menopause 2003; 10(6):526–33.

[16] Jones EC, Krohn PL. The relationship between age, numbers of oocytes and fertility in virgin and multiparous mice. J Endocrinol 1961;21:469–95.

[17] Singh RP, Carr DH. The anatomy and histology of XO human embryos and fetuses. Anat Rec 1966;155:369–81.

[18] Bione S, Sala C, Manzini C, et al. A human homologue of the Drosophila melanogaster diaphanous gene is disrupted in a patient with premature ovarian failure: evidence for conserved function in oogenesis and implications for human sterility. Am J Hum Genet 1998;62:533–41.

[19] Conway GS, Hettiarachi S, Murray A, et al. Fragile X premutation in familial premature ovarian failure. Lancet 1995;346:309–10.

[20] Marozzi A, Vegetti W, Manfredini E, et al. Association between idiopathic premature ovarian failure and fragile X premutation. Hum Reprod 2000;15(1):197–202.

[21] Hagerman RJ, Leavitt BR, Farzin F, et al. Fragile-X-associated tremor/ataxia syndrome (FXTAS) in females with the FMR1 premutation. Am J Hum Genet 2004;74(5): 1051–6.

[22] Sherman SL. Premature ovarian failure in the fragile X syndrome. Am J Med Genet 2000; 97(3):189–94.

[23] Day RW, Larson W, Wright SW. Clinical and cytogenetic studies on a group of females with XXX sex chromosome complements. J Pediatr 1964;64:24–33.

[24] Villanueva AL, Rebar RW. Triple-X syndrome and premature ovarian failure. Obstet Gynecol 1983;62:70S–3S.

[25] Biglieri EG, Herron MA, Brust N. 17-Hydroxylation deficiency in man. J Clin Invest 1966; 45:1946–54.

[26] Goldsmith O, Solomon DH, Horton R. Hypogonadism and mineralocorticoid excess, the 17-hydroxylase deficiency syndrome. N Engl J Med 1967;277:673–7.

[27] Mallin SR. Congenital adrenal hyperplasia secondary to 17-hydroxylase deficiency: two sisters with amenorrhea, hypokalemia, hypertension, and cystic ovaries. Ann Intern Med 1969; 70:69–75.

[28] Hoefnagel D, Wurster-Hili D, Child EL. Ovarian failure in galactosaemia. Lancet 1979;2: 1197.

[29] Kauffman FR, Kogut MD, Donnell GN, et al. Hypergonadotropic hypogonadism in female patients with galactosemia. N Engl J Med 1981;304:994–8.

[30] Crisponi L, Deiana M, Loi A, et al. The putative forkhead transcription factor FOXL2 is mutated in blepharophimosis/ptosis/epicanthus inversus syndrome. Nat Genet 2001;27: 159–66.

[31] Schiffmann R, Van der Knapp MS. The latest on leukodystrophies. Curr Opin Neurol 2004; 17:187–92.

[32] Fogli A, Gauthier-Barichard F, Shiffmann R, et al. Screening for known mutations in EIF2B genes in a large panel of patients with premature ovarian failure. BMC Womens Health 2004; 4(1):8–15.

[33] Shelling AN, Burton KA, Chand AL, et al. Inhibin: a candidate gene for premature ovarian failure. Hum Reprod 2000;15:2644–9.

[34] Laml T, Preyer O, Umek W, et al. Genetic disorders in premature ovarian failure. Hum Reprod Update 2002;8(4):483–91.

[35] Schlessinger D, Herrera L, Crisponi L, et al. Genes and translocations involved in POF. Am J Med Genet 2002;111:328–33.

[36] Di Pasquale E, Beck-Peccoz P, Persani L. Hypergonadotropic ovarian failure associated with an inherited mutation of human bone morphogenetic protein-15 (BMP15) gene. Am J Hum Genet 2004;75:106–11.

[37] Aittomaki K, Lucena JLD, Pakarinen P, et al. Mutation in the follicle-stimulating hormone receptor gene causes hereditary hypergonadotropic ovarian failure. Cell 1995;82:959–68.

[38] Layman LC, Made S, Cohen DP, et al. The Finnish follicle-stimulating hormone receptor gene mutation is rare in North American women with 46,XX ovarian failure. Fertil Steril 1998;69:300–2.

[39] Beau I, Touraine P, Meduri G, et al. A novel phenotype related to partial loss of function mutations of the follicle stimulating hormone receptor. J Clin Invest 1998;102:1352–9.

[40] Latronico AC, Anasti J, Arnhold IJ, et al. Brief report: testicular and ovarian resistance to luteinizing hormone caused by inactivating mutations of the luteinizing hormone-receptor gene. N Engl J Med 1996;334:507–12.

[41] Sluss PM, Schneyer AL. Low molecular weight follicle-stimulating hormone receptor binding inhibitor in sera from ovarian failure patients. J Clin Endocrinol Metab 1992;74:1242–6.

[42] Gulyas BJ, Hodgen GD, Tullner WW, et al. Effects of fetal or maternal hypophysectomy on endocrine organs and body weight in infant rhesus monkeys (Macaca mulatto): with particular emphasis on oogenesis. Biol Reprod 1977;16:216–7.

[43] Silva de Sa MF, Matthews MJ, Rebar RW. Altered forms of immunoreactive urinary FSH and LH in premature ovarian failure. Infertility 1988;11:1–11.

[44] LaBarbera AR, Miller MM, Ober C, et al. Autoimmune etiology in premature ovarian failure. Am J Reprod Immunol Microbiol 1988;16:115–22.

[45] Bakalov VK, Vanderhoof VH, Bondy CA, et al. Adrenal antibodies detect asymptomatic auto-immune adrenal insufficiency in young women with spontaneous premature ovarian failure. Hum Reprod 2002;17(8):2096–100.

[46] Chiauzzi V, Cigorraga S, Escobar ME, et al. Inhibition of follicle-stimulating hormone receptor binding by circulating immunoglobulins. J Clin Endocrinol Metab 1982;54:1221–8.

[47] Rebar RW. The thymus gland and reproduction: do thymic peptides influence reproductive lifespan in females? J Am Geriatr Soc 1982;30:603–6.

[48] Miller ME, Chatten J. Ovarian changes in ataxia telangiectasia. Acta Paediatr Scand 1967; 56:559–61.

[49] Healy DL, Bacher J, Hodgen GD. Thymic regulation of primate fetal ovarian–adrenal differentiation. Biol Reprod 1985;32:1127–33.

[50] Verp MS. Environmental causes of ovarian failure. Semin Reprod Endocrinol 1983;1: 101–11.

[51] Ash P. The influence of radiation on fertility in man. Br J Radiol 1980;53:271–8.
[52] Siris ES, Leventhal BG, Vaitukaitis JL. Effects of childhood leukemia and chemotherapy on puberty and reproductive function in girls. N Engl J Med 1976;294:1143–6.
[53] Stillman RJ, Schiff I, Schinfeld J. Reproductive and gonadal function in the female after therapy for childhood malignancy. Obstet Gynecol Surv 1982;37:385–93.
[54] Whitehead E, Shalet SM, Blackledge G, et al. The effect of combination chemotherapy on ovarian function in women treated for Hodgkin's disease. Cancer 1983;52:988–93.
[55] Morrison JC, Givens JR, Wiser WL, et al. Mumps oophoritis: a cause of premature menopause. Fertil Steril 1975;26:655–9.
[56] Jick H, Porter J, Morrison AS. Relation between smoking and age of natural menopause. Lancet 1977;1:1354–5.

ENDOCRINOLOGY
AND METABOLISM
CLINICS
OF NORTH AMERICA

Endocrinol Metab Clin N Am
34 (2005) 935–955

ELSEVIER
SAUNDERS

Mechanisms of Hypoandrogenemia in Healthy Aging Men

Peter Y. Liu, MBBS, PhD[a], Ali Iranmanesh, MD[b,c],
Ajay X. Nehra, MD[d], Daniel M. Keenan, PhD[e],
Johannes D. Veldhuis, MD[a],*

[a]Endocrine Research Unit, Department of Internal Medicine, Mayo School of Graduate
Education, General Clinical Research Center, Mayo Clinic, Rochester, MN, USA
[b]Endocrine Service, Medical Section Salem, Veterans Affairs Medical Center,
Salem, VA, USA
[c]University of Virginia School of Medicine, Charlottesville, VA, USA
[d]Department of Urology, Mayo Medical and Graduate Schools of Medicine,
Mayo Clinic, Rochester, MN, USA
[e]Department of Statistics, University of Virginia, Charlottesville, VA, USA

Increasing longevity in developed economies creates a need to foster safe and effective medical approaches that prolong independent, enjoyable living as long as possible. Longitudinal studies indicate that key functional determinants such as muscle strength and bone mineral density decline by 1% to 2% and less than 1% per year between the fifth and ninth decades, respectively. Furthermore, aging is associated with increased visceral fat, insulin resistance, falls, and fractures, and decreased muscle mass, muscle strength, physical performance, physical activity, bone mineral density, and libido [1–8]. This ensemble of clinical features, although individually nonspecific, is reminiscent of organic androgen deficiency. Testosterone replacement in young androgen-deficient men reverses the foregoing signs and symptoms [9]. Whether comparable improvements are achievable safely in older men

Dr. Liu was supported by fellowships from the National Health and Medical Research Council of Australia (grant ID 262025) and Royal Australasian College of Physicians. Support was provided by Grants K01 AG19164 and R01 AG23133 from the National Institutes of Health (Bethesda, MD); DMS-0107680, a National Science Foundation Interdisciplinary Grant in the Mathematical Sciences (Washington, DC); and M01 RR00585 from the National Center for Research Resources.

* Corresponding author. Mayo Medical and Graduate Schools of Medicine, Mayo Clinic, Rochester, MN 55905.

E-mail address: veldhuis.johannes@mayo.edu (J.D. Veldhuis).

remains to be established by health outcome-oriented randomized placebo-controlled studies [10,11].

Impoverishment of anabolic drive probably contributes to physical frailty and diminished quality of life in older individuals [12–14]. Nonetheless, the increased prevalence of prostatic disease, cardiovascular disease, and obstructive sleep apnea, and the likelihood that male-predominant/exclusive diseases are androgen-sensitive imply that even small detrimental effects of androgens on these endpoints in an older at-risk population could limit or negate benefits. For these reasons, guidelines to promote appropriate and curb unnecessary androgen prescription in older men are available, but they continue to evolve [15,16].

The systemic availability of testosterone falls by 35% to 50% after the sixth decade of life in healthy men [17,18]. Longitudinal [19–22] and large population-based cross-sectional [23–28] studies from various cohorts throughout the world consistently report an annual 1% to 2% decline in blood total testosterone concentrations between the fifth and ninth decades (Fig. 1). Intercurrent illness, trauma, surgery, stress, weight loss, diverse medications, and institutionalization reduce testosterone concentrations further. In parallel with therapeutic trials, mechanistic studies dissecting the bases for testosterone depletion with age should facilitate the development of preventive strategies and optimize replacement therapy. The fundamental mechanisms that force hypoandrogenemia in the aging male remain unknown, however [29]. As highlighted in Fig. 2, organic testosterone deficiency must be identified or excluded in all symptomatic older men before concluding that relative androgen depletion is age-related.

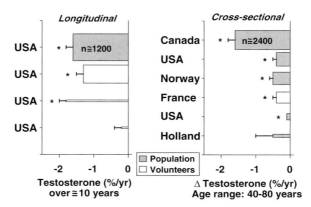

Fig. 1. Age-related fall in total testosterone concentrations. Cohorts of representative populations (gray) and volunteers (white) examined longitudinally (left) or cross-sectionally (right) consistently exhibit a 1%–2% annual decline in total serum testosterone concentrations. The larger studies are shown at the top of the graph, with proportionally smaller studies indicated by the relative width of the bar. Data are the mean ± SEM. Individual estimates that are significantly nonzero are indicated by the asterisk.

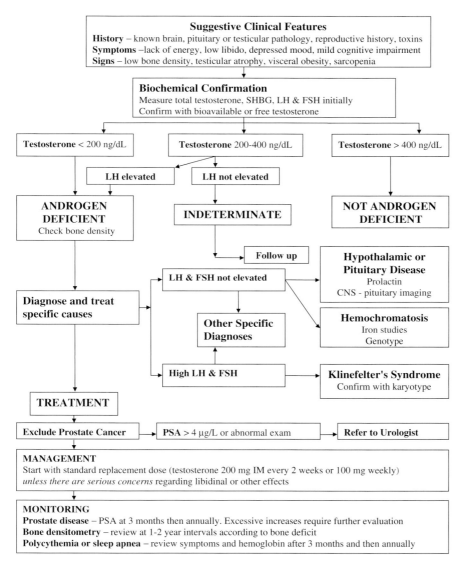

Fig. 2. Simplified assessment algorithm. (*Adapted from* Liu PY, Swerdloff RS, Veldhuis JD. The rationale, efficacy, and safety of androgen therapy in older men: future research and current practice recommendations. J Clin Endocrinol Metab 2004;89:4793; with permission.)

Recent clinical investigations offer new clues to the mechanistic bases of testosterone depletion in older men. In particular, aging-related reduction in androgen availability is marked jointly by:

- High-frequency and low-amplitude pulses of pituitary luteinizing hormone (LH) (Appendix 1)

- Quantifiably disorderly LH release, consistent with feedback disruption
- Normal or heightened LH secretion following single or repeated stimulation with the hypothalamic peptide, gonadotropin-releasing hormone (GnRH)
- Reduced testosterone secretory burst mass
- Impaired Leydig-cell testosterone production in response to secreted LH (stimulated by flutamide, tamoxifen, GnRH or anastrozole) and infused recombinant human (rh) LH [18,29]

The foregoing interconnected findings allow the integrative postulate that androgen deprivation in the older male reflects multi-site failure in the GnRH-LH-testosterone axis.

Extent and pace of relative hypoandrogenemia in older men

Albeit recognized biochemically nearly 50 years ago, testosterone depletion in aging is an increasingly pertinent clinical issue [12,29,30]. In part, this medical focus reflects the epidemiologic associations between hypoandrogenemia and sarcopenia, osteopenia, reduced physical stamina, sexual dysfunction, impaired quality of life, and (possibly) depressive mood and cognitive impairment [13,14,29,31,32]. Still, the primary cause of testosterone depletion and the indications for testosterone replacement are not known.

Impoverished testosterone availability in older men has been affirmed by: direct sampling of the spermatic vein, meta-analysis of cross-sectional data [33], and longitudinal investigations in healthy cohorts [20,21,34]. A 15-year prospective analysis in New Mexico reported that total testosterone concentrations fall by approximately 110 ng/dL per decade in men after the age of 60 years. The Senior European (SENIEUR) and Massachusetts Male Aging Cohort studies forecast a 0.8% to 1.3% annual decrement in bioavailable (non–sex hormone-binding globulin [SHBG]–bound) testosterone concentrations, and, the Baltimore Longitudinal Study of Aging predicted an annual decline of 4.9 pmol testosterone/nmol SHBG [20,21,34]. In the last study, the age-related prevalence of hypogonadal serum testosterone/SHBG ratios by young adult normative criteria exceeded 20%, 30%, and 50% at ages 60, 70, and 80 years, respectively [20]. Comorbidity in aged individuals exacerbates androgen deficiency markedly. Comorbid factors include chronic systemic disease, institutionalization, intercurrent acute illness, severe stress, weight loss, hospitalization, and the use of certain drugs [12,29,30,33,34].

Mechanistic bases of testosterone depletion

The primary mechanisms mediating hypoandrogenemia in older men have not been elucidated. Indeed, a unified mechanistic concept has been difficult to develop. In part, this challenge arises from the incremental nature of aging-related adaptations and emerging clinical evidence of multi-site rather than single-locus impairment in the gonadal axis. The latter includes reduced hypothalamic GnRH outflow, impaired testicular responsiveness to hCG/LH, and altered androgenic negative feedback [17,29,30,35,36]. An unresolved issue is whether presumptive mechanisms arise independently or emerge from ensemble connectivity among GnRH, LH, and testosterone.

Fig. 3 shows the ensemble concept of the male gonadal axis. An important unifying perspective is achieved by formalizing key feedback and feedforward interactions among GnRH, LH, and testosterone [37–39]. A broader vantage of the gonadal axis as a whole requires clarification of the nature of aging-related adaptations in each of the primary signals, GnRH, LH, and testosterone. The overall clinical expectation is to develop a simple, clear thematic understanding of the principal adaptations that mediate reduced androgen availability in healthy older men [17,18,29]. This section presents evidence for multi-site changes in the aging male gonadal axis.

Putative role of intrinsic gonadotropin-releasing hormone deficiency in older men in mediating low-amplitude pulsatile luteinizing protein secretion

The longstanding intuition that hypothalamic outflow of GnRH is reduced in older men never has been established or refuted [17,29]. The

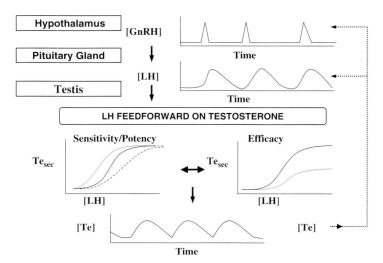

Fig. 3. Simplified schema of the male GnRH-LH-testosterone (hypothalamo-pituitary-Leydig cell) axis with key feedback (−, inhibitory) and feedforward (+, stimulatory) interactions. Implicit in vivo dose–response interfaces mediating LH-stimulated testosterone secretion (Tesec) are depicted at the bottom. Possible adaptations in feedforward sensitivity (steepness or slope), potency (one half-maximal stimulus concentration) (LH) and efficacy (maximal responsiveness) are illustrated by the interrupted curves.

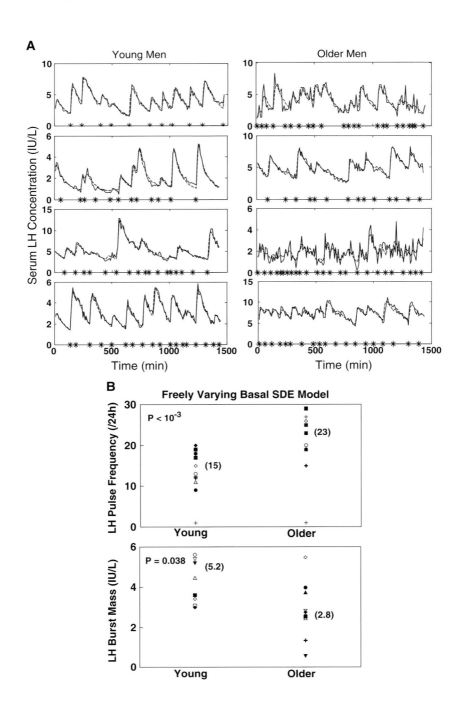

hypothesis is congruent with a significant repertoire of indirect clinical observations. Indirect evidence for impaired GnRH drive in aging men includes:

- Low-amplitude spontaneous LH pulses [35,38,39,41,48,69,70]
- Increased or normal LH secretory responsiveness to single or repeated (14-day) intravenous GnRH pulses, respectively [29,40,41,44,50]
- Blunted unleashing of pulsatile LH secretion under sex hormone feedback or opiate receptor blockade [48,65,66]
- Comparable young adult LH bioactivity in the unstimulated state [17,48,65,79,80]
- Quantifiably more disorderly patterns of LH release [38,39,41,66,67]
- Asynchrony of CNS-dependent neurohormone outflow with LH, follicle-stimulating hormone (FSH), prolactin, sleep-stage, and nocturnal penile tumescence (NPT) [68,78]
- Mathematical predictions based on an ensemble concept [37–39]

Pivotal findings are highlighted in Fig. 4. These include low spontaneous LH pulse amplitude (reduced mass of LH secreted per burst), which evolves in irregular patterns despite normal or heightened pituitary responses to GnRH [40,41]. Clinical inferences are nonexclusive, since some gainsaying studies have reported blunted gonadotrope responsivity to GnRH, increased LH pulse height, or diminished LH bioactivity in older men [34]. The foregoing discrepancies and the indirect nature of available observations highlight the need for more direct experimental appraisal of hypothalamic GnRH outflow in healthy older men. To this end, the authors recently monitored the degree of inhibition of endogenously driven (and fixed exogenous GnRH-induced) LH release by escalating doses of a potent and selective GnRH-receptor antagonist peptide (ganirelix) in 18 men aged 23 to 72 years to directly appraise hypothalamic GnRH outflow [42]. Age did not affect the inhibition of LH responses to a fixed exogenous submaximal GnRH stimulus, indicating consistent gonadotrope GnRH receptor–effector coupling. Increasing age, however, significantly potentiated the suppressive efficacy of any given serum ganirelix concentration on endogenously driven LH release. Given age-invariant competition between ganirelix and exogenous GnRH, these findings indicate that age reduces hypothalamic GnRH outflow (release and delivery) to gonadotrope cells.

Fig. 4. Age contrasts in LH secretion patterns. (*A*) Serum LH concentration profiles (*continuous lines*) measured by chemiluminescence assay in three young and three older men sampled every 10 minutes for 24 hours. Interrupted curves are predicted by an ensemble model of interlinked LH and testosterone secretion [37]. Discrete secretory bursts are marked by asterisks on the x-axis line. Older individuals show hypoandrogenemia and threefold alterations in GnRH/LH release with rapid-frequency, low-amplitude, and irregular (disorderly) patterns [38,39]. (*B*) Aging is marked by increased LH secretory burst frequency and reduced LH burst mass [39].

With due cognizance of potential species differences, basic laboratory experiments in the male rodent have delineated an important (but not exclusive) role of central hypogonadotropism in age-related hypoandrogenemia. Such evidence includes:

- Attenuated postcastration, anesthesia-stimulated and restraint stress-induced LH release, despite retention of acute gonadotrope secretory responsiveness to single GnRH stimuli [18,29,30,35,43–45]
- Diminished spontaneous in vivo LH pulse amplitude and reduced in vitro basal and neuroeffector-stimulated GnRH secretion by hypothalamic tissue [18,36,43,46,47]
- Altered GnRH neuronal synaptology [18]
- In one study, restoration of sexual activity in the impotent aged male by hypothalamic neuronal transplantation [18]

Enhanced gonadotrope luteinizing hormone secretory responsiveness to small amounts of gonadotropin-releasing hormone

Viewed mechanistically, impoverished LH secretory burst mass (which underlies reduced incremental LH pulse amplitude) in the aging male may denote diminished hypothalamic GnRH feedforward or impaired gonadotrope secretory responsiveness to available GnRH [29]. In relation to the latter consideration, prior studies based on a single (supramaximal) dose of GnRH in young and older men are divergent [29,30,35,36,44,48,49]. One recent dose–response study based on randomly ordered intravenous pulses of GnRH given on the same morning disclosed 1.6-fold higher GnRH-stimulated LH, FSH, and free-alpha-subunit concentrations in older compared with young men [40]. A second more extended dose–response analysis using separate morning, randomly ordered single-bolus intravenous doses spanning a 1000-fold range disclosed:

- Age invariance of maximal LH secretion (denoting equivalent GnRH efficacy)
- 1.8- to 2.1-fold accentuation of gonadotrope sensitivity (steeper slope of the dose–response) and GnRH potency (lower dose of GnRH required to stimulate one half-maximal LH secretion) in older men [50]

A third study administered intravenous pulses of GnRH (100 ng/kg) or saline every 90 minutes for 14 days in five young and five older men by portable infusion pump. Comparisons on the last day of intervention revealed comparable GnRH-stimulated LH secretion in the two cohorts but a 50% reduction in bioavailable and free testosterone concentrations achieved in the older group [41] (Fig. 5).

Heightened acute gonadotrope responsiveness to small amounts of GnRH (2.5, 10, and 25 ng/kg) in older men could reflect augmentation of releasable pituitary LH stores, upregulation of GnRH receptors, or less

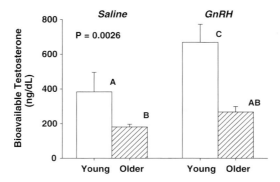

Fig. 5. Capability of 2 weeks of intravenous pulsatile GnRH stimulation to elevate bioavailable testosterone twofold more in young than older men, despite increasing 24-hour mean and pulsatile LH concentrations equally in the two age groups. (*Reprinted from* Mulligan T, Kerzner R, Demers LW, et al. Two-week pulsatile gonadotropin-releasing hormone infusion unmasks dual (hypothalamic and Leydig cell) defects in the healthy aging male gonadotropic axis. Eur J Endocrinol 1999;141:259; with permission.)

negative feedback because of lower concentrations of free and bioavailable testosterone in aging individuals. Available data do not distinguish among these mechanisms [17,18,29,30].

Apparent failure of Leydig cell steroidogenesis in older men

Administration of hCG fails to stimulate maximal young adult testosterone concentrations in many, but not all, aging men [12,30,36,51–54]. hCG injection paradigms, however, are difficult to interpret on experimental grounds:

- The extended half-life of hCG of 20 to 30 hours (compared with 0.75 to 1.5 hours for LH) does not mimic physiologically pulsatile gonadotropin stimulation of the testis [17,55–57].
- hCG demonstrably downregulates Leydig cell steroidogenesis in vivo and in vitro [58].
- Conventional hCG dosimetry explores maximal rather than physiologic Leydig cell responsiveness.

Furthermore, variable endogenous LH secretion, if not clamped, may be confounding. A pulsatile lutropic stimulus is mechanistically relevant to test the basis for relative hypoandrogenemia in healthy older men in as much as LH concentrations are normal or only minimally elevated [29].

One means to examine Leydig cell responsiveness to near physiologic lutropic drive entails pulsatile intravenous infusion of rh LH following injection of a GnRH receptor antagonist to suppress endogenous LH [59] (Fig. 6). Application of this paradigm for 14 hours in eight young and seven older men failed to increase bioavailable and free testosterone concentrations

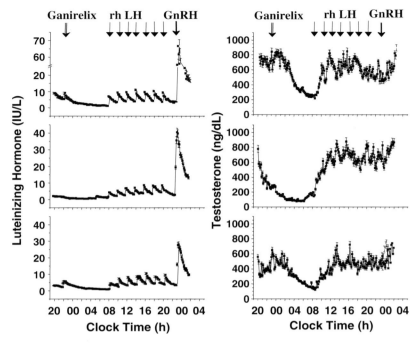

Fig. 6. Responses of three young men to overnight suppression of LH and testosterone concentrations by a single injection of a GnRH receptor antagonist (ganirelix) followed by seven consecutive intravenous pulses of recombinant human LH. Bolus GnRH (100 μg) injection after rh LH pulses documents the competitive nature of ganirelix inhibition. Ganirelix, rh LH pulses, and GnRH were administered at 120 minutes (*double arrow*), 720 minutes (*single arrow*), and 1620 minutes (*x axis*), respectively. Blood was sampled every 10 minutes for 32 hours. (*Adapted from* Veldhuis JD, Iranmanesh A. Pulsatile intravenous infusion of recombinant human luteinizing hormone under acute gonadotropin-releasing hormone receptor blockade reconstitutes testosterone secretion in young men. J Clin Endocrinol Metab 2004;89:4477; with permission.)

comparably in older men [90]. What remains uncertain is whether more extended delivery of LH pulses would drive young adult-like testosterone secretion. Experiments in the aged Brown-Norway rat point to fixed steroidogenic defects in Leydig cells in vitro or the perfused testis ex vivo [60]. Albeit plausible, the relevance of this animal model to human aging is not established.

Aging determines the feedback actions of testosterone on gonadotropin-releasing hormone and luteinizing hormone secretion

The nature of androgen-dependent negative feedback in older men remains indeterminate. First, three clinical studies noted excessive repression of LH concentrations in older men by short-term (4-day) intravenous infusion of testosterone, longer-term (11-day and 15-month) trans-scrotal replacement of testosterone, or transdermal delivery of 5 α-dihydrotestosterone (DHT) [44,61,62]. Second, two clinical investigations reported less suppression of LH concentrations in older compared with young subjects following intramuscular injection of testosterone [63,64]. Third, two other studies described abnormal LH secretory adaptations to short-term withdrawal of sex steroids in elderly men [65,66]. Fourth, a cross-correlation analysis inferred age-related attenuation of negative feedback by endogenous testosterone concentrations on time-varying LH release (Fig. 7). Fifth, model-based analyses of the ensemble axis (see Fig. 3) forecast threefold failure of GnRH secretion, testosterone production, and androgenic feedback on GnRH and LH output in the aging male [38,39]. Finally, histochemical analyses have quantitated reduced androgen–receptor expression in the brain and pituitary gland of the aged rat and in genital fibroblasts of the older human [29,45]. In principle, receptor depletion could contribute to attenuation of feedback efficacy in older men.

Definitive analyses are lacking of testosterone concentration-dependent feedback on the frequency, amplitude, and orderliness of pulsatile LH release. These three basic facets of regulated GnRH/LH release are significant, given that:

- Healthy older men maintain high-frequency, low-amplitude, and irregular LH secretion patterns [41,67–70].
- Experimental short-term hypoandrogenemia (induced by a steroidogenic-enzyme inhibitor) evokes anomalous LH secretion patterns in healthy young men, which mimic the baseline findings in older subjects [66,71].

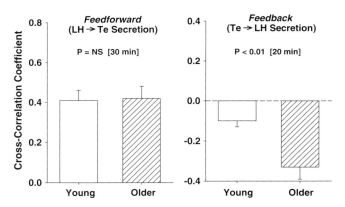

Fig. 7. Cross-correlation values (r) relating time-varying LH to testosterone (Te) concentrations (feedforward) and vice versa (feedback) in young and older men. Lower cross-correlation coefficients in older men signify reduced coupling of feedforward and feedback control between LH and testosterone in aging. (*Data from* Veldhuis JD, Iranmanesh A, Keenan DM. Erosion of endogenous testosterone-driven negative feedback on pulsatile LH secretion in healthy aging men. J Clin Endocrinol Metab 2004;89:5757.)

An important distinction is that acute testosterone or estradiol deprivation doubles the size of LH secretory bursts in young but not older men [66,71]. Therefore, low LH pulse amplitude in older men is not attributable to hypoandrogenemia, whereas more frequent and less orderly LH secretory bursts may be.

Clinical investigative strategies in aging men

Available data in older men point to simultaneous disruption of hypothalamic GnRH outflow, LH-stimulated Leydig cell steroidogenesis, and testosterone-dependent negative feedback (Fig. 8) [17,18,29,30,36,43,44,60]. Verifying interlinked adaptations in ensemble axis regulation, however, is difficult technically, in view of: the biologic interdependence of GnRH, LH, and testosterone and the need to quantitate time-evolving hormonal interactions without disturbing feedback or feedforward interactions. One approach to quantitating the net effect of multiple regulatory changes within an interlinked network like the gonadal axis is the approximate entropy (ApEn) measures [67,72–75] (Appendix 2). This statistic monitors the relative orderliness of subpatterns in hormone secretion (sample-by-sample pattern consistency, rather than pulses or circadian rhythms). Such analyses have disclosed less orderly secretion of LH and testosterone in older compared with young men [67]. As an extension of the ApEn metric, the cross-ApEn statistic measures the joint pattern synchrony of two coupled processes, thus helping to identify altered linkages between specifically paired signals [39,67]. Cross-ApEn analyses unmask prominent age-related

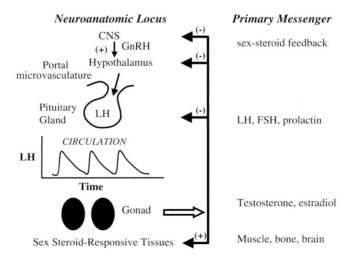

Fig. 8. Inferred sites and mechanisms that subserve relative testosterone deficiency in healthy older men.

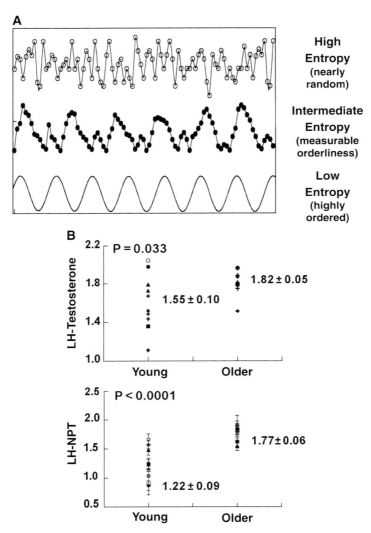

Fig. 9. (*A*) Notion of the approximate entropy (ApEn) statistic to quantitate the serial regularity or orderliness of subpatterns in a hormone time series. The bottom curve gives a cosine function (low ApEn or well-ordered pattern); the middle plot shows less regular serial data, and the top frame depicts an irregular profile (high ApEn). (*B*) Elevated cross-ApEn (X-ApEn) values in older men signify deterioration of joint synchrony between LH and testosterone release (*upper*) and LH and nocturnal penile tumescence (NPT) oscillations (*lower*). Data reflect 2.5 minute monitoring (overnight) in young and aging males. (*Adapted from* Veldhuis JD, Iranmanesh A, Mulligan T, et al. Disruption of the young adult synchrony between luteinizing hormone release and oscillations in follicle-stimulating hormone, prolactin, and nocturnal penile tumescence (NPT) in healthy older men. J Clin Endocrinol Metab 1999;84:3503; with permission.)

deterioration of coordinate LH and testosterone secretion, LH release and sleep-stage transitions, and oscillations in LH concentrations and NPT (Fig. 9) [38,39,67,68]. This is marked by greater testosterone–LH feedback coordination than LH–testosterone feedforward synchrony in healthy men of all ages, and significant and symmetric erosion of feedforward and feedback linkages in older individuals [76]. Such observations point to more general erosion of synchronous central neurohormone outflow in the older man.

New concepts in clinical investigation of the aging male gonadal axis include biomathematical constructs that encapsulate nonlinear, dose responsive and time-delayed feedforward and feedback coupling among GnRH, LH, and testosterone [37–39]. One may estimate dose–response properties noninvasively without injecting GnRH, LH, or testosterone or interrupting feedback linkages. Experimental validation of such strategies was by (1) repetitive direct sampling of cavernous sinus and internal jugular venous concentrations (and secretion rates) of GnRH, LH, and testosterone in the awake stallion and ram and (2) frequent simultaneous measurements of LH and spermatic vein testosterone concentrations in people [77]. Fig. 10 illustrates recent analytical reconstruction of the endogenous LH–testosterone

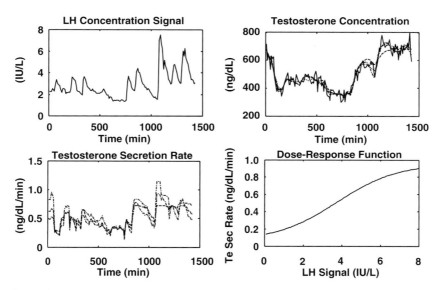

Fig. 10. Analytical reconstruction of pulsatile LH release profiles (LH signal, *upper left*), fluctuating testosterone concentrations (Te Conc, *upper right*), the free testosterone secretion rate (Te Sec tate, *bottom left*), and thereby the implicit (unobserved) dose–response function mediating spontaneous pulsatile LH-dependent testosterone secretion (*bottom right*) in a normal young man. LH and testosterone were sampled every 10 minutes for 24 hours without any intervention. (*Data from* Keenan DM, Veldhuis JD. Divergent gonadotropin–gonadal dose responsive coupling in healthy young and aging men. Am J Physiol 2004;286:R387; with permission.)

concentration–response function using paired peripheral measurements of the two hormones over 24 hours. Comparable analyses in 30 men predicted that aging selectively impairs endogenous LH efficacy (reduces maximally stimulated testosterone secretion).

Computer-assisted stimulation of gonadal axis adaptations in the older male illustrates that:

- A hypothesis of isolated failure of central GnRH drive would forecast only inappropriately low LH pulse amplitudes and attendant hypoandrogenemia.
- A notion of singular Leydig cell steroidogenic deficiency presages low testosterone but elevated LH concentrations.
- A tripartite postulate of impaired GnRH-dependent feedforward, blunted LH-stimulated testosterone secretion and reduced feedback by testosterone predicts hypoandrogenemia, attenuated LH pulse amplitude, accelerated LH pulse frequency, and disorderly LH release [37–39,67].

The crucial implication is that under basic model assumptions (see Fig. 3), no single defect explicates all the foregoing features of relative hypogonadotropic hypoandrogenemia in healthy older men.

Summary

Androgen deprivation adversely impacts libido and sexual potency, psychologic well being, mood and (possibly) cognition, exercise tolerance, muscle mass, bone mineral density, intra-abdominal adiposity, and lipid and carbohydrate metabolism [32,34]. Collective data identify presumptive impairment of hypothalamic GnRH outflow, reduction in pulsatile LH-stimulated testosterone synthesis, and decreased negative feedback in older men. Understanding the primary mechanistic bases of testosterone depletion in aging men may foster novel therapeutic strategies to maintain anabolism, enhance quality of life, and minimize physical frailty.

Acknowledgments

The authors thank Kris Nunez and Kandace Bradford for excellent assistance in text preparation and graphical illustrations.

Appendix 1. Feedback control of luteinizing pulse frequency

Intensive sampling paradigms consistently reveal an elevated LH pulse frequency in older compared with young men. A basic mechanistic issue is whether accelerated LH pulse frequency reflects a primary hypothalamic disturbance in the aging male or an expected feedback adjustment to lower systemic concentrations of free and bioavailable testosterone. In the latter regard, data in healthy young men establish that:

- Exposure to testosterone or nonaromatizable androgens (eg, 5 α-dihydrotestosterone or fluoxymesterone) suppresses LH pulse frequency [30,81].
- Conversely, administration of ketoconazole (which depletes testosterone) or flutamide (which inhibits androgen-receptor binding) accelerates LH pulse frequency [82].

Other studies indicate that more rapid pulsatile GnRH stimulation blunts incremental (and fractional) LH pulse amplitude. The latter reciprocal relationship (albeit not fully understood) indicates that hypoandrogenemia in aging, in principle, could mediate the elevated frequency and attenuated amplitude of LH pulses [41,69].

Appendix 2. Ensemble feedback/feedforward control: quantitation by the approximate entropy statistic

Pattern regularity is a quantifiable marker of adaptive feedback and feedforward control within an interlinked system [83–85]. The ApEn statistic measures this property. ApEn is calculated on a personal computer as a single number, which is an ensemble estimate of pattern consistency in any given time series. Higher ApEn values denote greater relative randomness (reduced orderliness) (see Fig. 9). In neuroendocrine studies, ApEn achieves sensitive (greater than 90%) and specific (greater than 90%) discrimination of subtle physiologic (and overt pathologic) adaptations in feedback and feedforward control [67,84–89]. Thus, elevated ApEn of LH concentration profiles in the elderly male denotes disruption of feedforward and/or feedback control within the interlinked GnRH-LH-testosterone [38,39,67].

References

[1] Hughes VA, Frontera WR, Roubenoff R, et al. Longitudinal changes in body composition in older men and women: role of body weight change and physical activity. Am J Clin Nutr 2002;76:473–81.
[2] Rantanen T, Masaki K, Foley D, et al. Grip strength changes over 27 yr in Japanese American men. J Appl Physiol 1998;85:2047–53.
[3] Santavirta S, Konttinen YT, Heliovaara M, et al. Determinants of osteoporotic thoracic vertebral fracture. Screening of 57,000 Finnish women and men. Acta Orthop Scand 1992;63: 198–202.
[4] Incidence of vertebral fracture in Europe: results from the European Prospective Osteoporosis Study (EPOS). J Bone Miner Res 2002;17:716–24.
[5] Fink RI, Kolterman OG, Griffin J, et al. Mechanisms of insulin resistance in aging. J Clin Invest 1983;71:1523–35.
[6] Nguyen TV, Eisman JA, Kelly PJ, et al. Risk factors for osteoporotic fractures in elderly men. Am J Epidemiol 1996;144:255–63.

[7] Davidson JM, Chen JJ, Crapo L, et al. Hormonal changes and sexual function in aging men. J Clin Endocrinol Metab 1983;57:71–7.

[8] Frontera WR, Hughes VA, Fielding RA, et al. Aging of skeletal muscle: a 12-yr longitudinal study. J Appl Physiol 2000;88:1321–6.

[9] Zitzmann M, Nieschlag E. Hormone substitution in male hypogonadism. Mol Cell Endocrinol 2000;161:73–88.

[10] Liu PY, Swerdloff RS, Veldhuis JD. The rationale, efficacy and safety of androgen therapy in older men: future research and current practice recommendations. J Clin Endocrinol Metab 2004;89:4789–96.

[11] Liu PY, Death AK, Handelsman DJ. Androgens and cardiovascular disease. Endocr Rev 2003;24:313–40.

[12] Stearns EL, MacDonald JA, Kaufman BJ, et al. Declining testicular function with age, hormonal, and clinical correlates. Am J Med 1974;57:761–6.

[13] Liu PY, Wishart SM, Handelsman DJ. A double-blind, placebo-controlled, randomized clinical trial of recombinant human chorionic gonadotropin on muscle strength and physical function and activity in older men with partial age-related androgen deficiency. J Clin Endocrinol Metab 2002;87:3125–35.

[14] Cunningham GR, Hirshkowitz M, Korenman SG, et al. Testosterone replacement therapy and sleep-related erections in hypogonadal men. J Clin Endocrinol Metab 1990;70:792–7.

[15] Conway AJ, Handelsman DJ, Lording DW, et al. Use, misuse and abuse of androgens. The Endocrine Society of Australia consensus guidelines for androgen prescribing. Med J Aust 2000;172:220–4.

[16] Cunningham G, Swerdloff RS. Endocrine Society Consensus Meeting statement. Chevy Chase (MD): The Endocrine Society; 2001.

[17] Urban RJ, Evans WS, Rogol AD, et al. Contemporary aspects of discrete peak detection algorithms. I. The paradigm of the luteinizing hormone pulse signal in men. Endocr Rev 1988; 9:3–37.

[18] Veldhuis JD, Iranmanesh A, Keenan DM. An ensemble perspective of aging-related hypoandrogenemia in men. In: Winters SJ, editor. Male hypogonadism: basic, clinical, and theoretical principles. Totowa (NJ): Humana Press; 2004. p. 261–84.

[19] Feldman HA, Longcope C, Derby CA, et al. Age trends in the level of serum testosterone and other hormones in middle-aged men: longitudinal results from the Massachusetts male aging study. J Clin Endocrinol Metab 2002;87:589–98.

[20] Harman SM, Metter EJ, Tobin JD, et al. Longitudinal effects of aging on serum total and free testosterone levels in healthy men. Baltimore Longitudinal Study of Aging. J Clin Endocrinol Metab 2001;86:724–31.

[21] Morley JE, Kaiser FE, Perry HM 3rd, et al. Longitudinal changes in testosterone, luteinizing hormone, and follicle-stimulating hormone in healthy older men. Metab Clin Exp 1997;46: 410–3.

[22] Zmuda JM, Cauley JA, Kriska A, et al. Longitudinal relation between endogenous testosterone and cardiovascular disease risk factors in middle-aged men. A 13-year follow-up of former Multiple Risk Factor Intervention Trial participants. Am J Epidemiol 1997;146: 609–17.

[23] Svartberg J, Midtby M, Bonaa KH, et al. The associations of age, lifestyle factors and chronic disease with testosterone in men: the Tromso Study. Eur J Endocrinol 2003;149:145–52.

[24] van den Beld AW, De Jong FH, Grobbee DE, et al. Measures of bioavailable serum testosterone and estradiol and their relationships with muscle strength, bone density, and body composition in elderly men. J Clin Endocrinol Metab 2000;85:3276–82.

[25] Dhandapani KM, Brann DW. The role of glutamate and nitric oxide in the reproductive neuroendocrine system. Biochem Cell Biol 2000;78:165–79.

[26] Simon D, Charles MA, Nahoul K, et al. Association between plasma total testosterone and cardiovascular risk factors in healthy adult men: the Telecom Study. J Clin Endocrinol Metab 1997;82:682–5.

[27] Belanger A, Candas B, Dupont A, et al. Changes in serum concentrations of conjugated and unconjugated steroids in 40- to 80-year-old men. J Clin Endocrinol Metab 1994;79: 1086–90.

[28] Gray A, Feldman HA, McKinlay JB, et al. Age, disease, and changing sex hormone levels in middle-aged men: results of the Massachusetts Male Aging Study. J Clin Endocrinol Metab 1991;73:1016–25.

[29] Veldhuis JD, Johnson ML, Keenan D, et al. The ensemble male hypothalamo-pituitary-gonadal axis. In: Timiras PS, editor. Physiological basis of aging and geriatrics. 3rd edition. Boca Raton (FL): CRC Press; 2003. p. 213–31.

[30] Baker HWG, Burger HG, de Kretser DM, et al. Changes in the pituitary–testicular system with age. Clin Endocrinol (Oxf) 1976;5:349–72.

[31] Wang C, Alexander G, Berman N, et al. Testosterone replacement therapy improves mood in hypogonadal men—a clinical research center study. J Clin Endocrinol Metab 1996;81: 3578–83.

[32] Barrett-Connor E, Goodman-Gruen D, Patay B. Endogenous sex hormones and cognitive function in older men. J Clin Endocrinol Metab 1999;84:3681–5.

[33] Gray A, Berlin JA, McKinlay JB, et al. An examination of research design effects on the association of testosterone and male aging: results of a meta-analysis. J Clin Epidemiol 1991; 44:671–84.

[34] Madersbacher S, Stulnig T, Huber LA, et al. Serum glycoprotein hormones and their free α-subunit in a healthy elderly population selected according to the SENIEUR protocol. Analyses with ultrasensitive time resolved fluoroimmunoassays. Mech Aging Devel 1993; 71:223–33.

[35] Vermeulen A, Deslypere JP, De Meirleir K. A new look at the andropause: altered function of the gonadotrophs. J Steroid Biochem 1989;32:163–5.

[36] Winters SJ, Troen P. Episodic luteinizing hormone (LH) secretion and the response of LH and follicle-stimulating hormone to LH-releasing hormone in aged men: evidence for coexistent primary testicular insufficiency and an impairment in gonadotropin secretion. J Clin Endocrinol Metab 1982;55:560–5.

[37] Keenan DM, Veldhuis JD. A biomathematical model of time-delayed feedback in the human male hypothalamic-pituitary-Leydig cell axis. Am J Physiol 1998;275:E157–76.

[38] Keenan DM, Veldhuis JD. Hypothesis testing of the aging male gonadal axis via a biomathematical construct. Am J Physiol 2001;280:R1755–71.

[39] Keenan DM, Veldhuis JD. Disruption of the hypothalamic luteinizing-hormone pulsing mechanism in aging men. Am J Physiol 2001;281:R1917–24.

[40] Zwart AD, Urban RJ, Odell WD, et al. Contrasts in the gonadotropin-releasing dose–response relationships for luteinizing hormone, follicle-stimulating hormone, and alpha-subunit release in young versus older men: appraisal with high-specificity immunoradiometric assay and deconvolution analysis. Eur J Endocrinol 1996;135:399–406.

[41] Mulligan T, Iranmanesh A, Kerzner R, et al. Two-week pulsatile gonadotropin releasing hormone infusion unmasks dual (hypothalamic and Leydig cell) defects in the healthy aging male gonadotropic axis. Eur J Endocrinol 1999;141:257–66.

[42] Takahashi PY, Liu PY, Roebuck PD, et al. Graded inhibition of pulsatile luteinizing hormone secretion by a selective gonadotropin-releasing hormone (GnRH)-receptor antagonist in healthy men: evidence that age attenuates hypothalamic GnRH outflow. J Clin Endocrinol Metab 2005;90:2768–74.

[43] Gruenewald DA, Naai MA, Hess DL, et al. The Brown Norway rat as a model of male reproductive aging: evidence for both primary and secondary testicular failure. J Gerontol 1994;49:B42–50.

[44] Deslypere JP, Kaufman JM, Vermeulen T, et al. Influence of age on pulsatile luteinizing hormone release and responsiveness of the gonadotrophs to sex hormone feedback in men. J Clin Endocrinol Metab 1987;64:68–73.

[45] Haji M, Kato KI, Nawata H, et al. Age-related changes in the concentrations of cytosol receptors for sex steroid hormones in the hypothalamus and pituitary gland of the rat. Brain Res 1980;204:373–86.

[46] Mitchell R, Hollis S, Rothwell C, et al. Age-related changes in the pituitary–testicular axis in normal men; lower serum testosterone results from decreased bioactive LH drive. Clin Endocrinol (Oxf) 1995;42:501–7.

[47] Coquelin AW, Desjardins C. Luteinizing hormone and testosterone secretion in young and old male mice. Am J Physiol 1982;243:E257–63.

[48] Urban RJ, Veldhuis JD, Blizzard RM, et al. Attenuated release of biologically active luteinizing hormone in healthy aging men. J Clin Invest 1988;81:1020–9.

[49] Snyder PJ, Reitano JF, Utiger RD. Serum LH and FSH responses to synthetic gonadotropin-releasing hormone in normal men. J Clin Endocrinol Metab 1975;41:938–45.

[50] Veldhuis JD, Iranmanesh A, Mulligan T. Age and testosterone feedback jointly control the dose-dependent actions of gonadotropin-releasing hormone in healthy men. J Clin Endocrinol Metab 2005;90(1):302–9.

[51] Reubens R, Dhondt M, Vermeulen A. Further studies on Leydig cell response to human choriogonadotropin. J Clin Endocrinol Metab 1976;39:40–5.

[52] Harman SM, Tsitouras PD. Reproductive hormones in aging men. I. Measurement of sex steroids, basal luteinizing hormone, and Leydig cell response to human chorionic gonadotropin. J Clin Endocrinol Metab 1980;51:35–40.

[53] Longcope C. The effect of human chorionic gonadotropin on plasma steroid levels in young and old men. Steroids 1973;21:583–92.

[54] Nankin HR, Lin T, Murono EP. The aging Leydig cell III. Gonadotropin stimulation in men. J Androl 1981;2:181–6.

[55] Veldhuis JD, King JC, Urban RJ, et al. Operating characteristics of the male hypothalamo-pituitary-gonadal axis: pulsatile release of testosterone and follicle-stimulating hormone and their temporal coupling with luteinizing hormone. J Clin Endocrinol Metab 1987;65:929–41.

[56] Foresta C, Bordon P, Rossato M, et al. Specific linkages among luteinizing hormone, follicle-stimulating hormone, and testosterone release in the peripheral blood and human spermatic vein: evidence for both positive (feed-forward) and negative (feedback) within-axis regulation. J Clin Endocrinol Metab 1997;82:3040–6.

[57] Winters SJ, Troen PE. Testosterone and estradiol are co-secreted episodically by the human testis. J Clin Invest 1986;78:870–2.

[58] Glass AR, Vigersky RA. Resensitization of testosterone production in men after human chorionic gonadotropin-induced desensitization. J Clin Endocrinol Metab 1980;51:1395–400.

[59] Veldhuis JD, Iranmanesh A. Pulsatile intravenous infusion of recombinant human luteinizing hormone under acute gonadotropin-releasing hormone receptor blockade reconstitutes testosterone secretion in young men. J Clin Endocrinol Metab 2004;89:4474–9.

[60] Grzywacz FW, Chen H, Allegretti J, et al. Does age-associated reduced Leydig cell testosterone production in Brown Norway rats result from understimulation by luteinizing hormone? J Androl 1998;19:625–30.

[61] Winters SJ, Atkinson L. Serum LH concentrations in hypogonadal men during transdermal testosterone replacement through scrotal skin: further evidence that aging enhances testosterone negative feedback. Clin Endocrinol (Oxf) 1997;47:317–22.

[62] Winters SJ, Sherins RJ, Troen P. The gonadotropin-suppressive activity of androgen is increased in elderly men. Metabolism 1984;33:1052–9.

[63] Gentili A, Mulligan T, Godschalk M, et al. Unequal impact of short-term testosterone repletion on the somatotropic axis of young and older men. J Clin Endocrinol Metab 2002;87:825–34.

[64] Muta K, Kato K, Akamine Y, et al. Age-related changes in the feedback regulation of gonadotrophin secretion by sex steroids in men. Acta Endocrinol (Copenh) 1981;96:154–62.

[65] Veldhuis JD, Urban RJ, Dufau ML. Differential responses of biologically active LH secretion in older versus young men to interruption of androgen negative feedback. J Clin Endocrinol Metab 1994;79:1763–70.

[66] Veldhuis JD, Zwart A, Mulligan T, et al. Muting of androgen negative feedback unveils impoverished gonadotropin-releasing hormone/luteinizing hormone secretory reactivity in healthy older men. J Clin Endocrinol Metab 2001;86:529–35.

[67] Pincus SM, Mulligan T, Iranmanesh A, et al. Older males secrete luteinizing hormone and testosterone more irregularly, and jointly more asynchronously, than younger males. Proc Natl Acad Sci USA 1996;93:14100–5.

[68] Veldhuis JD, Iranmanesh A, Godschalk M, et al. Older men manifest multifold synchrony disruption of reproductive neurohormone outflow. J Clin Endocrinol Metab 2000;85: 1477–86.

[69] Veldhuis JD, Urban RJ, Lizarralde G, et al. Attenuation of luteinizing hormone secretory burst amplitude is a proximate basis for the hypoandrogenism of healthy aging in men. J Clin Endocrinol Metab 1992;75:52–8.

[70] Mulligan T, Iranmanesh A, Gheorghiu S, et al. Amplified nocturnal luteinizing hormone (LH) secretory burst frequency with selective attenuation of pulsatile (but not basal) testosterone secretion in healthy aged men: possible Leydig cell desensitization to endogenous LH signaling—a clinical research center study. J Clin Endocrinol Metab 1995;80:3025–31.

[71] Veldhuis JD, Iranmanesh A. Short-term aromatase enzyme blockade unmasks impaired feedback adaptations in luteinizing hormone and testosterone secretion in older men. J Clin Endocrinol Metab 2005;90(1):211–8.

[72] Pincus SM. Approximate entropy as a measure of system complexity. Proc Natl Acad Sci USA 1991;88:2297–301.

[73] Pincus SM, Kalman RE. Not all (possibly) random sequences are created equal. Proc Natl Acad Sci USA 1997;94:3513–8.

[74] Pincus SM, Goldberger AL. Physiological time-series analysis: what does regularity quantify? Am J Physiol 1994;266:H1643–H656.

[75] Veldhuis JD, Johnson ML. Operating characteristics of the human male hypothalamo-pituitary-gonadal axis: circadian, ultradian and pulsatile release of prolactin, and its temporal coupling with luteinizing hormone. J Clin Endocrinol Metab 1988;67:116–23.

[76] Liu PY, Pincus SM, Keenan DM, et al. Analysis of bidirectional pattern synchrony of concentration-secretion pairs: implementation in the human testicular and adrenal axes. Am J Physiol Regul Integr Comp Physiol 2005;288(2):R440–6.

[77] Keenan DM, Alexander SL, Irvine CHG, et al. Reconstruction of in vivo time-evolving neuroendocrine dose-response properties unveils admixed deterministic and stochastic elements in interglandular signaling. Proc Natl Acad Sci USA 2004;101:6740–5.

[78] Veldhuis JD, Iranmanesh A, Mulligan T, et al. Disruption of the young-adult synchrony between luteinizing hormone release and oscillations in follicle-stimulating hormone, prolactin, and nocturnal penile tumescence (NPT) in healthy older men. J Clin Endocrinol Metab 1999;84:3498–505.

[79] Veldhuis JD, Urban RJ, Beitins I, et al. Pathophysiological features of the pulsatile secretion of biologically active luteinizing hormone in man. J Steroid Biochem 1989;33:739–50.

[80] Veldhuis JD, Dufau ML. Estradiol modulates the pulsatile secretion of biologically active luteinizing hormone in man. J Clin Invest 1987;80:631–8.

[81] Wang C, Berman N, Veldhuis JD, et al. Graded testosterone infusions distinguish gonadotropin negative feedback responsiveness in Asians and white men—a clinical research center study. J Clin Endocrinol Metab 1998;83:870–6.

[82] Urban RJ, Davis MR, Rogol AD, et al. Acute androgen receptor blockade increases luteinizing hormone secretory activity in men. J Clin Endocrinol Metab 1988;67:1149–55.

[83] Pincus SM. Quantifying complexity and regularity of neurobiological systems. Methods in Neuroscience 1995;28:336–63.

[84] Veldhuis JD, Johnson ML, Veldhuis OL, et al. Impact of pulsatility on the ensemble order-liness (approximate entropy) of neurohormone secretion. Am J Physiol 2001;281:R1975–85.

[85] Veldhuis JD, Straume M, Iranmanesh A, et al. Secretory process regularity monitors neuro-endocrine feedback and feedforward signaling strength in humans. Am J Physiol 2001;280:R721–9.

[86] Veldhuis JD, Pincus SM. Orderliness of hormone release patterns: a complementary measure to conventional pulsatile and circadian analyses. Eur J Endocrinol 1998;138:358–62.

[87] Veldhuis JD, Metzger DL, Martha PM Jr, et al. Estrogen and testosterone, but not a nonar-omatizable androgen, direct network integration of the hypothalamo–somatotrope (growth hormone)-insulin-like growth factor I axis in the human: evidence from pubertal pathophys-iology and sex-steroid hormone replacement. J Clin Endocrinol Metab 1997;82:3414–20.

[88] Pincus SM, Gevers E, Robinson ICAF, et al. Females secrete growth hormone with more process irregularity than males in both human and rat. Am J Physiol 1996;270:E107–15.

[89] Pincus SM, Hartman ML, Roelfsema F, et al. Hormone pulsatility discrimination via coarse and short time sampling. Am J Physiol 1999;277:E948–57.

[90] Veldhuis JD, Veldhuis NJ, Keenan DM, et al. Age diminishes the testicular steroidogenic re-sponse to repeated intravenous pulses of recombinant human LH during acute GnRH-receptor blockade in healthy men. Am J Physiol Endocrinol Metab 2005;288:E775–81.

ELSEVIER
SAUNDERS

Endocrinol Metab Clin N Am
34 (2005) 957–972

ENDOCRINOLOGY
AND METABOLISM
CLINICS
OF NORTH AMERICA

Relative Testosterone Deficiency in Older Men: Clinical Definition and Presentation

Peter Y. Liu, MD, PhD[a], Ronald S. Swerdloff, MD[a,b], Christina Wang, MD[b,c,*]

[a]*Division of Endocrinology, Department of Medicine, Los Angeles Biomedical Research Institute, Harbor–University of California at Los Angeles Medical Center, Torrance, CA, USA*
[b]*David Geffen School of Medicine, University of California at Los Angeles, Los Angeles, CA, USA*
[c]*General Clinical Research Center, Los Angeles Biomedical Research Institute, Harbor–University of California at Los Angeles Medical Center, Torrance, CA, USA*

The increased longevity observed in many communities worldwide has created a need to foster healthy aging. Devising safe and effective medical approaches that prolong healthy, independent, and enjoyable living is therefore a priority for health care providers. Androgen replacement therapy for older men holds promise in this regard, because systemic levels of testosterone fall by 1% to 2% each year, creating a state of relative (compared with young men) androgen deficiency [1,2]. Furthermore, many aspects of aging resemble features of organic androgen deficiency in younger men in whom testosterone replacement is an accepted therapy and widely regarded as safe, affordable, and effective [3,4] (Table 1).

In contrast, androgen replacement therapy in older men remains controversial for numerous reasons [5,6]. First, rigorous data confirming age-specific benefits over potential long-term adverse effects are limited. Second,

Dr. Liu was supported by grants from the Lalor Foundation and National Health and Medical Research Council of Australia. Drs. Swerdloff and Wang were jointly supported by National Institutes of Health (NIH) training Grant T32 DK07571-17. Dr. Wang was supported by Grant NIH-MO1 RR00425 to the General Clinical Research Center at Harbor–University of California.

* Corresponding author. General Clinical Research Center, Los Angeles Biomedical Research Institute, Harbor–University of California at Los Angeles Medical Center, 1000 West Carson Street, Torrance, CA 90509.

E-mail address: wang@labiomed.org (C. Wang).

Table 1
Clinical features of androgen deficiency and comparison of effect of androgen administration in organic androgen deficiency and aging

Criteria	Features	Reversal by androgen	
		Organic androgen deficiency	Aging
Muscle mass	↓	Yes	Yes
Muscular strength	↓	Yes	Yes
Fat mass	↑	Yes	Yes
Physical function	↓	Yes	?
Bone density	↓	Yes	Yes
Hair/skin	↓	Yes	?
Cognition/mood	↓	Yes	?
Libido	↓	Yes	?
Quality of life	↓	Yes	?

many older men may have serum testosterone levels that are only modestly below the young healthy male range, and thus the chemical abnormality may not be sufficient to warrant replacement. Third, concerns about risk-to-benefit ratios that are age-specific (ie, prostate and cardiovascular disease) remain in the critiques of many clinicians. Finally, many of the clinical features attributed to relative androgen deficiency are subtle and nonspecific and conceivably could be caused by many etiologies, including other hormonal deficiencies (particularly growth hormone and possibly, estradiol), mitochondrial dysfunction, increased cytokines, and oxidative stress. This confounds the clinical presentation of relative testosterone deficiency. For these reasons, the efficacy and safety of androgen therapy in older men will remain undefined until additional data from adequately powered randomized placebo-controlled studies become available to validate or refute the clinical significance and interventional potential for this putative syndrome.

Relative androgen deficiency in older men: the questions

Does it exist?

There are overwhelming indirect data showing that relative androgen deficiency exists and that the merits and risks of replacement therapy are worthy of consideration. Aging is associated with specific and multiple alterations throughout the entire hypothalamo–pituitary testicular axis. Such changes in luteinizing hormone (LH) and testosterone secretion characteristics and their integrative feedforward and feedback regulation [7] strongly implicate the relevance of testicular axis alterations in the pathogenesis of a subtle clinical syndrome. These changes associated with aging orchestrate the irrefutable decline in systemic testosterone exposure (measured as total, free or bioavailable testosterone) with age that has been confirmed in many representative longitudinal and large cross-sectional cohorts worldwide (see Liu and colleagues elsewhere in this issue). This decline likely explains at least some of the symptoms and signs such as lethargy, sexual dysfunction, decreased muscle, osteopenia, and increased fat commonly observed in older men. Relative testosterone deficiency in older men? The term adequately describes the phenomenon that serum testosterone concentrations fall with age. Multiple alternatives such as viropause, partial androgen deficiency of aging men (PADAM), androgen deficiency of aging men (ADAM), senile hypogonadism, and, most recently, late-onset hypogonadism have been used to describe this same clinical syndrome. Other terms such as andropause or male menopause may be less satisfactory, because they draw an inappropriate analogy with the female menopause, which in contrast is a clear-cut and well-defined clinical syndrome associated with the cessation of menses. The plethora of so many descriptive terms may reflect the ill-defined nature of any putative clinical syndrome of age-specific relative androgen deficiency.

Ideally, the clinical syndrome (symptoms, signs, and simple laboratory investigations) should identify a group of older men who are more likely to favorably respond to androgen therapy (ie, have more beneficial effects or fewer adverse effects), or predict a group of men who are likely to undergo accelerated functional decline. In either group, testosterone (or some other adjunctive therapies) may benefit the patient. Unfortunately, no such definition is available. Although the degree of androgen deficiency, as assessed by baseline systemic testosterone exposure, is a predictor of androgen responsiveness in older men [8], the utility of defining a syndrome [9,10] that simply correlates with low serum testosterone concentrations is of limited usefulness given the ease with which blood can be obtained and analyzed. Any such definition should include a serum concentration testosterone or specific testosterone fraction measurement [5,11–13], and a threshold level for the chemical diagnosis is required. Estimates of prevalence rates based on testosterone concentrations are premature given the uncertain response relationship between serum testosterone concentrations and any clinical syndrome [2,14,15].

Best practice guidelines provide a definition based on low serum concentrations of total testosterone or its non–sex hormone-binding globulin (SHBG) bound component (ie, free or bioavailable testosterone) in combination with a compatible clinical picture [5,11–13]. Such a definition is premised upon extrapolating the clinical syndrome of organic androgen deficiency of young men into the older population. Which testosterone cutoff to employ (using which testosterone measurement) and which complex of symptoms and signs define the disorder remain controversial, however. Furthermore, the extrapolation of clinical symptomatology in particular is confounded by differing comorbidities.

Should relative androgen deficiency of older men be treated?

Considerable evidence shows that hypogonadism in younger men responds favorably in many distinct clinical domains to testosterone treatment

[3,4]. The possibility that older men may fail to respond or be less responsive to testosterone treatment compared with young men has been highlighted by some investigators. To the contrary, recent data have shown equivalent increases in muscular mass and strength and comparable decreases in fat mass in response to short-term testosterone treatment irrespective of age [16]. These data, showing no age-associated worsening in testosterone responsiveness strongly imply that the age-related relative decrease in systemic testosterone concentration has real and reversible effects on skeletal muscle and adipose tissue and inferentially suggest similar relationships with other androgen-responsive tissues. Because muscular mass and strength are known determinants of physical function, disability, and quality of life, these data suggest that theses effects of androgen replacement therapy in the older male may have other widespread nonmuscular effects. Thus androgens could improve physical functioning by preventing the frailty, falls, and fractures in older men that mar quality of life and threaten independent living. The definitive demonstration of functional improvement and decreased morbidity and mortality of testosterone treatment of age-related androgen deficiency are awaited.

    Even if testosterone treatment is effective in older men, this may be negated by increased risks. The speculation that older men are more prone to adverse effects of testosterone treatment (in particular prostate disease, raised hematocrit, and fluid retention) has been confirmed directly [16]. It may be that a clinical syndrome of relative androgen deficiency exists, but treating all older men nonselectively with androgens could cause more harm than good. This is a potential problem for many therapeutic interventions and can be solved partly by vigilant monitoring and dose titration. Also, combining interventional strategies such as appropriate exercise with other anabolic agents may enhance effect and allow lower dosing.

Putative clinical definition of relative androgen deficiency in older men

Testosterone cutoff

    At present, there are only limited data to show that a particular testosterone cutoff level separates older men by testosterone responsiveness or risk of disability. This is in stark contrast with well-demarcated cardiovascular risk-defined partition levels for diastolic blood pressure [17] or efficacy-defined division levels for blood glucose control [18]. Epidemiologic information linking chemical levels and symptom complex is accumulating slowly [19–21], and available data suggest a linear rather than bimodal relationship [8]. More information is needed [6]. Until this occurs, the segregation level of serum testosterone for diagnosing relative testosterone deficiency in older men has been defined statistically using normative ranges obtained from healthy young men. In such a population, the 95% confidence interval of serum total testosterone ranges from 300 to 1000 ng/dL (10 to 35 nmol/L), provided that blood is sampled in the morning. In other words, 2.5% of all young men have blood concentrations below 300 ng/dL. Given the uncertainty of androgen therapy in older men, however, a more stringent 98% confidence interval may be applied, which corresponds to a blood testosterone concentration of about 250 ng/dL (8.7 nmol/L). Approximately 1% of healthy young men will have a serum testosterone concentration of less than 250 ng/dL. Such a threshold defining male hypogonadism has been adopted almost universally throughout the world [5,11–13]. As an example, the United States-based Endocrine Society has made the following recommendations [12]:

> "If the serum testosterone level is above 350 ng/dL (12.1 nmol/L), then most likely the man does not have relative androgen deficiency. Values in between 250 and 350 ng/mL warrant a repeat serum level and further assessment of the unbound testosterone measured as free testosterone using equilibrium dialysis or ultracentrifugation to separate the free steroid from testosterone bound to proteins. If the testosterone levels are below 250 ng/dL on repeated samples, then the patient is likely androgen-deficient."

Non-SHBG–bound (bioavailable) testosterone, which comprises the free and albumin-bound fractions, can be measured directly after ammonium sulfate precipitation. Either free or non-SHBG–bound testosterone can be calculated from concentration of total testosterone, and SHBG can be measured usually by immunoassays using the law of mass action (formula available at http://www.issam.ch). Bioavailable or free testosterone may help clarify the clinical picture in men with symptoms or signs suggestive of androgen deficiency and borderline total testosterone concentrations. Nevertheless, how androgen deficiency is defined and confirmed by which testosterone measurement remains unresolved, because empirical validation of these measures against independent biologic markers of androgen action in man is lacking [22].

Compatible clinical presentation

In younger men with organic androgen deficiency, commonly self-reported symptoms include lack of energy, diminished libido, erectile dysfunction, loss of motivation, cantankerous mood, sleepiness after lunch, and inability to concentrate [23]. Other symptoms such as hot flushes, slowed beard growth, and muscular aches also have been reported, but less frequently. These symptoms are putative markers of relative testosterone deficiency in older men, and variations thereof have been used both in the Androgen Deficiency in Aging Males (ADAM) and Aging Males' Symptoms (AMS) scale questionnaires (Box 1 and Fig. 1) [10,24–26]. The development of these questionnaires reflects two differing approaches to defining the presumptive clinical syndrome. The ADAM questionnaire was a screening questionnaire validated primarily against serum testosterone concentrations, and hence, it

---

Box 1. Androgen deficiency in aging males questionnaire

1. Do you have a decrease in libido (sex drive)?
2. Do you have a lack of energy?
3. Do you have a decrease in strength and/or endurance?
4. Have you lost weight?
5. Have you noticed a decreased enjoyment of life?
6. Are you sad and/or grumpy?
7. Are your erections less strong?
8. Have you noted a recent deterioration in your ability to play sports?
9. Are you falling asleep after dinner?
10. Has there been a recent deterioration in your work performance?

   A positive response is a yes answer to questions 1, 7, or any three other questions.

   Modified from Morley JE, et al. Validation of a screening questionnaire for androgen deficiency in aging males. Metabolism 2000;49(9):1239–42; with permission.

---

can be viewed as a noninvasive method to screen for this outcome. The AMS questionnaire in contrast was not developed as a screening test for low testosterone concentrations, and it has not been compared against serum testosterone concentrations. Instead, it was designed as a quality-of-life questionnaire, for which population-based normative data derived from large samples from many different countries have been collected, and internal reliability and psychologic, somatic, and sexual subscale agreement have been verified [25]. Each component of the AMS (psychologic, somatic, and sexual symptomatology) has been shown in a limited unblinded study to improve with testosterone administration in older men [26]. In this study, however, only 40% of subjects enrolled were over the age of 60; placebo controls were not included in the study design, and the treatment was for only 3 months.

Sexual symptoms

   Diminished sexual function is an important feature of organic androgen deficiency, and it universally is included as part of the clinical definition of relative age-dependent androgen deficiency [9,10,25]. The usefulness of this criterion in the aging male, however, is limited, because both components of sexual dysfunction (erectile dysfunction and reduced libido) occur commonly with increasing age, as demonstrated in numerous representative population-based studies (n = 28,000 men) [27–37]. Furthermore, this decline is unlikely to be related solely to the modest declines observed with age,

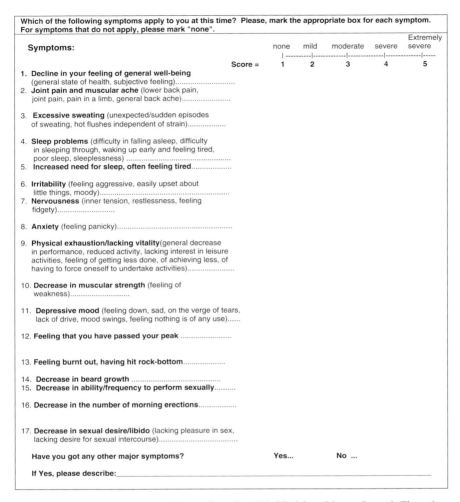

Fig. 1. Aging males symptoms scale questionnaire. (*Modified from* Moore C, et al. The aging males' symptoms scale (AMS) as outcome measure for treatment of androgen deficiency. Eur Urol 2004;46(1):85; with permission.)

because the blood testosterone threshold for maintaining male sexual function is low [16,38,39]. The inability of serum testosterone to fully predict sexual dysfunction is illustrated further by analysis of a large twin database that showed that nonheritable factors account for no more than 70% of the variance in erectile dysfunction [40].

Nevertheless, primarily libido, and secondarily erectile function, are testosterone-sensitive parameters [38,39,41–43]. Although testosterone-sensitive, erectile dysfunction in older men is multi-factorial in origin and cannot often be explained simply by organic androgen deficiency [44]. Hence the discriminatory utility of screening men with sexual dysfunction for relative androgen deficiency is limited, and positive identification is likely to be confined to men who are more severely androgen deficient.

Somatic symptoms

Somatic features related to symptoms of decreased muscular strength, fatigue, and energy; clinical signs of reduced lean mass and increased adiposity; and reduced beard growth are all features of organic androgen deficiency. These characteristics also have been incorporated universally into the clinical definition of age-related relative androgen deficiency [9,10,25]. Body compositional changes, however, are known to occur with aging itself, which may or may not be related to age-related declines in serum testosterone concentrations. Longitudinal studies using hydrodensitometry have shown that fat mass decreases, and lean mass increases during childhood and puberty (when adjusted for stature) [45], followed by an increase in fat and a decrease in lean mass during adulthood [46–49] and very old age [50]. These and other large longitudinal [51,52] studies of at least 100 men are summarized in Table 2, and they collectively show a loss of 0.1 to 0.2 kg/y of lean mass and an increase of 0.1 to 0.6 kg/y of fat mass. Because total weight increases up to the age of 60 and then declines in more than 60% of men, the accumulation of fat mass must occur predominately during midlife [53–55]. The midlife increase in fat mass, which is predominantly abdominal/central, is associated with the metabolic syndrome and is a critical predictor of all-cause mortality [56–58]. How these age-specific body compositional changes relate to changes in serum testosterone, or to changes in integrative gonadotropin axis signaling, is undefined. Hence, although these body compositional changes commonly are considered part of the

Table 2
Age-related changes in body composition

First author, year [Ref.]	N	Baseline age range (y)	Follow-up (y)	Method	Approximate Δfat (kg/y) mean ± SEM	Approximate Δmuscle (kg/y) mean ± SEM
Siervogel, 1998 [46]	202	≈ 35 (18–65)	≈ 10	Hydrodensitometry	↑ 0.4 ± 0.1	↔
Guo, 1999 [47]	102	44 (40–58)	9 (1–20)	Hydrodensitometry	↑ 0.4 ± 0.06	↔
Keys, 1973 [48]	58	22 (18–26)	19	Hydrodensitometry	↑ 0.6 ± ?	↓ 0.1 ± ?
Hughes, 2002 [50]	53	61 (46–80)	9 (5–12)	Hydrodensitometry	↑ 0.1 ± 0.04	↓ 0.1 ± 0.03
Chien, 1975 [49]	27	32 (21–44)	12	Hydrodensitometry	↑ 0.6 ± 0.02	↔
Flynn, 1989 [52]	564	≈ 50 (28–60)	< 18	Total body potassium	↔	↔
Jackson, 1995 [51]	153	46 (25–70)	4	Skinfold thickness	↔	↓ 0.1 ± 0.03

clinical definition of relative androgen deficiency, their diagnostic utility remains unclear.

Similarly, other important somatic features such as muscular strength are known to decline with age. Studies of at least 100 subjects examining the effect of age on upper limb [55,59–62] and lower limb [63,64] strength are summarized in Tables 3 and 4. These show that maximal dynamic force production declines with age in the upper and lower limbs. Furthermore, increasing age seems to be associated with an even greater reduction in percentage strength. Although there are no large series examining the longitudinal decline in lower limb strength (Table 4), smaller longitudinal [65–68] and population-based cross-sectional studies [69] confirm a similar 1% to 3% decrease in strength per year.

All of these somatic features decline with age, irrespective of gender. They often are used in the clinical definition of relative androgen deficiency, but they are unlikely to be useful as currently used. Markers of physical performance such as gait speed [70,71], manual performance [72], ability to stand up from a chair [71] and balance [71] decline with age in longitudinal studies and have been shown in longitudinal [73–78] and cross-sectional [79–81] studies to predict a range of important outcomes (Table 5). These declines also are not universal [71], suggesting the possibility that selective preventative strategies are feasible. Thus these physical performance characteristics may be of paramount importance in selecting subpopulations of older men who comprise the at-risk population likely to become disabled and therefore most likely to benefit from androgen therapy. Such verification

Table 3
Age-related changes in upper limb muscle strength

First author, year [Ref.]	N	Baseline age range (y)	Follow-up (y)	Population	Method	Strength (% decline/y)
Rantanen, 1998 [55]	3741	≈ 55 (45–68)	27	Representative	Handgrip	1 ± 0.01
Metter, 1997 [60]	837	≈ 35 (18–65)	10 (9–57)	Volunteer	Isokinetic	1 ± 0.2
Clement, 1974 [62]	369	≈ 60 (16–90)	10 (5–15)	Representative	Handgrip	1.2
Bassey, 1993 [61]	240	72 (64–94)	4	Representative	Handgrip	3 ± 0.3
Clement, 1974 [62]	1139	≈ 60 (16–90)	0	Representative	Handgrip	0.8
Metter, 1997 [60]	993	≈ 35 (18–65)	0	Volunteer	Isokinetic	< 1
Bassey, 1993 [61]	354	74 (> 60)	0	Representative	Handgrip	2
Baumgartner, 1999 [59]	121	77 (65–97)	0	Volunteer	Handgrip	< 1

Table 4
Age-related changes in lower limb muscle strength

First author, year [Ref.]	N	Baseline age range (y)	Follow-up (y)	Population	Method	Strength (% decline/y)
Lindle, 1997 [63]	346	≈ 55 (20–93)	0	Volunteer	Isometric	< 1
Fisher, 1990 [97]	116	≈ 40 (20–79)	0	Volunteer	Isometric	< 1
Larson, 1979 [64]	114	≈ 40 (11–70)	0	Volunteer	Isometric	< 1

will require large randomized placebo-controlled studies examining baseline somatic characteristics in careful prospectively planned analyses to identify an androgen responsive subgroup, or specific and strict entry criteria based on physical performance.

Psychologic and cognitive symptoms

Depressed mood, irritability, inability to concentrate, and other mild and subtle psychologic and cognitive disturbances are reported universally in men with organic androgen deficiency. Such features also are used to determine relative androgen deficiency in older men [9,10,25]. Interpretation is convoluted, because depression increases with age, even in very old age [82]. Secondly, either dysthymia or major depression may suppress serum testosterone concentrations modestly in older men [83]. A further complication arises from varying androgen receptor polymorphisms, because systemic testosterone predicts depression, but only in the subgroup of men with shorter CAG repeats [84]. Although these data suggest the importance of testosterone in depression, randomized trials examining the effect of testosterone therapy on mood in depressed men with lower serum testosterone concentrations

Table 5
Poor physical performance leads to disability

First author, year [Ref.]	N	Age (y)	Follow-up (y)	Physical function	Predicts
Dargent-Molina, 1996 [75]	7575	> 75	2	Gait, dynamic balance	Hip fracture
Penninx, 2000 [73]	3381	> 70	4	Gain, balance, chair rise	Hospitalization
Guralnik, 1995 [76]	1122	> 70	4	Gait, balance, chair rise	Disability
Tinetti, 1988 [78]	336	> 70	1	Gait, balance, chair rise	Falls
Vellas, 1997 [74]	316	> 60	3	Static balance	Injurious falls
Reuben, 1992 [77]	149	> 70	2	Gait, physical performance	Mortality and nursing home placement
Guralnik, 1994 [81]	5174	> 70	0	Gait, balance, chair rise	Mortatlity
Ferrucci, 2000 [79]	3381	> 70	0	Gait, balance, chair rise	Hip fracture
Judge, 1996 [80]	2190	> 65	0	Gait, balance, chair rise	Disability

have shown no benefit [85]. This indicates that selecting responsiveness solely on systemic testosterone exposure may not correctly identify the androgen-responsive population with relative androgen deficiency.

The use of psychologic outcomes for assessing relative androgen deficiency is also problematic, because accurate assessments are made difficult by the low motivation of severe depression and the disorganized thought of anxiety-related illness, either of which may be present to some degree in older men. When the underlying psychiatric disorder improves, self-perception is likely to change independent of objective changes. For these reasons, the use of psychologic outcomes in the definition of relative androgen deficiency is especially uncertain.

Similarly, in older men, lower testosterone concentrations are associated with poorer cognitive function [86,87] and predict faster decline in visual memory [87]. There is growing evidence that androgens, possibly after local aromatization, are important for spatial cognition and some aspects of memory in older men. Whether differences are caused by subtle differences in testing procedures, duration and dose of administration, baseline androgen status, or baseline cognitive ability is unknown. The detrimental effects of androgen therapy on spatial cognition only have been detected at higher doses [88,89], whereas beneficial [90–92] or no [93–95], effects only have been shown at lower doses. This observation is coherent with the putative U-shaped relationship between serum testosterone and spatial cognitive abilities reported in cross-sectional studies in men [96]. These uncertainties and the relative difficulty in assessing these cognitive functions in clinical practice makes it seem improbable that any of these features can be used alone to adequately define relative androgen deficiency. Although these psychologic and cognitive symptoms are unlikely to be useful diagnostically, their utility in monitoring treatment has not been studied adequately.

Summary

Serum total, free, and non-SHBG–bound testosterone concentrations decline progressively with age. In many older men, the resulting testosterone levels fall below the normal reference range established in healthy young men, therefore demonstrating statistically definable relative testosterone deficiency. Many older men have symptoms indicative of organic testosterone deficiency. The classical clinical features of organic testosterone deficiency, however, have limited specificity in the older man because of multiple coexisting etiologies. Individual symptoms are androgen responsive; none of the sexual, somatic, or psychologic features commonly used are sensitive or specific for androgen deficiency. For example, even questionnaires developed to screen on the basis of low serum testosterone concentrations have poor sensitivity (ranging from 75% to 90%) and specificity (ranging from 50% to 60%) for this outcome [9,10]. Furthermore, whether this inaccuracy can be improved by combining multiple symptoms has not been studied adequately.

Future research exploring the putative clinical syndrome of relative androgen deficiency in older men should be focused primarily on randomized clinical trials that unequivocally demonstrate health outcome benefits with androgen therapy. This will help establish the parameters that will identify those who are most likely to benefit from androgen therapy. At this stage, the clinician will have to be vigilant in identifying cases, because many of the sexual, somatic, and psychologic indicators are nonspecific. Future research also should focus on identifying those at risk of disability (particularly by examining specific somatic features) and elucidating simple clinical biomarkers of testosterone response (possibly in the psychologic and cognitive domains). To this end, monitoring a single symptom or a limited collection of related symptoms, which may differ from person to person, may be more useful than a wide-ranging questionnaire with multiple endpoints, some of which are likely to be irrelevant to any given person. Until more answers become available, clinicians are left with best practice guidelines and recommendations for future research [5,6].

References

[1] Feldman HA, Longcope C, Derby CA, et al. Age trends in the level of serum testosterone and other hormones in middle-aged men: longitudinal results from the Massachusetts male aging study. J Clin Endocrinol Metab 2002;87(2):589–98.
[2] Harman SM, Metter EJ, Tobin JD, et al. Longitudinal effects of aging on serum total and free testosterone levels in healthy men. Baltimore Longitudinal Study of Aging. J Clin Endocrinol Metab 2001;86(2):724–31.
[3] Wang C, Swerdloff RS. Androgen replacement therapy in hypogonadal men. In: Winters SJ, editor. Male hypogonadism: basic, clinical and therapeutic principles. 2nd edition. Totowa (NJ): The Humana Press; 2003. p. 353–70.
[4] Zitzmann M, Nieschlag E. Hormone substitution in male hypogonadism. Mol Cell Endocrinol 2000;161:73–88.
[5] Liu PY, Swerdloff RS, Veldhuis JD. The rationale, efficacy and safety of androgen therapy in older men: future research and current practice recommendations. J Clin Endocrinol Metab 2004;89(10):4789–96.
[6] Liverman CT, Blazer DG, editors. Testosterone and aging: clinical research directions. Washington (DC): National Academies Press; 2003.
[7] Liu PY, Pincus SM, Keenan DM, et al. Analysis of bidirectional pattern synchrony of concentration–secretion pairs: implementation in the human testicular and adrenal axes. Am J Physiol Regul Integr Comp Physiol 2005;288(2):R440–6.
[8] Snyder PJ, Peachey H, Hannoush P, et al. Effect of testosterone treatment on bone mineral density in men over 65 years of age. J Clin Endocrinol Metab 1999;84(6):1966–72.
[9] Smith KW, Feldman HA, McKinlay JB. Construction and field validation of a self-administered screener for testosterone deficiency (hypogonadism) in ageing men. Clin Endocrinol (Oxf) 2000;53(6):703–11.
[10] Morley JE, Charlton E, Patrick P, et al. Validation of a screening questionnaire for androgen deficiency in aging males. Metabolism 2000;49(9):1239–42.
[11] McLachlan RI, Robertson DM, Pruysers E, et al. Relationship between serum gonadotropins and spermatogenic suppression in men undergoing steroidal contraceptive treatment. J Clin Endocrinol Metab 2004;89(1):142–9.

[12] Cunningham G, Swerdloff RS. Endocrine Society consensus statement. Chevy Chase (MD): Endocrine Society; 2001.

[13] Conway AJ, Handelsman DJ, Lording DW, et al. Use, misuse and abuse of androgens. The Endocrine Society of Australia consensus guidelines for androgen prescribing. Med J Aust 2000;172(5):220–4.

[14] McLachlan RI, Allan CA. Defining the prevalence and incidence of androgen deficiency in aging men: where are the goal posts? J Clin Endocrinol Metab 2004;89(12):5916–9.

[15] Araujo AB, O'Donnell AB, Brambilla DJ, et al. Prevalence and incidence of androgen deficiency in middle-aged and older men: estimates from the Massachusetts male aging study. J Clin Endocrinol Metab 2004;89(12):5920–6.

[16] Bhasin S, Woodhouse L, Casaburi R, et al. Older men are as responsive as young men to the anabolic effects of graded doses of testosterone on the skeletal muscle. J Clin Endocrinol Metab 2005;90(2):678–88.

[17] Vasan RS, Larson MG, Leip EP, et al. Impact of high-normal blood pressure on the risk of cardiovascular disease. N Engl J Med 2001;345(18):1291–7.

[18] Writing Team for the Diabetes Control Complications Trial/Epidemiology of Diabetes Interventions Complications Research Group. Sustained effect of intensive treatment of type 1 diabetes mellitus on development and progression of diabetic nephropathy: the Epidemiology of Diabetes Interventions and Complications (EDIC) study. JAMA 2003;290(16): 2159–67.

[19] Szulc P, Claustrat B, Marchand F, et al. Increased risk of falls and increased bone resorption in elderly men with partial androgen deficiency: the MINOS study. J Clin Endocrinol Metab 2003;88(11):5240–7.

[20] Vermeulen A. Androgen replacement therapy in the aging male—a critical evaluation. J Clin Endocrinol Metab 2001;86(6):2380–90.

[21] Vermeulen A, Verdonck L, Kaufman JM. A critical evaluation of simple methods for the estimation of free testosterone in serum. J Clin Endocrinol Metab 1999;84(10):3666–72.

[22] Liu PY, Death AK, Handelsman DJ. Androgens and cardiovascular disease. Endocr Rev 2003;24(3):313–40.

[23] Kelleher S, Conway AJ, Handelsman DJ. Blood testosterone threshold for androgen deficiency symptoms. J Clin Endocrinol Metab 2004;89(8):3813–7.

[24] Heinemann LAJ, Zimmermann T, Vermeulen A, et al. A new aging males symptoms rating scale. Aging Male 1999;2:105–14.

[25] Daig I, Heinemann LA, Kim S, et al. The Aging Males Symptoms (AMS) scale: review of its methodological characteristics. Health Qual Life Outcomes 2003;1(1):77.

[26] Moore C, Huebler D, Zimmermann T, et al. The Aging Males Symptoms scale (AMS) as outcome measure for treatment of androgen deficiency. Eur Urol 2004;46(1):80–7.

[27] Macfarlane GJ, Botto H, Sagnier PP, et al. The relationship between sexual life and urinary condition in the French community. J Clin Epidemiol 1996;49(10):1171–6.

[28] Laumann EO, Paik A, Rosen RC. Sexual dysfunction in the United States: prevalence and predictors. JAMA 1999;281(6):537–44.

[29] Blanker MH, Bohnen AM, Groeneveld FP, et al. Correlates for erectile and ejaculatory dysfunction in older Dutch men: a community-based study. J Am Geriatr Soc 2001;49(4): 436–42.

[30] Shiri R, Koskimaki J, Hakama M, et al. Effect of chronic diseases on incidence of erectile dysfunction. Urology 2003;62(6):1097–102.

[31] Pinnock CB, Stapleton AM, Marshall VR. Erectile dysfunction in the community: a prevalence study. Med J Aust 1999;171(7):353–7.

[32] Morillo LE, Diaz J, Estevez E, et al. Prevalence of erectile dysfunction in Colombia, Ecuador, and Venezuela: a population-based study (DENSA). Int J Impot Res 2002;14(Suppl 2): S10–8.

[33] Moreira ED Jr, Lbo CF, Diament A, et al. Incidence of erectile dysfunction in men 40- to 69-years old: results from a population-based cohort study in Brazil. Urology 2003;61(2):431–6.

[34] Johannes CB, Araujo AB, Feldman HA, et al. Incidence of erectile dysfunction in men 40- to 69-years old: longitudinal results from the Massachusetts male aging study. J Urol 2000; 163(2):460–3.

[35] Panser LA, Rhodes T, Girman CJ, et al. Sexual function of men ages 40 to 79 years: the Olmsted County Study of Urinary Symptoms and Health Status Among Men. J Am Geriatr Soc 1995;43(10):1107–11.

[36] Akkus E, Kadioglu A, Esen A, et al. Prevalence and correlates of erectile dysfunction in Turkey: a population-based study. Eur Urol 2002;41(3):298–304.

[37] Rosen R, Altwein J, Boyle P, et al. Lower urinary tract symptoms and male sexual dysfunction: the multi-national survey of the aging male (MSAM-7). Eur Urol 2003;44(6): 637–49.

[38] Buena F, Swerdloff RS, Steiner BS, et al. Sexual function does not change when serum testosterone levels are pharmacologically varied within the normal male range. Fertil Steril 1993;59(5):1118–23.

[39] Bagatell CJ, Heiman JR, Rivier JE, et al. Effects of endogenous testosterone and estradiol on sexual behaviour in normal young men. J Clin Endocrinol Metab 1994;78(3):711–6.

[40] Fischer ME, Vitek ME, Hedeker D, et al. A twin study of erectile dysfunction. Arch Intern Med 2004;164(2):165–8.

[41] Penson DF, Ng C, Cai L, et al. Androgen and pituitary control of penile nitric oxide synthase and erectile function in the rat. Biol Reprod 1996;55(3):567–74.

[42] Morelli A, Filippi S, Mancina R, et al. Androgens regulate phosphodiesterase type 5 expression and functional activity in corpora cavernosa. Endocrinology 2004;145(5):2253–63.

[43] Aversa A, Isidori AM, Spera G, et al. Androgens improve cavernous vasodilation and response to sildenafil in patients with erectile dysfunction. Clin Endocrinol (Oxf) 2003;58(5): 632–8.

[44] Kandeel FR, Koussa VK, Swerdloff RS. Male sexual function and its disorders: physiology, pathophysiology, clinical investigation, and treatment. Endocr Rev 2001;22(3):342–88.

[45] Siervogel RM, Maynard LM, Wisemandle WA, et al. Annual changes in total body fat and fat-free mass in children from 8 to 18 years in relation to changes in body mass index. The Fels Longitudinal Study. Ann N Y Acad Sci 2000;904:420–3.

[46] Siervogel RM, Wisemandle W, Maynard LM, et al. Serial changes in body composition throughout adulthood and their relationships to changes in lipid and lipoprotein levels. The Fels Longitudinal Study. Arterioscler Thromb Vasc Biol 1998;18(11):1759–64.

[47] Guo SS, Zeller C, Chumlea WC, et al. Aging, body composition, and lifestyle: the Fels Longitudinal Study. Am J Clin Nutr 1999;70(3):405–11.

[48] Keys A, Taylor HL, Grande F. Basal metabolism and age of adult man. Metabolism 1973; 22(4):579–87.

[49] Chien S, Peng MT, Chen KP, et al. Longitudinal measurements of blood volume and essential body mass in human subjects. J Appl Physiol 1975;39(5):818–24.

[50] Hughes VA, Frontera WR, Roubenoff R, et al. Longitudinal changes in body composition in older men and women: role of body weight change and physical activity. Am J Clin Nutr 2002;76(2):473–81.

[51] Jackson AS, Beard EF, Wier LT, et al. Changes in aerobic power of men, ages 25–70 yr. Med Sci Sports Exerc 1995;27(1):113–20.

[52] Flynn MA, Nolph GB, Baker AS, et al. Total body potassium in aging humans: a longitudinal study. Am J Clin Nutr 1989;50(4):713–7.

[53] Flegal KM, Carroll MD, Kuczmarski RJ, et al. Overweight and obesity in the United States: prevalence and trends, 1960–1994. Int J Obes 1998;22(1):39–47.

[54] Bennett SA, Magnus P. Trends in cardiovascular risk factors in Australia. Results from the National Heart Foundation's Risk Factor Prevalence study, 1980–1989. Med J Aust 1994; 161(9):519–27.

[55] Rantanen T, Masaki K, Foley D, et al. Grip strength changes over 27 yr in Japanese American men. J Appl Physiol 1998;85(6):2047–53.

[56] Lee I, Manson JE, Hennekens CH, et al. Body weight and mortality: a 27-year follow-up of middle-aged men. JAMA 1993;270(23):2823–8.

[57] Stevens J, Cai J, Pamuk ER, et al. The effect of age on the association between body-mass index and mortality. N Engl J Med 1998;338(1):1–7.

[58] Ford ES, Giles WH, Dietz WH. Prevalence of the metabolic syndrome among US adults: findings from the third National Health and Nutrition Examination survey. JAMA 2002; 287(3):356–9.

[59] Baumgartner RN, Waters DL, Gallagher D, et al. Predictors of skeletal muscle mass in elderly men and women. Mech Ageing Dev 1999;107(2):123–36.

[60] Metter EJ, Conwit R, Tobin J, et al. Age-associated loss of power and strength in the upper extremities in women and men. J Gerontol A Biol Sci Med Sci 1997;52(5):B267–76.

[61] Bassey EJ, Harries UJ. Normal values for handgrip strength in 920 men and women aged over 65 years, and longitudinal changes over 4 years in 620 survivors. Clin Sci 1993;84(3): 331–7.

[62] Clement FJ. Longitudinal and cross-sectional assessments of age changes in physical strength as related to sex, social class, and mental ability. J Gerontol 1974;29(4): 423–9.

[63] Lindle RS, Metter EJ, Lynch NA, et al. Age and gender comparisons of muscle strength in 654 women and men aged 20–93 yr. J Appl Physiol 1997;83(5):1581–7.

[64] Larsson L, Grimby G, Karlsson J. Muscle strength and speed of movement in relation to age and muscle morphology. J Appl Physiol 1979;46(3):451–6.

[65] Hughes VA, Frontera WR, Wood M, et al. Longitudinal muscle strength changes in older adults: influence of muscle mass, physical activity, and health. J Gerontol A Biol Sci Med Sci 2001;56(5):B209–17.

[66] Frontera WR, Hughes VA, Fielding RA, et al. Aging of skeletal muscle: a 12-yr longitudinal study. J Appl Physiol 2000;88(4):1321–6.

[67] Rantanen T, Era P, Heikkinen E. Physical activity and the changes in maximal isometric strength in men and women from the age of 75 to 80 years. J Am Geriatr Soc 1997;45(12): 1439–45.

[68] Grimby G. Muscle performance and structure in the elderly as studied cross-sectionally and longitudinally. J Gerontol A Biol Sci Med Sci 1995;50:17–22.

[69] Sunnerhagen KS, Hedberg M, Henning GB, et al. Muscle performance in an urban population sample of 40- to 79-year-old men and women. Scand J Rehabil Med 2000;32(4): 159–67.

[70] Gibbs J, Hughes S, Dunlop D, et al. Predictors of change in walking velocity in older adults. J Am Geriatr Soc 1996;44(2):126–32.

[71] Seeman TE, Charpentier PA, Berkman LF, et al. Predicting changes in physical performance in a high-functioning elderly cohort: MacArthur studies of successful aging. Journal of Gerontology: Medical Sciences 1994;49(3):M97–108.

[72] Hughes S, Gibbs J, Dunlop D, et al. Predictors of decline in manual performance in older adults. J Am Geriatr Soc 1997;45(8):905–10.

[73] Penninx BW, Ferrucci L, Leveille SG, et al. Lower extremity performance in nondisabled older persons as a predictor of subsequent hospitalization. J Gerontol A Biol Sci Med Sci 2000;55(11):M691–7.

[74] Vellas BJ, Wayne SJ, Romero L, et al. One-leg balance is an important predictor of injurious falls in older persons. J Am Geriatr Soc 1997;45:735–8.

[75] Dargent-Molina P, Favier F, Grandjean H, et al. Fall-related factors and risk of hip fracture: the EPIDOS prospective study. Lancet 1996;348(9021):145–9.

[76] Guralnik JM, Ferrucci L, Simonsick EM, et al. Lower-extremity function in persons over the age of 70 years as a predictor of subsequent disability. N Engl J Med 1995;332: 556–61.

[77] Reuben DB, Siu AL, Kimpau S. The predictive validity of self-report and performance-based measures of function and health. J Gerontol 1992;47(4):M106–10.

[78] Tinetti ME, Speechley M, Ginter SF. Risk factors for falls among elderly persons living in the community. N Engl J Med 1988;319:1701–7.

[79] Ferrucci L, Penninx BW, Leveille SG, et al. Characteristics of nondisabled older persons who perform poorly in objective tests of lower extremity function. J Am Geriatr Soc 2000;48(9): 1102–10.

[80] Judge JO, Schechtman K, Cress E. The relationship between physical performance measures and independence in instrumental activities of daily living. The FICSIT Group. Frailty and injury: cooperative studies of intervention trials. J Am Geriatr Soc 1996;44(11):1332–41.

[81] Guralnik JM, Simonsick EM, Ferrucci L, et al. A short physical performance battery assessing lower extremity function: association with self-reported disability and prediction of mortality and nursing home admission. J Gerontol 1994;49(2):M85–94.

[82] Skoog I. Psychiatric epidemiology of old age: the H70 study—the NAPE lecture 2003. Acta Psychiatr Scand 2004;109(1):4–18.

[83] Seidman SN, Araujo AB, Roose SP, et al. Low testosterone levels in elderly men with dysthymic disorder. Am J Psychiatry 2002;159(3):456–9.

[84] Seidman SN, Araujo AB, Roose SP, et al. Testosterone level, androgen receptor polymorphism, and depressive symptoms in middle-aged men. Biol Psychiatry 2001;50(5):371–6.

[85] Seidman SN, Spatz E, Rizzo C, et al. Testosterone replacement therapy for hypogonadal men with major depressive disorder: a randomized, placebo-controlled clinical trial. J Clin Psychiatry 2001;62(6):406–12.

[86] Barrett-Connor E, Goodman-Gruen D, Patay B. Endogenous sex hormones and cognitive function in older men. J Clin Endocrinol Metab 1999;84(10):3681–5.

[87] Moffat SD, Zonderman AB, Metter EJ, et al. Longitudinal assessment of serum free testosterone concentration predicts memory performance and cognitive status in elderly men. J Clin Endocrinol Metab 2002;87(11):5001–7.

[88] O'Connor DB, Archer J, Hair WM, et al. Activational effects of testosterone on cognitive function in men. Neuropsychologia 2001;39(13):1385–94.

[89] Wolf OT, Preut R, Hellhammer DH, et al. Testosterone and cognition in elderly men: a single testosterone injection blocks the practice effect in verbal fluency, but has no effect on spatial or verbal memory. Biol Psychiatry 2000;47(7):650–4.

[90] Cherrier MM, Asthana S, Plymate S, et al. Testosterone supplementation improves spatial and verbal memory in healthy older men. Neurology 2001;57(1):80–8.

[91] Janowsky JS, Chavez B, Orwoll E. Sex steroids modify working memory. J Cogn Neurosci 2000;12(3):407–14.

[92] Janowsky JS, Oviatt SK, Orwoll ES. Testosterone influences spatial cognition in older men. Behav Neurosci 1994;108(2):325–32.

[93] Cherrier MM, Anawalt BD, Herbst KL, et al. Cognitive effects of short-term manipulation of serum sex steroids in healthy young men. J Clin Endocrinol Metab 2002;87(7):3090–6.

[94] Ly LP, Jimenez M, Zhuang TN, et al. A double-blind, placebo-controlled, randomized clinical trial of transdermal dihydrotestosterone gel on muscular strength, mobility, and quality of life in older men with partial androgen deficiency. J Clin Endocrinol Metab 2001;86(9): 4078–88.

[95] Sih R, Morley JE, Kaiser FE, et al. Testosterone replacement in older hypogonadal men: a 12-month randomized controlled trial. J Clin Endocrinol Metab 1997;82(6):1661–7.

[96] Moffat SD, Hampson E. A curvilinear relationship between testosterone and spatial cognition in humans: possible influence of hand preference. Psychoneuroendocrinology 1996; 21(3):323–37.

[97] Fisher NM, Pendergast DR, Calkins EC. Maximal isometric torque of knee extension as a function of muscle length in subjects of advancing age. Arch Phys Med Rehabil 1990; 71(10):729–34.

ELSEVIER
SAUNDERS

Endocrinol Metab Clin N Am
34 (2005) 973–992

ENDOCRINOLOGY
AND METABOLISM
CLINICS
OF NORTH AMERICA

Thyrotropin-Axis Adaptation in Aging and Chronic Disease

Marius Stan, MD, John C. Morris, MD*

Division of Endocrinology, Mayo Clinic College of Medicine, Rochester, MN, USA

Aging has been described as a genetically programmed, slowly progressive, irreversible change that involves cell loss and replacement events and adaptation to them [1]. Identifying the changes associated with aging is a challenging task, because aging mechanisms are not well defined and because diseases can influence the aging process and age may influence disease progression. Although much work has been completed, the process and physiology of aging and its effect on the function of the hypothalamic-pituitary-thyroid (HPT) axis has not yet been characterized clearly. Primary aging was labeled by researchers as the inherent effect of time on cell function, which is different than the effects of disease, which have been termed secondary aging. This distinction is imperfect, because the effect of aging on disease progression is not clear.

The thyroid conditions that commonly affect elderly persons may present differently than in younger individuals and include apathetic thyrotoxicosis, unsuspected hypothyroidism, and aggressive spread of differentiated tumors [1]. Thyroid disease in elderly patients may present without classic signs and symptoms. Nonspecific symptoms, even in the absence of thyroid dysfunction, are common in this age group, including fatigue, loss of motivation, anorexia, weight loss, failure to rehabilitate, failure to thrive, and difficulty concentrating [2]. These nonspecific symptoms frequently confound clinicians, who may interpret them inaccurately as being thyroid related or be misled by their masking of symptoms that may truly represent abnormalities of thyroid function. Symptoms of aging can be confused easily with hypothyroidism, and in past decades, decreased thyroid function was believed to be a hallmark of aging. The interpretation of thyroid function tests is also cumbersome in aged individuals because of the difficulty in differentiating physiologic age-associated changes from alterations secondary to acute

---

* Corresponding author.
E-mail address: morris.john@mayo.edu (J.C. Morris).

0889-8529/05/$ - see front matter © 2005 Elsevier Inc. All rights reserved.
doi:10.1016/j.ecl.2005.07.012   *endo.theclinics.com*

or chronic nonthyroidal illness (NTI) or drugs often administered to patients.

In this article we review the changes that have been described in the function of the HPT axis in the aging process. Animal studies and human studies are discussed. We also review the differences in thyroid diseases that are observed in elderly patients as compared with younger individuals.

Changes in hypothalamic-pituitary-thyroid physiology with age

Animal studies

Most animal studies published to date have reported a decrease in circulating free thyroxine (T4) levels with increasing age [3–5]. The findings with respect to serum thyroid-stimulating hormone (TSH) and free triiodothyronine (T3) levels suggest gender, strain, and perhaps species differences [5,6].

The finding of normal TSH levels in aged rats despite low free T4 levels has been explained by increased intrapituitary 5′ deiodinase (5′DI) and resulting enhanced local production of T3 [4]. This finding is similar to the response noted in hypothyroidism except that only type II 5′DI seems to be increased [4]. The modulation of the pituitary activity of 5′DI during neonatal development and adulthood and during aging [7–11] may represent an adaptive mechanism that seeks to preserve, as much as possible, intrapituitary concentrations of T3 in the face of the widely varying thyroid hormone levels [12].

In contrast to the studies outlined previously, other groups have reported decreased activity of intrapituitary 5′DI in female rats [13,14]. One group also reported variations in DI activities between young and old animals in different periods of the year [14]. These findings suggest that directly or through decreased thyrotropin-releasing hormone (TRH) stimulus from the hypothalamus, the aged thyrotrophs were unable to respond efficiently to the decreased hormone levels [13]. In contrast to the findings in the preceding paragraph, intrathyroidal DI activity was reduced in male rats, although it was not significantly decreased in female rats [4].

In trying to assess whether these differences were gender and strain related, a study with paired within-strain male and female rats was performed. The study assessed the functional activity of HPT axis at baseline and during stress [15]. Increased age in female rats was associated with a fall in plasma-free T3 and total T4 with unchanged TSH, TSH mRNA, and pre-pro TRH mRNA. Aging in male rats revealed decreased total T4, similar free T3 but lower TSH mRNA and TRH mRNA. Between genders, lower TSH and TSH mRNA was noted with similar free T3, total T4, and TRH mRNA in young female rats, whereas TSH levels were higher in aged female rats with similar T3, T4, and pre-pro TRH mRNA. Increased prolactin levels also were noted in female rats compared with male rats. Stress failed to influence any aspect of the HPT axis function in old female rats and decreased

TSH mRNA only in old male rats, without any significant difference between old female and male rats [15].

In summary, gender disparity was present in the effects of age on baseline HPT function but not in the response to stress. At baseline, aging seems to be associated with central hypothyroidism in both genders, although the magnitude of this alteration was less in old female than in old male rats. Of note, TSH and TSH mRNA were higher in young male rats than in female rats, but in old rats no gender differences were found, which suggested that TSH level differences may be attributed to testosterone [13]. Some researchers suggest that pituitary responsiveness to TRH is maintained in aged animals based on basal and TRH-stimulated TSH levels in young and old rats [16]. Other researchers reported that aging seems to be associated with central hypothyroidism in both genders but less so in female subjects, possibly secondary to relationship of TRH response with serum testosterone [13].

Stress-mediated inhibition of TRH was attenuated in old rats by deficient stress-induced activation of norepinephrine, a stimulatory neurotransmitter to the corticotropin-releasing hormone neuron [17]. Corticotropin-releasing hormone stimulates somatostatin, which in turn may inhibit TRH production [18,19]. A direct reciprocal TRH inhibition by corticotropin-releasing hormone also may occur [20].

Several age-related changes within the thyroid itself have been described in animals. The effect of TSH on the thyroid with age may be altered in rats. Aged rats demonstrated up to 50% reduction in the concentration of TSH receptors on thyroid cells and reduced responsiveness to TSH. The postreceptor cAMP system seemed to be unaltered by age [21]. Further thyroglobulin endocytosis gradually slows down with age [22]. Thyroidal lysosomal function was analyzed in aged cream hamsters by van den Hove and colleagues (Fig. 1) [23]. They identified the presence of two morphologic changes specific to old female thyroids: the existence of most large follicles with flat epithelium (related to compression by colloid accumulation in the setting of age-related endocytosis failure) and the presence of amyloid deposition in the interfollicular space. With the help of ^{125}I and ^{127}I kinetics, they observed slow thyroglobulin turnover in large follicles, likely related to reduced capacity of late endosomes to mature into or fuse with dense lysosomes, which is speculated as related to docking or motion problems with late endosomes [23].

The marked decrease in thyroid peroxidase mRNA that was observed in aged rats was postulated to be caused by decreased testosterone production, because in female rats thyroid peroxidase mRNA and thyroglobulin mRNA levels were not affected by aging and were lower than in young male rats [13,24–26]. Despite low thyroid peroxidase and Tg mRNA expression, normal T4 levels in young female rats suggested that other factors were involved in control of thyroid function, however, and that in both sexes the aged thyroid becomes less responsive to circulating TSH [13].

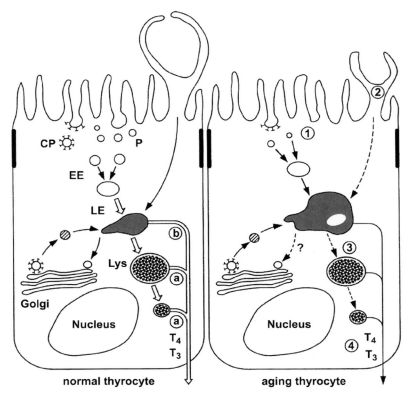

Fig. 1. Endocytic pathways in normal and aging thyrocytes of cream hamsters. In normal thyrocytes (*left panel*), thyroglobulin is endocytosed either by micropinocytosis via clathrin-coated (CP) or uncoated (P) pits into early endosomes (EE) or by macropinocytosis. Internalized Tg transits through late endosomes (LE, *gray*) that contain lysosomal enzymes and is finally transported to dense lysosomes, where acid hydrolases are most concentrated (Lys, *black*). Hormones (T3 and T4) not only are liberated in dense lysosomes (a) but also can be released selectively before Tg transfer into lysosomes (b). With aging (*right panel*), (1) Tg endocytosis gradually slows down and (2) colloid macopinocytosis in response to an acute TSH stimulation is reduced. Van den Hove and colleagues reported a third age-related defect (3), a delay in the progression of thyroglobulin toward dense lysosomes. It is proposed that the transfer from late endosomes to lysosomes becomes rate limiting and contributes to the reduction ion T4 and T3 secretion (4). (*From* Van den Hove, Couvreur M, Authelet M, et al. Age delays thyroglobulin progression toward dense lysosomes in the cream hamster thyroid. Cell and Tissue Research 1998;294(1):125–35; with permission.)

Regarding peripheral tissues, basal expression of thyroid hormone responsive protein mRNA increases, whereas the thyroid hormone responsive protein mass decreases in aging rats, which suggests that cerebral responsiveness to thyroid hormone was reduced with aging [27]. In contrast to the adenohypophysis, the activity of type I $5'DI$ decreased with age in the thyroid gland and in the liver of the same animals, which indicated impaired thyroid hormone disposal and action in peripheral tissues [4]. It seems that aging that affects the pituitary, thyroid, and liver DI activity in animals induces changes in the thyroid gland function and regulation and that some of these changes are gender related.

Animal studies suggest that changes occur in the function of the HPT axis with aging at all levels but may be species, gender, and strain specific. Translation of these studies to humans is difficult, at best.

Human studies

Several studies have examined age-related changes in the HPT axis in healthy individuals, although some reported results are conflicting. T3, T4, TSH, and TRH-stimulated TSH response have been found to be reduced, normal, or increased in different studies [28,29]. Some studies also reported a sex-related variation. In one group of 124 healthy Italian volunteers, only free T4 varied inversely with age and then only in male subjects [30]. In contrast, in 51 healthy elderly Indian men, T3 and TSH levels were significantly lower, whereas the T4 level was significantly higher in men older than 60 years versus young controls [31]. In a carefully selected population of aging individuals (healthy centenarians and 65- to 80-year-old subjects who met the Eurage Senieur criteria), thyroid function was well preserved until the eighth decade of life [28], although free T3 and TSH were found to be significantly lower with advancing age (consistently with centenarians) (Fig. 2) [28,32–35]. This same result was observed in TSH level variation in hypothyroid patients (avoiding the negative feedback of T4) [36]. Free T3/free T4 ratio also was progressively lower with advancing age; the opposite was true for reverse T3 [31,34]. The lack of compensation by an increase in TSH level suggests a decrease in the feedback mechanism of the HPT axis.

Evidence exists for reduced hypothalamic and pituitary responsiveness in the regulation of the HPT axis with aging. Several groups have agreed that individuals of all ages responded to TRH stimulation, but elderly persons responded significantly less so [33,37–40]. Circadian modulation of TSH secretion was found to be preserved until the eighth decade, although probably at a lower level in the elderly population, and was lost thereafter [33,41]. Similar findings were reported by other groups [38,41]. Regarding the thyroid, the earliest changes with age seem to be a delayed T4 response and a reduction of the height of the peak thyroid hormone release after the nocturnal TSH surge, which suggests slower response from the thyroid [42]. A combination of these defects seems likely with aging.

The increase in dopamine content in the brain with aging [43,44] and the increased sensitivity to dopamine with aging [44] could play a role in the reduced TSH and prolactin (PRL) response to TRH stimulation [39,44–48]. Another cause for reduced basal and TRH-stimulated TSH could be an adaptation to the reduced metabolic demands of old age, leading to the

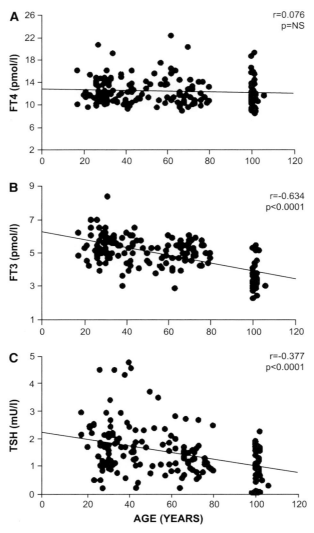

Fig. 2. Age-dependent variations in (*A*) free T4 (FT4), (*B*) free T3 (FT3), and (*C*) TSH in healthy subjects. (*From* Mariotti S, Barbesino G, Caturegli P, et al. Complex alteration of thyroid function in healthy centenarians. J Clin Endocrinol Metab 1993;77(5):1130–4; with permission.)

maintenance of a progressively lower euthyroid state during senescence [33]. Along these lines, it is questionable if the basal metabolic rate decreases or is unchanged with aging when fat-free body mass is considered [49]. This question is difficult to settle because in basal metabolic rate studies one must stratify for weight and thyroid status, which is not uniformly accomplished.

Leptin, growth hormone, and androgen levels, which also change with age, also affect basal metabolic rate [42].

A decrease in the free T3/free T4 ratio is a marker of decreased peripheral 5'DI activity, and increased reverse T3 with aging also has been reported [4,35,49]. This occurrence could be age dependent (age-related increase in cytokines may have a pathogenetic role; tumor necrosis factor alpha, interleukin-1, and interleukin-6 have been described to play inhibitory roles on 5'DI), linked to NTI, caused by decreased TSH stimulation, or a combination of all these events [44,48,50–52]. 5'DI is a selenium-containing enzyme, and in elderly patients a direct association was found between selenium and free T3 and selenium and free T3/free T4 ratio, which suggests that selenium levels may affect thyroid hormone levels [53].

Exercise seems to increase the T3 value regardless of age [54]. Physically less active individuals had significantly lower TSH values than active individuals [54]; other studies reported unchanged, increased, or decreased T3 levels in trained elderly men compared with sedentary men [55–57]. A compounding factor in the interpretation of these studies is the effect of nonthyroidal illness. For example, one study reported that the major determinant in decreased free T3 with age was poor health status (by the predictive value of body mass index, prealbumin, and hemoglobin) [12]. The finding of normal reverse T3 levels in their subjects raises the question of whether poor health was defined appropriately.

In summary, changes in hypothalamic function and resetting of the pituitary threshold for the TSH feedback accompanied by changes in the peripheral hormones levels secondary to their altered metabolism (including decreased peripheral 5'DI activity) are observed commonly in elderly individuals.

Incidence of thyroid disease with age

Hypothyroidism

The reported prevalence of hypothyroidism in the elderly population varies with the definition of hypothyroidism that has been used in studies that have examined the problem. One screening study reported 17.8% of their 3015 elderly patients with abnormal thyroid function test results, which indicated hypothyroidism of varying degrees, as opposed to the reported clinical prevalence for the population at only 1.6% [58]. The difference was presumed to be the biochemical expression of the changes in HPT axis function of aging and not evidence of disease [58]. Many studies have confirmed a predisposition to hypothyroidism with advancing age in women [59–62]. The prevalence reported by different studies varies, however, probably because of differences in the evaluation of patients (eg, the use of variable methods of assessment), inclusion or exclusion of subclinical disease, and the iodine status of studied population. The Rosses survey found that

8.6% of individuals over age 50 had overt (TSH > 10 mIU/L), spontaneous hypothyroidism, and a further 0.9% had subclinical hypothyroidism (TSH 4–10 mIU/L), in sharp contrast to persons aged 18 to 50, in whom the prevalence was 0.9% [63]. This figure is comparable to the 7.7% prevalence reported in the Whickham study in women older than age 60 (Fig. 3) [64]. Similarly, subclinical hypothyroidism has been reported at higher frequency in elderly persons [65,66].

As in younger individuals, autoimmune thyroiditis is the most common mechanism of hypothyroidism in elderly individuals [67]. Hypothyroidism secondary to treated hyperthyroidism and other forms of drug-induced thyroid dysfunction is also commonly observed, however [61]. The diagnosis of hypothyroidism sometimes is hampered in elderly persons by the influence of certain drugs (eg, steroids and dopamine) on TSH levels and by the increase in TSH levels observed during recovery from NTI [68].

In a recent study that evaluated physically impaired elderly women [69], a twofold risk of cognitive decline was found in the women in the lowest tertile compared with the women in the highest tertile of T4 values (all within the normal range). This finding suggested that thyroid hormone levels may have contributed to cognitive impairment in physically impaired women. In stark contrast to this finding is a recent report of increased longevity in otherwise healthy elderly individuals with mild and subclinical hypothyroidism as compared with elderly individuals with normal TSH and free T4 levels [70]. Clearly the issue of the importance of mild changes in thyroid function on cognitive, cardiovascular, and metabolic functions remains open for investigation.

Hyperthyroidism

In elderly persons, hyperthyroidism can present differently than in young persons, the classic clinical picture of "apathetic hyperthyroidism" described

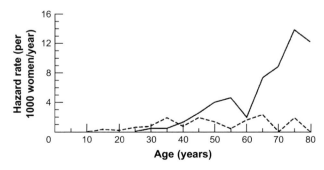

Fig. 3. The age-specific hazard rates for development of hypothyroidism (*solid line*) and hyperthyroidism (*dotted line*) in women. (*From* Vanderpump M, Tunbridge W, French J, et al. The incidence of thyroid disorders in the community: a twenty-year follow up of the Whickham Survey. Clin Endocrinol 1995;43:55–68; with permission.)

by Lahey [71] being dominated by fatigue and apathy. Failure to thrive, generalized wasting, congestive heart failure, and atrial fibrillation are also more common presenting symptoms and signs than in younger patients. Hyperthyroidism, reported to range between 0.5% and 2.3% in the elderly population, was most commonly caused by toxic multinodular goiter in areas with low iodine intake and Graves' disease in iodine-sufficient regions [72]. Iatrogenic thyrotoxicosis can be seen with high-level iodine exposure, through iodinated contrast, for example, (especially in iodine-deficient areas [73]), or in patients treated for many years with the same dose of thyroid hormone in the setting of age-related decrease in the T4 clearance.

The prevalence of subclinical hyperthyroidism—normal free T4 and T3 with low TSH levels—among elderly persons ranges from 1.5% to 12.5% [65,74,75]. High rates of progression to overt hyperthyroidism have been noted in patients with autonomously functioning thyroid adenoma (4% per year) and multinodular goiters (9%–30% in 1–7 years) in iodine-deficient areas [75,76], whereas in iodine-sufficient areas "subclinical" Graves' disease is the most common cause [75]. Cardiovascular and bone-related complications of subclinical hyperthyroidism are more likely in the elderly population, and intervention rather than observation seems to be uniformly agreed upon [73], especially when the TSH level falls below 0.1 mIU/L [77].

Considering the data presented on TRH stimulation testing, it seems that the rarely used TRH stimulation test must be interpreted with caution in the elderly population, because subnormal responses may be seen in many elderly individuals without evidence of thyrotoxicosis.

Autoimmune thyroid disease

The prevalence of autoimmune thyroid disease is increased in the elderly, although this increase is caused exclusively by an increase in the incidence of primary hypothyroidism (Fig. 3) [64,78,79]. An age-related trend to reduction in prevalence and titers of antithyroid autoantibodies has been reported in Graves' disease and, to a lesser extent, in Hashimoto's thyroiditis [80,81] in this population. The prevalence of positivity for thyroid autoantibodies varies with the selected group of elderly patients studied. In centenarians, several studies reported a lower incidence of antithyroid antibody positivity than in healthy 65- to 80-year-old subjects [35,82]. If strict criteria are used to identify healthy elderly individuals (as in the Eurage Senieur study [83,84]), the prevalence of thyroid autoantibodies is not increased when compared with that in younger normal controls [28,34]. It should be noted that in control populations, thyroid peroxidase antibody positivity in most cases was not accompanied by elevation of the serum TSH level [35]. The few studies published that examined hospitalized geriatric patients found that euthyroid patients had a significantly higher occurrence of autoantibodies, with the thyroid peroxidase antibody positivity rate in female subjects ranging to 36% [85,86]. The nonthyroidal pathology of euthyroid patients did not correlate with antibody prevalence [85]. In hospitalized geriatric patients, antibody positivity is nonspecific in euthyroid subjects and has a low positive predictive value in detecting thyroid dysfunction in this population. Antibody status should be determined only when TSH measurement reveals abnormal results, because subclinical hypothyroidism with positive antibodies is prone to develop into clinical hypothyroidism [87].

Based on these data it seems that the aging process per se is not associated with increased production of antithyroid autoantibodies. Rather, the different nonthyroidal illnesses that might accompany aging in a given individual seem to be associated with thyroid autoimmune phenomena. Based on this concept, it has been speculated that if an unusually efficient immune system is an important prerequisite for longevity, then appearance of organ-specific antibodies at senescence may be a predictor of shorter life expectancy [82].

Evidence exists for a direct interaction between pituitary-thyroid hormones and the immune system through the presence of receptors for thyrotropin (TSH) and thyroid hormones on lymphocytes or changes in immune function in physiologic and pathologic fluctuations of thyroid hormones. Immune derived products, such as lymphokines and monokines, have been shown to influence the pituitary thyroid axis, modulating either thyroid hormone levels or the hormone/cytokines production by thyrocytes [88–90]. Low plasma thymosin levels, which were found in thyroidectomized or propylthiouracil-treated mice, were restored to normal values within a few days of treatment with thyroid hormones [91,92]. Patients who have hypothyroidism have decreased plasma thymosin levels that normalized with treatment [93]. In hyperthyroidism of Graves' disease, thymus hypertrophy is noted followed by reduction to normal size with treatment and by reduced autoimmune phenomena, such as autoantibody titers in some cases [78,88,94]. In these studies a direct correlation was found between thymosin concentration and T3, which suggested that T3 may represent the thyroid hormone acting on the thymus. Based on these data, the age-related changes in the function of HPT axis might be relevant to the decreased immune response that elderly persons seem to be able to generate when challenged by infections. Further study is needed to define this event more completely.

The involvement of thyroid function in the regulation of immune system is also demonstrated by the significant correlation observed between the serum total T3 level and the natural killer cell activity in elderly individuals [95]. Lymphocytes from elderly patients with T3 levels at the low end of the reference range demonstrated improvement in natural killer cell activity when exposed to T3 in vitro, whereas cells from young individuals with low T3 levels did not respond with increased natural killer cell activity. In contrast, lymphocytes from young or older individuals with normal T3 concentrations did not alter their natural killer cell activity in response to T3 exposure [95]. This finding suggests that in elderly persons this aspect is more strongly affected by altered thyroid function.

Thyroid nodules

Thyroid nodularity increases with age, especially in iodine-deficient areas but also in iodine-sufficient areas. Clinically relevant (palpable) nodules are found in approximately 5% of patients at age 60, but autopsy studies reveal 90% of women over the age of 70 and 60% of men over the age of 80 have a nodular thyroid [49]. The prevalence reaches almost 100% in women after the age of 90 [96]. By ultrasound examination, the prevalence rate for thyroid nodules is 50% at the age of 50 [97] and increases further with advancing age. The risk of malignancy is approximately 10% in cold, single nodules and is highest if these nodules are found in men older than age 70 [98]. Grossly the aging thyroid decreases little—if at all—in size and weight [99].

By light microscopic examination, virtually all old subjects show an enlargement of thyroid follicles, with retention of colloid and flattening of the lining epithelium and an increase in interstitial fibrous tissue, compared with glands from younger individuals [100]. With the electron microscope, the lining epithelium of the follicle demonstrates flattening of the villi at the apical (luminal) surface, where normally there are lysosomes representing the site of enzymatic cleavage of thyroglobulin to thyroid hormones. In old age these lysosomes become large and irregular and acquire lipid droplets, a change associated with reduced thyroglobulin cleavage [100]. These changes are consistent with a decrease in thyroid hormone secretions and they are found in laboratory animals and in humans. The increase in fibrous tissue may account for some of the gross nodularity. With advancing age, however, there is an increase in the prevalence of follicular (retention) cysts, which appear to represent a progression of the normal aging change and may account for some of the gross nodularity. In general there is a decline with age in the frequency of normal thyroids and an increase in those with lesions. In almost all groups this decline is greater in women than men [100].

Thyroid cancer

The overall annual age-specific incidence rate of clinical and occult differentiated thyroid carcinoma does not increase with age, but some age-related differences in its clinical expression do exist. Papillary to follicular carcinoma ratio is 2:1 in elderly versus 3:1 to 4:1 in young patients [101]. The gender difference in incidence rates seen in younger individuals in favor of higher rates in women is less prominent in the elderly population [102]. Anaplastic thyroid carcinoma is observed almost exclusively in patients over the age of 65. Sarcomas and primary thyroid lymphomas are also seen more frequently in elderly persons. In one study from Sicily, the thyroid nodules harbored carcinoma six times more frequently in men older than age 60 than in middle-aged patients [98]. Another characteristic of thyroid carcinoma in elderly persons is the increased aggressiveness of the tumors. Cause-specific mortality rates for thyroid cancer are clearly much higher with advanced age even after correction for other tumor-specific variables, such as size, extent, presence of metastatic disease, and histologic subtype [103–105]. To improve outcome it is important that efforts be directed at earlier diagnosis (only 18 of 145 well-differentiated thyroid carcinomas were diagnosed in stage 1 [102]), with any significant mass in the thyroid bed evaluated expeditiously by fine-needle aspiration and cytologic examination in this at-risk population.

Drug effects on aging thyroid

Many medications that have influence on thyroid function are used with increasing frequency in the elderly population. Well known among this group are lithium (20% incidence of overt hypothyroidism [106]) and amiodarone, as well as interferon alpha or interleukin-2, both of which can produce hypo- and hyperthyroidism. Many more are known to alter thyroid function tests, without major changes in thyroid status [73]. In elderly patients with untreated or inadequately treated hypothyroidism, the metabolism and excretion of some drugs (eg, insulin, vitamin K, morphine, digoxin, and steroids) may be retarded, which may result in accumulation and side effects [107]. Screening by careful history taking for these drugs is an important and efficient first step in evaluating thyroid dysfunction in elderly persons.

Nonthyroidal illness

NTI is seen more often in elderly persons, which is no surprise considering that the overall number of comorbidities increases with age. The classic presentation of the syndrome commonly termed the *euthyroid-sick syndrome* includes low T3, normal to low T4, normal to low TSH, and increased reverse T3 [108]. In severely ill individuals, the amplitude of these changes correlates with survival rates [109]. T4 is normal in most studies, except in cases of severe illness, in which free T4 is low regardless of the testing method [110]. Much of the change in thyroid function in this syndrome is centrally mediated, as demonstrated by a study that examined severely ill intensive care unit patients (mean age, 67 years) and found the abnormal circadian variability of TSH in elderly persons to be even further impaired [111]. TSH and thyroid hormones were suppressed along with growth hormone, insulin-like growth factor (IGF)-1, testosterone, and dehydroepiandrosterone (DHEA). The only partial response to gonadotropin-releasing hormone (GnRH) administration pointed to a combined hypothalamo-pituitary-gonadal dysfunction, which suggested the need for further investigation with growth hormone and TSH secretagogues. Because of this, the differential diagnosis of thyroid dysfunction in elderly individuals with NTI can be challenging and is best delayed, when at all possible, until the NTI resolves.

Influence of iodine intake in the elderly population

It is remarkable that no differences can be found in iodine excretion in patients with and without goiter, in contrast to studies in young adults, which suggest that factors other than iodine intake, such as nodularity and the amount of autonomously functioning thyroid tissue, may have more of an effect on thyroid size in old age [97]. More of the nodules are autonomously functioning in older thyroid glands, which may be a prerequisite for iodine-induced thyrotoxicosis, a feared situation in elderly persons [97,112].

An increased incidence of clinical goiter, hyperthyroidism, and suppressed TSH was found in an aged population from a low iodine intake area (with 1 in 30 elderly women having unrecognized hyperthyroidism) in comparison with a similar population from a high iodine intake area [72]. In concert with this, an increased incidence of subclinical hypothyroidism was found in elderly persons from the high iodine intake area, presumably because of increased susceptibility of elderly persons to the inhibitory effects of high iodine on the hormonal synthesis when compared with young adults [113] or the worsening of autoimmune thyroiditis by high iodine intake, as supported by some data [72,114–116]. The difference in the type of iodine dysfunction and iodine intake is supported by data from iodine-sufficient individuals who participated in the Framingham study [117], with 4.4% of elderly subjects with TSH > 10 mIU/L versus 0.9% in Italy [118] and 1.5% in Germany [119], both countries with low iodine intake. This phenomenon is also observed in the frequency of adverse effects of the anti-arrhythmic and iodine-containing drug amiodarone because it most commonly induces hyperthyroidism in Italy as opposed to hypothyroidism in the United States [120].

It is clear that the iodine status of a population plays an important role in the thyroid pathology of the elderly population, which should be considered when designing screening, epidemiologic, or other research studies of thyroid diseases in this population.

Summary

Existing data suggest that healthy elderly humans experience a decline in thyroid function similar (but smaller in magnitude) to that observed in what may otherwise be termed central hypothyroidism–reduced TSH, reduced TSH response to TRH stimulation, decreased free T3, and decreased T4 secretion by the thyroid, but little or no change in circulating T4 levels. The changes in T3 levels are also mediated by decreased peripheral conversion from T4 because of decreased activity of peripheral 5'DI. This phenomenon also contributes to the preservation of circulating T4 levels (Box 1) [121–123].

The incidence of subclinical and clinical hypothyroidism increases with age. The frequency of hyperthyroidism appears unchanged, although toxic multinodular disease is a more common cause of thyrotoxicosis than in younger individuals and, in regions of iodine, deficiency may represent the most common etiology. Serum TSH is the most important screening test

---

Box 1. Changes in HPT axis with aging

TSH
No change to slight decrease in basal level (centenarians) [28,32–35,67,121,122]
Decreased response to TRH stimulation [33,40–47]
Decreased amplitude to absent (centenarians) circadian variation [33,38,41,42]

Thyroxine
Normal serum level [28,32–35,122]
Decreased secretion [2,123]
Decreased degradation [2,123]

T3
Slight decrease in serum level [28,32–35,122]
Decreased production [2,49,73]
Decreased (peripheral) and increased (thyroid?) T4/T3 conversion (5′DI activity) [34,35,122]
Increased RT3 [4,31,34,35,49]

Thyroglobulin
Increased (within normal limits) [31]

Antithyroid Antibodies
Increased chronic disease/number of hospitalized patients [35,82,85]
Normal healthy elderly [28,34,35,82]

---

in elderly persons to detect thyroid dysfunction. Because low TSH is much more common in elderly individuals, obtaining a full thyroid panel (ie, free T4 and free or total T3) before diagnosing hyperthyroidism is necessary.

Changes in HPT axis function with age were observed in healthy well-functioning elderly persons, so it is difficult to describe them as pathologic. Rather, we believe that they are better regarded as the result of a new balance between the metabolic requirement for thyroid hormone and the mechanisms regulating hormone production [28,84]. Further evaluation of these phenomena is needed to answer this question more carefully.

References

[1] Kowal J, Cheng B. General principles of endocrine function after the sixth decade. Curr Ther Endocrinol Metab 1994;5:579–84.
[2] Hornick TR, Kowal J. Clinical epidemiology of endocrine disorders in the elderly. Endocrinol Metab Clin North Am 1997;26(1):145–63.

[3] Klug TL, Adelman RC. Altered hypothalamic-pituitary regulation of thyrotropin in male rats during aging. Endocrinology 1979;104(4):1136–42.

[4] Donda A, Lemarchand-Beraud T. Aging alters the activity of 5'-deiodinase in the adenohypophysis, thyroid gland, and liver of the male rat. Endocrinology 1989;124(3): 1305–9.

[5] Greeley GH Jr, Lipton MA, Kizer JS. Serum thyroxine, triiodothyronine, and TSH levels and TSH release after TRH in aging male and female rats. Endocr Res Commun 1982; 9(3–4):169–77.

[6] Pekary AE, Hershman JM, Sugawara M, et al. Preferential release of triiodothyronine: an intrathyroidal adaptation to reduced serum thyroxine in aging rats. J Gerontol 1983;38(6): 653–9.

[7] Naito K, Inada M, Mashio Y, et al. Modulation of T4 5'-monodeiodination in rat anterior pituitary and liver homogenates by thyroid states and fasting. Endocrinol Jpn 1981;28(6): 793–8.

[8] Visser TJ, Kaplan MM, Leonard JL, et al. Evidence for two pathways of iodothyronine 5'-deiodination in rat pituitary that differ in kinetics, propylthiouracil sensitivity, and response to hypothyroidism. J Clin Invest 1983;71(4):992–1002.

[9] van Doorn J, Roelfsema F, van der Heide D. Contribution from local conversion of thyroxine to 3,5,3'-triiodothyronine to intracellular 3,5,3'-triiodothyronine in several organs in hypothyroid rats at isotope equilibrium. Acta Endocrinol (Copenh) 1982; 101(3):386–96.

[10] Cheron RG, Kaplan MM, Larsen PR. Divergent changes of thyroxine-5'-monodeiodination in rat pituitary and liver during maturation. Endocrinology 1980;106(5):1405–9.

[11] El-Zaheri MM, Braverman LE, Vagenakis AG. Enhanced conversion of thyroxine to triiodothyronine by the neonatal rat pituitary. Endocrinology 1980;106(6):1735–9.

[12] Goichot B, Schlienger JL, Grunenberger F, et al. Thyroid hormone status and nutrient intake in the free-living elderly: interest of reverse triiodothyronine assessment. Eur J Endocrinol 1994;130(3):244–52.

[13] da Costa VM, Moreira DG, Rosenthal D. Thyroid function and aging: gender-related differences. J Endocrinol 2001;171(1):193–8.

[14] Correa da Costa VM, Rosenthal D. Effect of aging on thyroidal and pituitary T4–5'-deiodinase activity in female rats. Life Sci 1996;59(18):1515–20.

[15] Cizza G, Brady LS, Esclapes ME, et al. Age and gender influence basal and stress-modulated hypothalamic-pituitary-thyroidal function in Fischer 344/N rats. Neuroendocrinology 1996; 64(6):440–8.

[16] Borges PP, Curty FH, Pazos-Moura CC, et al. Effect of testosterone propionate treatment on thyrotropin secretion of young and old rats in vitro. Life Sci 1998;62(22):2035–43.

[17] Cizza G, Pacak K, Kvetnansky R, et al. Decreased stress responsivity of central and peripheral catecholaminergic systems in aged 344/N Fischer rats. J Clin Invest 1995;95(3): 1217–24.

[18] Rivier C, Vale W. Involvement of corticotropin-releasing factor and somatostatin in stress-induced inhibition of growth hormone secretion in the rat. Endocrinology 1985;117(6): 2478–82.

[19] Martin JB, Reichlin S. Clinical neuroendocrinology. Philadelphia: FA Davis; 1987. p. 116–20.

[20] Hisano S, Fukui Y, Chikamori-Aoyama M, et al. Reciprocal synaptic relations between CRF-immunoreactive- and TRH-immunoreactive neurons in the paraventricular nucleus of the rat hypothalamus. Brain Res 1993;620(2):343–6.

[21] Reymond F, Denereaz N, Lemarchand-Beraud T. Thyrotropin action is impaired in the thyroid gland of old rats. Acta Endocrinol (Copenh) 1992;126(1):55–63.

[22] Gerber H, Peter HJ, Studer H. Age-related failure of endocytosis may be the pathogenetic mechanism responsible for "cold" follicle formation in the aging mouse thyroid. Endocrinology 1987;120(5):1758–64.

[23] van den Hove MF, Couvreur M, Authelet M, et al. Age delays thyroglobulin progression towards dense lysosomes in the cream hamster thyroid. Cell Tissue Res 1998;294(1):125–35.

[24] Frolkis VV, Verzhikovskaya NV, Valueva GV. The thyroid and age. Exp Gerontol 1973; 8(5):285–96.

[25] Wong CC, Dohler KD, Atkinson MJ, et al. Influence of age, strain and season on diurnal periodicity of thyroid stimulating hormone, thyroxine, triiodothyronine and parathyroid hormone in the serum of male laboratory rats. Acta Endocrinol (Copenh) 1983;102(3): 377–85.

[26] Azizi F. Changes in pituitary and thyroid function with increasing age in young male rats. Am J Physiol 1979;237(3):E224–6.

[27] Mooradian AD, Li J, Shah GN. Age-related changes in thyroid hormone responsive protein (THRP) expression in cerebral tissue of rats. Brain Res 1998;793(1–2):302–4.

[28] Mariotti S, Barbesino G, Caturegli P, et al. Complex alteration of thyroid function in healthy centenarians. J Clin Endocrinol Metab 1993;77(5):1130–4.

[29] Ohara H, Kobayashi T, Shiraishi M, et al. Thyroid function of the aged as viewed from the pituitary-thyroid system. Endocrinol Jpn 1974;21(5):377–86.

[30] Ognibene A, Petruzzi E, Troiano L, et al. Age-related changes of thyroid function in both sexes. J Endocrinol Invest 1999;22(10 Suppl):38–9.

[31] Chakraborti S, Chakraborti T, Mandal M, et al. Hypothalamic-pituitary-thyroid axis status of humans during development of ageing process. Clin Chim Acta 1999;288(1–2): 137–45.

[32] Tietz NW, Shuey DF, Wekstein DR. Laboratory values in fit aging individuals: sexagenarians through centenarians. Clin Chem 1992;38(6):1167–85.

[33] Monzani F, Del Guerra P, Caraccio N, et al. Age-related modifications in the regulation of the hypothalamic-pituitary-thyroid axis. Horm Res 1996;46(3):107–12.

[34] Magri F, Cravello L, Fioravanti M, et al. Thyroid function in old and very old healthy subjects. J Endocrinol Invest 2002;25(10 Suppl):60–3.

[35] Magri F, Muzzoni B, Cravello L, et al. Thyroid function in physiological aging and in centenarians: possible relationships with some nutritional markers. Metabolism 2002;51(1): 105–9.

[36] Wiener R, Utiger RD, Lew R, et al. Age, sex, and serum thyrotropin concentrations in primary hypothyroidism. Acta Endocrinol (Copenh) 1991;124(4):364–9.

[37] Snyder PJ, Utiger RD. Response to thyrotropin releasing hormone (TRH) in normal man. J Clin Endocrinol Metab 1972;34(2):380–5.

[38] van Coevorden A, Laurent E, Decoster C, et al. Decreased basal and stimulated thyrotropin secretion in healthy elderly men. J Clin Endocrinol Metab 1989;69(1):177–85.

[39] Jacques C, Schlienger JL, Kissel C, et al. TRH-induced TSH and prolactin responses in the elderly. Age Ageing 1987;16(3):181–8.

[40] Erfurth EM, Norden NE, Hedner P, et al. Normal reference interval for thyrotropin response to thyroliberin: dependence on age, sex, free thyroxin index, and basal concentrations of thyrotropin. Clin Chem 1984;30(2):196–9.

[41] Barreca T, Franceschini R, Messina V, et al. 24-hour thyroid-stimulating hormone secretory pattern in elderly men. Gerontology 1985;31(2):119–23.

[42] Leitol H, Behrends J, Brabant G. The thyroid axis in ageing. Novartis Found Symp 2002; 242:193–204.

[43] Greenspan SL, Klibanski A, Rowe JW, et al. Age alters pulsatile prolactin release: influence of dopaminergic inhibition. Am J Physiol 1990;258(5 Pt 1):E799–804.

[44] Greenspan SL, Sparrow D, Rowe JW. Dopaminergic regulation of gonadotropin and thyrotropin hormone secretion is altered with age. Horm Res 1991;36(1–2):41–6.

[45] Cooper DS, Klibanski A, Ridgway EC. Dopaminergic modulation of TSH and its subunits: in vivo and in vitro studies. Clin Endocrinol (Oxf) 1983;18(3):265–75.

[46] Ben-Jonathan N. Dopamine: a prolactin-inhibiting hormone. Endo Rev 1985;6(4):564–89.

[47] Samuels MH, Veldhuis JD, Henry P, et al. Pathophysiology of pulsatile and copulsatile re-lease of thyroid-stimulating hormone, luteinizing hormone, follicle-stimulating hormone, and alpha-subunit. J Clin Endocrinol Metab 1990;71(2):425–32.

[48] Olsson T, Viitanen M, Hagg E, et al. Hormones in "young" and "old" elderly: pituitary-thyroid and pituitary-adrenal axes. Gerontology 1989;35(2–3):144–52.

[49] Mariotti S, Franceschi C, Cossarizza A, et al. The aging thyroid. Endo Rev 1995;16(6): 686–715.

[50] Herrmann J, Rusche HJ, Kroll HJ, et al. Free triiodothyronine (t3)- and thyroxine (t4) se-rum levels in old age. Horm Metab Res 1974;6(3):239–40.

[51] Bermudez F, Surks MI, Oppenheimer JH. High incidence of decreased serum triiodothyro-nine concentration in patients with nonthyroidal disease. J Clin Endocrinol Metab 1975; 41(1):27–40.

[52] Kabadi UM. Thyroid disorders and the elderly. Compr Ther 1989;15(6):53–65.

[53] Ravaglia G, Forti P, Maioli F, et al. Blood selenium levels and thyroid function in subjects aged 80 years and over. J Endocrinol Invest 1999;22(10 Suppl):47–8.

[54] Ravaglia G, Forti P, Maioli F, et al. Regular moderate intensity physical activity and blood concentrations of endogenous anabolic hormones and thyroid hormones in aging men. Mech Ageing Dev 2001;122(2):191–203.

[55] Poehlman ET, McAuliffe TL, Van Houten DR, et al. Influence of age and endurance training on metabolic rate and hormones in healthy men. Am J Physiol 1990;259: E66–72.

[56] Hagberg JM, Seals DS, Yerg JE, et al. Metabolic response to exercise in young and older athletes and sedentary men. J Appl Physiol 1988;65:900–8.

[57] Lee MS, Kang CW, Shin YS, et al. Acute effects of chundosunbup qi-training on blood con-centrations of TSH, calcitonin, PTH and thyroid hormones in elderly subjects. Am J Chin Med 1998;26(3–4):275–81.

[58] Maugeri D, Speciale S, Santangelo A, et al. Altered laboratory thyroid parameters in el-derly people. J Endocrinol Invest 1999;22(10 Suppl):37.

[59] Bagchi N, Brown TR, Parish RF. Thyroid dysfunction in adults over age 55 years: a study in an urban US community. Arch Intern Med 1990;150(4):785–7.

[60] Parle JV, Franklyn JA, Cross KW, et al. Prevalence and follow-up of abnormal thyrotro-phin (TSH) concentrations in the elderly in the United Kingdom. Clin Endocrinol (Oxf) 1991;34(1):77–83.

[61] Robuschi G, Safran M, Braverman LE, et al. Hypothyroidism in the elderly. Endocr Rev 1987;8(2):142–53.

[62] Laurberg P, Bulow Pedersen I, Pedersen KM, et al. Low incidence rate of overt hypothy-roidism compared with hyperthyroidism in an area with moderately low iodine intake. Thy-roid 1999;9(1):33–8.

[63] Bonar BD, McColgan B, Smith DF, et al. Hypothyroidism and aging: the Rosses' survey. Thyroid 2000;10(9):821–7.

[64] Vanderpump MP, Tunbridge WM, French JM, et al. The incidence of thyroid disorders in the community: a twenty-year follow-up of the Whickham Survey. Clin Endocrinol (Oxf) 1995;43:55–68.

[65] Jayme JJ, Ladenson PW. Subclinical thyroid dysfunction in the elderly. Trends Endocrinol Metab 1994;5:79–86.

[66] Surks MI, Ocampo E. Subclinical thyroid disease. Am J Med 1996;100:217–23.

[67] Mokshagundam S, Barzel US. Thyroid disease in the elderly. J Am Geriatr Soc 1993;41(12): 1361–9.

[68] Stockigt JR. Guidelines for diagnosis and monitoring of thyroid disease: nonthyroidal ill-ness. Clin Chem 1996;42(1):188–92.

[69] Volpato S, Guralnik JM, Fried LP, et al. Serum thyroxine level and cognitive decline in eu-thyroid older women. Neurology 2002;58(7):1055–61.

[70] Gussekloo J, van Exel E, de Craen AJM, et al. Thyroid status, disability and cognitive function, and survival in old age. JAMA 2004;292(24):2591–9.

[71] Lahey FA. Non-activated (apathetic) type of hyperthyroidism. N Engl J Med 1931; 204:747.

[72] Laurberg P, Pedersen KM, Hreidarsson A, et al. Iodine intake and the pattern of thyroid disorders: a comparative epidemiological study of thyroid abnormalities in the elderly in Iceland and in Jutland, Denmark. J Clin Endocrinol Metab 1998;83(3):765–9.

[73] Chiovato L, Mariotti S, Pinchera A. Thyroid diseases in the elderly. Baillieres Clin Endocrinol Metab 1997;11(2):251–70.

[74] Wiersinga WM. Subclinical hypothyroidism and hyperthyroidism: I. Prevalence and clinical relevance. Neth J Med 1995;46:197–204.

[75] Haden ST, Marqusee E, Utiger RD. Subclinical hypothyroidism. Endocrinologist 1996;6: 322–7.

[76] Tenerz A, Forberg R, Jansson J. Is a more active attitude warranted in patients with subclinical thyrotoxicosis. J Intern Med 1990;228:229–33.

[77] Surks MI, Ortiz E, Daniels GH, et al. Subclinical thyroid disease: scientific review and guidelines for diagnosis and management. JAMA 2004;291(2):228–38.

[78] Volpe R, Clarke PV, Row VV. Relationship of age-specific incidence rates to immunological aspects of Hashimoto's thyroiditis. Can Med Assoc J 1973;109:898–901.

[79] Tunbridge WM, Evered DC, Hall R, et al. Lipid profiles and cardiovascular disease in the Wickham area with particular reference to thyroid disease. Clin Endocrinol (Oxf) 1977;7: 495–508.

[80] Aizawa T, Ishihara M, Hashizume K, et al. Age-related changes of thyroid function and immunologic abnormalities in patients with hyperthyroidism due to Graves' disease. J Am Geriatr Soc 1989;37(10):944–8.

[81] Nakamura S, Hattori J, Ogawa T, et al. Thyroid hormone autoantibodies in patients with untreated Graves' disease: with special reference to age. Endocr J 1993;40(3):337–42.

[82] Pinchera A, Mariotti S, Barbesino G, et al. Thyroid autoimmunity and ageing. Horm Res 1995;43(1–3):64–8.

[83] Ligthart GJ, Corberand JX, Fournier C, et al. Admission criteria for immunogerontological studies in man: the SENIEUR protocol. Mech Ageing Dev 1984;28(1):47–55.

[84] Ligthart GJ, Corberand JX, Geertzen HG, et al. Necessity of the assessment of health status in human immunogerontological studies: evaluation of the SENIEUR protocol. Mech Ageing Dev 1990;55(1):89–105.

[85] Szabolcs I, Bernard W, Horster FA. Thyroid autoantibodies in hospitalized chronic geriatric patients: prevalence, effects of age, nonthyroidal clinical state, and thyroid function. J Am Geriatr Soc 1995;43(6):670–3.

[86] Moulias R, Proust J, Wang A, et al. Age-related changes in autoantibodies. Lancet 1984;i: 1128–9.

[87] Rosenthal MJ, Hunt WC, Garry PJ, et al. Thyroid failure in the elderly: microsomal antibodies as discriminant for therapy. JAMA 1987;258(2):209–13.

[88] Mariotti S, Pinchera A. Role of the immune system in the control of thyroid function. In: Greer MA, editor. The thyroid gland. New York: Raven Press; 1990. p. 147–219.

[89] Pekonen F, Weintraub BD. Thyrotropin binding to cultured lymphocytes and thyroid cells. Endocrinology 1978;103:1668–77.

[90] Lemarchand-Beraud T, Holm AC, Scazziga BR. Triiodothyronine and thyroxine nuclear receptors in lymphocytes from normal, hyper- and hypothyroid patients. Acta Endocrinol (Copenh) 1977;85:44–51.

[91] Fabris N, Mocchegiani E. Endocrine control of thymic serum factor production in young-adult and old mice. Cell Immunol 1985;91:325–35.

[92] Salvino W, Wolf B, Aratan-Spire S, et al. Thymic hormone containing cells. IV. Fluctuations in the thyroid hormone levels "in vivo" can modulate the secretion of thymulin by the epithelial cells of young mouse thymus. Clin Exp Immunol 1984;55:629–35.

[93] Fabris N, Mocchegiani E, Mariotti S, et al. Thyroid function modulates thymus endocrine activity. J Clin Endocrinol Metab 1986;62:474–8.

[94] Fabris N, Mocchegiani E, Provinciali M. Pituitary-thyroid axis and immune system: a reciprocal neuroendocrine-immune interaction. Horm Res 1995;43(1–3):29–38.

[95] Kmiec Z, Mysliwska J, Rachon D, et al. Natural killer activity and thyroid hormone levels in young and elderly persons. Gerontology 2001;47(5):282–8.

[96] Denham MJ, Wills EJ. A clinico-pathological survey of thyroid glands in old age. Gerontology 1980;26(3):160–6.

[97] Hintze G, Windeler J, Baumert J, et al. Thyroid volume and goitre prevalence in the elderly as determined by ultrasound and their relationships to laboratory indices. Acta Endocrinol (Copenh) 1991;124(1):12–8.

[98] Belfiore A, La Rosa GL, La Porta GA, et al. Cancer risk in patients with cold thyroid nodules: relevance of iodine intake, sex, age, and multinodularity. [see comment] Am J Med 1992;93(4):363–9.

[99] Hegedus L, Perrild H, Poulsen LR, et al. The determination of thyroid volume by ultrasound and its relationship to body weight, age, and sex in normal subjects. J Clin Endocrinol Metab 1983;56(2):260–3.

[100] Blumenthal HT, Perlstein IB. The aging thyroid. I. A description of lesions and an analysis of their age and sex distribution. J Am Geriatr Soc 1987;35(9):843–54.

[101] Thoresen SO, Akslen LA, Glattre E, et al. Survival and prognostic factors in differentiated thyroid cancer: a multivariate analysis of 1,055 cases. Br J Cancer 1989;59(2):231–5.

[102] Lin JD, Chao TC, Chen ST, et al. Characteristics of thyroid carcinomas in aging patients. Eur J Clin Invest 2000;30(2):147–53.

[103] Hay ID, Bergstralh EJ, Goellner JR, et al. Predicting outcome in papillary thyroid carcinoma: development of a reliable prognostic scoring system in a cohort of 1779 patients surgically treated at one institution during 1940 through 1989. Surgery 1993;114:1050–8.

[104] Mazzaferri EL, Young RL. Papillary thyroid carcinoma: a 10 year follow-up report of the impact of therapy in 576 patients. Am J Med 1981;70:511–8.

[105] McConahey WM, Hay ID, Wollner LB, et al. Papillary thyroid cancer treated at the Mayo Clinic 1946 through 1970 initial manifestations, pathologic finding, therapy, and outcome. Mol Cell Proteomics 1986;61:978–96.

[106] Surks MI, Sievert R. Drugs and thyroid function. N Engl J Med 1995;100:217–23.

[107] Franklyn JA. Metabolic changes in hypothyroidism. In: Braverman LE, Utiger RD, editors. The thyroid. 8th edition. Philadelphia: Lippincott; 2000. p. 833–6.

[108] Wersinga WM. Nonthyroidal illness. In: Braverman LE, Utiger RD, editors. The thyroid. 8th edition. Philadelphia: Lippincott; 2000. p. 281–95.

[109] Wartofsky L. The low T3 or "sick euthyroid syndrome". Endocr Rev 1994;3:248–51.

[110] Rae P, Farrar J, Beckett G, et al. Assessment of thyroid function in the elderly. BMJ 1993; 307:177–80.

[111] van den Berghe G, Weekers F, Baxter RC, et al. Five-day pulsatile gonadotropin-releasing hormone administration unveils combined hypothalamic-pituitary-gonadal defects underlying profound hypoandrogenism in men with prolonged critical illness. J Clin Endocrinol Metab 2001;86(7):3217–26.

[112] Bahre M, Hilgers R, Lindemann C, et al. Thyroid autonomy sensitive detection in vivo and estimation of its functional relevance using quantified high-resolution scintigraphy. Acta Endocrinol (Copenh) 1988;117:145–53.

[113] Paul T, Meyers B, Witorsch RJ, et al. The effect of small increases in dietary iodine on thyroid function in euthyroid subjects. Metabolism 1988;37(2):121–4.

[114] Sundick R, Bagchi N, Brown TR. The role of iodine in thyroid autoimmunity: from chickens to humans [review]. Autoimmunity 1992;13:61–8.

[115] Weaver DK, Batsakis JG, Nishiyama RH. Relationship of iodine to lymphocytic goiters. Arch Surg 1969;98:183–6.

[116] Harach HR, Williams ED. Thyroid cancer and thyroiditis in the goitrous region of Salta, Argentina before and after iodine prophylaxis. Clin Endocrinol (Oxf) 1995;43:701–6.

[117] Sawin CT, Castelli WP, Hershman JM, et al. The aging thyroid: thyroid deficiency in the Framingham Study. Arch Intern Med 1985;145(8):1386–8.

[118] Roti E, Gardini E, Minelli R, et al. Prevalence of anti-thyroid peroxidase antibodies in serum in the elderly: comparison with other tests for anti-thyroid antibodies. Clin Chem 1992; 38(1):88–92.

[119] Hintze G, Burghardt U, Baumert J, et al. Prevalence of thyroid dysfunction in elderly subjects from the general population in an iodine deficiency area. Aging 1991;3:325–31.

[120] Martino E, Safran M, Aghini-Lombardi F, et al. Environmental iodine intake and thyroid dysfunction during chronic amiodarone therapy. Ann Intern Med 1984 Jul;101AIM 1984; 101(1):28–34.

[121] Sawin CT, Bigos ST, Land S, et al. The aging thyroid: relationship between elevated serum thyrotropin level and thyroid antibodies in elderly patients. Am J Med 1985;79(5):591–5.

[122] Urban RJ. Neuroendocrinology of aging in the male and female. Endocrinol Metab Clin North Am 1992;21(4):921–31.

[123] Fisher DA. Physiological variations in thyroid hormones: physiological and pathophysiological considerations. Clin Chem 1996;42(1):135–9.

ENDOCRINOLOGY
AND METABOLISM
CLINICS
OF NORTH AMERICA

ELSEVIER
SAUNDERS

Endocrinol Metab Clin N Am
34 (2005) 993–1014

Aging-Related Adaptations in the Corticotropic Axis: Modulation by Gender

Johannes D. Veldhuis, MD[a],*, Daniel M. Keenan, PhD[b],
Ferdinand Roelfsema, MD[c],
Ali Iranmanesh, MD[d,e]

[a]Endocrine Research Unit, Department of Internal Medicine, Mayo School of Graduate
Medical Education, Mayo Clinic, Rochester, MN, USA
[b]Department of Statistics, University of Virginia, Charlottesville, VA, USA
[c]Department of Endocrinology, Leiden University Medical Center, Leiden, The Netherlands
[d]Endocrine Section, Medical Service Salem, Veterans Affairs Medical Center,
Salem, VA, USA
[e]University of Virginia School of Medicine, Charlottesville, VA, USA

Mechanisms that mediate aging-related disruption of neuroendocrine axes are difficult to parse. The clinical investigative challenge stems in part from the incremental nature of the aging process and the ensemble regulatory properties of homeostatic systems [1–4]. Strongly interlinked signal exchange dictates that no single effector acts alone or can be interpreted in isolation. For example, in the stress-adaptive corticotropic axis, pituitary adrenocorticotropic hormone (ACTH) secretion is the tripartite consequence of feedforward (stimulation) by ACTH-releasing hormone (CRH) and arginine vasopressin (AVP) and feedback (inhibition) by cortisol. ACTH promotes adrenal secretion of cortisol, which represses CRH, AVP, and ACTH outflow. Thus, modifying any one regulatory locus perforce influences the output of all interconnected sites. The latter insight has

This work was supported in part by a Merit Award from the Veterans Affairs Administration, Grants K01 AG19164 and R01 DK60717 from the National Institutes of Health (Bethesda, MD), DMS-0107680 Interdisciplinary Grant in the Mathematical Sciences from the National Science Foundation (Washington, DC), and M01 RR00585 to the General Clinical Research Center of the Mayo Clinic and Foundation from the National Center for Research Resources (Rockville, MD).

* Corresponding author. Endocrine Research Unit, Department of Internal Medicine, Mayo School of Graduate Medical Education, Mayo Clinic, 200 First Street SW, Rochester, MN 55905.
E-mail address: veldhuis.johannes@mayo.edu (J.D. Veldhuis).

motivated innovative analytic methods and interventional experiments to dissect multipathway mechanisms driving cortisol production [1,5,6].

Aging limits adrenal-androgen secretion

The zona reticularis of the adrenal cortex is the primary source of dehydroepiandrosterone (DHEA) and its sulfate (DHEAS). The half-life of the sulfated form is prolonged, thus allowing stable estimates of serum concentrations. Cross-sectional and longitudinal studies document a uniform decline in DHEA and DHEAS production after young adulthood in men and women. DHEA/DHEAS concentrations at 80 years of age are < 10% of young adult values [7,8]. In one cross-sectional study, maximal serum DHEAS concentrations in 981 men and 481 women 11 to 89 years of age occurred at ages 20 to 24 and 15 to 19 years, respectively [7]. Despite a parallel decline thereafter, values remained higher in men than in women. A 13-year longitudinal study of DHEAS concentrations in 97 healthy men (32–83 years of age) in the Baltimore Longitudinal Study of Aging identified a fall in 67%, no change in 13%, and an increase in 20% of individuals [8].

The mechanisms that mediate the age-related decrease in adrenal androgens are not understood. ACTH stimulates DHEA production acutely, and diurnal rhythms of DHEA and cortisol are similar [9]. However, the prominent adrenarchal rise and adult decline in adrenal androgens occur without corresponding changes in ACTH or cortisol production [9]. No adrenal stimulatory hormone specific for DHEA synthesis has been cloned. Anatomic studies show age-dependent atrophy of the zona reticularis, putatively due to a reduction in cell number rather than size [8,10]. Developmental age determines the activity of the androgen-biosynthetic enzymes, 17α-hydroxylase/17,20-desmolase and 3β-hydroxysteroid dehydrogenase isomerase (3β-HSD) [11,12]. Liu and colleagues [11] estimated the activity of adrenal enzymes indirectly in a group of postmenopausal women by calculating relevant product/precursor concentrations ratios. Although apparent enzymatic activities of 3β-HSD and 17α-hydroxylase were similar in postmenopausal and young women, the inferred activity of 17,20-desmolase was lower after the menopause. In a combined cohort of men and women, the response to ACTH injection suggested attenuation of 3β-HSD activity [13]. The aggregate data are consistent with the failure of CRH and ACTH administration to normalize DHEA concentrations despite stimulating cortisol secretion in older adults [13,14].

Diurnal variations in cortisol and putatively DHEA concentrations arise from 24-hour regulation of the frequency or amplitude of burst-like secretion of each [11,15,16]. One study in 10 young women (21–34 years of age) and 10 postmenopausal women (50–60 years of age) inferred decreased DHEA pulse amplitude and normal cortisol pulsatility in the aged cohort [11].

Hypothalamic-pituitary-glucocorticoid axis

Concepts of a physiologic ensemble

An axiom in multipathway biologic systems is that homeostasis is maintained by repeated incremental signaling adjustments among all components of the axis so as to maintain the physiologic mean [1]. Fig. 1 exemplifies this theme for the hypothalamo-pituitary-adrenal (HPA) axis. Direct sampling of hypothalamo-pituitary portal blood in the rat, sheep, and horse indicates that CRH and AVP are secreted in discrete pulses of varying amplitudes and temporal concordance [17–19]. These potent agonists exert individual and joint (synergistic) stimulation of ACTH synthesis and release [20,21]. The second-messenger signaling pathways driven by CRH (cAMP-protein kinase A) and AVP (Ca^{2+} and protein kinase C) putatively converge to mediate synergy in dually CRH/AVP-responsive corticotropes [22]. Pulses of ACTH in turn stimulate burst-like cortisol secretion by the adrenal zona fasciculata [15]. Cortisol acts via negative feedback to oppose feedforward drive. The set of interactions maintains glucocorticoid homeostasis.

Tissue actions of gluco- and mineralocorticoids

Cortisol acts upon diverse target tissues, which include the central nervous system and the pituitary gland. Significant but non-exclusive

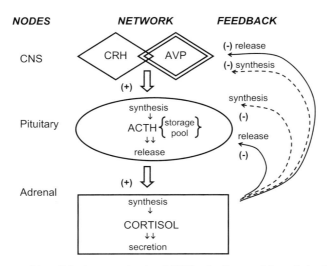

Fig. 1. Schema of interlinked stress-adaptive ACTH axis. Bursts of hypothalamic AVP and CRH individually and jointly stimulate (+) pulsatile release of pituitary ACTH. Blood-borne ACTH drives adrenal secretion of cortisol, which feeds back (−) centrally on CRH/AVP and ACTH output. (*From* Keenan DM, Licinio J, Veldhuis JD. A feedback-controlled ensemble model of the stress-responsive hypothalamo-pituitary-adrenal axis. Proc Natl Acad Sci USA 2001;98:4028–33; with permission.)

transduction is via nuclear type I (mineralocorticoid) and type II (glucocorticoid) receptors [9,23]. Mineralocorticoid receptors (MRs) and glucocorticoid receptors (GRs) have nominal dissociation constants for cortisol in the human of 0.14 and 2.3 μg/dL (4 and 63 nmol/L), respectively [24]. Given that only 6% of total plasma cortisol is free (protein-unbound) [5], nadir and peak free cortisol concentrations are about 0.3 and 1.4 μg/dL. Such estimates predict >90% and >50% occupancies of MRs in the early morning and late evening, respectively, and < 35% occupancy of GRs in the unstressed state. Major surgery elevates total and free cortisol concentrations by 2- and 7-fold, respectively (thus, free levels are 8–12 μg/dL), which saturates GRs and MRs.

Local (target-cell) regulation of cortisol action

The concentration-dependent effects of cortisol are target-tissue and cell specific. For example, for corticosterone in the rat, one half maximally effective concentrations (μg/dL) are approximately 1 for CRH repression, 2 for thymus involution, and 5 for AVP inhibition [25]. This 5-fold range reflects the relative density of GRs and MRs and possible antagonism by GR-β [26]. Glucocorticoid activity is controlled further at the cellular level by 11β-hydroxysteroid dehydrogenase type I (converting inactive cortisone to active cortisol) and type II (the reverse or cortisol-inactivating enzyme) [27]. In addition to local receptor expression and activation/deactivation reactions, GR polymorphisms may modify tissue effects [28]. Box 1 summarizes these and other factors that modulate the stress response. How age governs each regulatory mechanism in the human has not been defined.

Negative feedback

Autoinhibition is a physiologic hallmark of regulated systems. Negative feedback by excessive amounts of 11-desoxycorticosterone results in atrophy of the adrenal gland, as recognized in 1940 by Selye [32]. Glucocorticoid- and mineralocorticoid-dependent negative feedback are demonstrable in humans. In particular, administration of canrenoate in the late day or mifepristone (RU 486) in the morning to selectively

---

Box 1. Factors determining stress responsivity in humans

Glucocorticoid-receptor haplotype [29]
Glucocorticoid-receptor polymorphisms [28]
Corticosteroid-binding globulin concentrations
11β-Hydroxysteroid dehydrogenase activity (type I activates
    cortisone → cortisol) [30]
Progesterone (augments stress response) [31]

antagonize MRs or GRs, respectively, stimulates cortisol secretion [33,34]. Sites of feedback restraint in the rat include the lateral septum, hippocampus (dentate gyrus) via MRs and GRs, and the parvocellular paraventricular nucleus (PVN), locus caeruleus, and corticotrope cells (principally via GRs). Collective data in the human, monkey, rat, and cat indicate that hippocampal sites mediate negative feedback to CRH neurons and in lesser measure to AVP neurons in the PVN [35,36]. A study limited to five patients disclosed that direct electrical simulation of the hippocampus can inhibit, and of the amygdala enhance, cortisol secretion in the conscious human [37]. CRH and AVP neurons express GRs, and their gene promoters are repressed by glucocorticoids [38,39]. In addition, glucocorticoids inhibit CRH- and AVP-stimulated corticotrope secretion noncompetitively (reduced efficacy) in vitro and in vivo [20,40]. Direct pituitary repression is consistent with the fact that 99% of corticotropes express GRs.

Box 2 highlights the foregoing and other mechanisms of negative feedback. For example, glucocorticoids may inhibit adrenal steroidogenesis directly via local GRs [41]. Steroid hormones may also modulate central neurotransmission to CRH and AVP neurons by rapid (nongenomic) effects on membrane-associated receptors [42,43].

Day/night contrasts in adrenocorticotropic hormone and cortisol secretion

Circadian rhythms of cortisol secretion are endowed conjointly by diurnal rhythmicity of hypothalamic CRH and AVP gene expression, ACTH secretion, and adrenal responsiveness to ACTH [44,45]. The first two rhythms persist after adrenalectomy and the last after hypophysectomy. Rhythmicity

---

Box 2. Sites of sustained cortisol negative feedback

Reduced ACTH secretion directly
Reduced AVP gene in PVN
Reduced CRH gene in PVN
Reduced pituitary CRH-R1
Reduced glucocorticoid and mineralocorticoid receptors
Reduced adrenal cortisol secretion directly

Long-term effect is reduced corticotrope and adrenal size. PVN denotes the parvocellular region of the paraventricular nucleus.

Data from Erkut ZA, Pool C, Swaab DF. Glucocorticoids suppress corticotropin-releasing hormone and vasopressin expression in human hypothalamic neurons. J Clin Endocrinol Metab 1998;83:2066–73; and Sakai K, Horiba N, Sakai Y, et al. Regulation of corticotropin-releasing factor receptor messenger ribonucleic acid in rat anterior pituitary. Endocrinology 1996;137:1758–63.

is supervised by neural signals from the suprachiasmatic nucleus, which reach the paraventricular nucleus via local inputs and the adrenal gland via splanchnic nerves [45]. In the human, the mass and the shape (waveform) of underlying ACTH secretory bursts exhibit prominent diurnal adaptations (Fig. 2) [5,6]. The mean mass of ACTH bursts increases from 46 to 82 ng/L (and that of cortisol by 2.5-fold) at night, and their shape is abbreviated by > 50%. These analytic inferences point to highly precise diurnal regulation of CRH and AVP action and glucocorticoid negative feedback on the corticotrope secretory process.

Peptide-receptor and agonist specificity

Genetic studies have unveiled specific subclasses of AVP and CRH receptors (eg, V1b [V3] and CRH-R1 in the pituitary gland) [46,47]. Elucidating receptor subtypes should identify more precise targets for novel

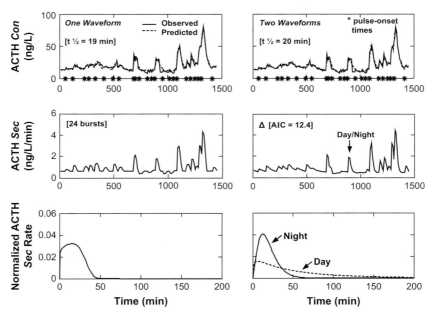

Fig. 2. Illustrative plasma ACTH concentration (*con*) time series obtained by sampling blood every 10 minutes for 24 hours in one healthy adult. Left and right columns give representations achieved by the single and dual ACTH *sec*-burst models, respectively. The panels depict (*top*) measured ACTH *con* (continuous curves) and predicted ACTH *con* (interrupted curves, wherein time zero denotes 0800 hours clocktime); (*middle*) estimated instantaneous ACTH secretion (*sec*) rates; and (*bottom*) the reconstructed three-parameter ACTH *sec*-burst waveform (shape). Asterisks on the *x* axes of ACTH *con* mark a priori estimates of pulse-onset times. The boldface day/night arrow (*right middle*) identifies the analytic changepoint (demarcation time between the day/night waveforms). The positive Akaike information coefficient (AIC) difference (*right middle*) denotes a significantly enhanced precision of fit under statistical penalty for the two- versus one-waveform model of ACTH *sec* bursts.

pharmacologic antagonists [48,49]. Clinical goals would be to limit excessive CRH, ACTH, and cortisol production and action; to reduce heightened sympathetic outflow; and to suppress stress-related anxiety. Conversely, urocortin-1 is a natural agonist of CRH-R1 and R2 that stimulates ACTH and thereby cortisol secretion in the human [50]. Other peptidyl regulators remain to be studied definitively, such as atriopeptin, adrenomedullin, Orexin (hypocretin), ghrelin, and neuropeptide Y.

Free cortisol hypothesis

Free (ie, protein-unbound) and CBG- and albumin-bound cortisol constitute about 6%, 80%, and 14%, respectively, of total plasma cortisol in the human [5,24]. Significant indirect evidence supports the biologic relevance of the free moiety. In particular, free glucocorticoid concentrations predict hippocampal GR occupancy, in vivo negative feedback, and fractional hepatic extraction of corticosterone in the rat and cerebrospinal fluid concentrations of cortisol in the human [51–54]. Age and gender do not seem to affect free cortisol concentrations [5,55].

Cortisol and adrenocorticotropic hormone kinetics

At physiologic CBG concentrations, the half-life of total cortisol is 35 to 65 minutes [5,6,15,56]. Longer half-lives reflect relatively higher CBG concentrations (eg, in young women compared with men) [57]. Distribution-volume estimates differed markedly among earlier methods (from 4–115 L) but have approached 8 to 10 L/m^2 in recent studies [56]. Whether the distribution volume or metabolic elimination of total cortisol changes in the elderly population is not clear. Model-based analyses in 32 adults indicated that the median half-life of elimination of free cortisol is 4.1 minutes and does not vary with age, gender, or time of day (Fig. 3A) [5]. However, the metabolic clearance of total cortisol is higher in the morning than in the evening [58]. This dichotomy is readily explained by greater total cortisol availability at the circadian maximum. Analyses indicate that cortisol infusions at this time may exceed the binding capacity of high-affinity CBG and thereby increase free (and weakly albumin-bound) cortisol concentrations (Fig. 3B). In this regard, estrogen increases CBG concentrations, whereas insulin, obesity, and testosterone decrease CBG concentrations [59].

The half-life of ACTH is 8 to 25 minutes by bioassay and immunoassay [5,6,60]. Rapid disappearance imposes a requirement for frequent blood sampling to monitor ACTH pulsatility accurately [61–63]. Data derived from 5- and 10-minute sampling protocols indicate that unstressed adults secrete 2 to 5 μg of ACTH per day [6,60,63,64]. Like other large proteins, ACTH is distributed primarily in the plasma volume of 30 to 50 mL/kg. Whether aging affects the distribution volume or elimination kinetics of ACTH remains undetermined.

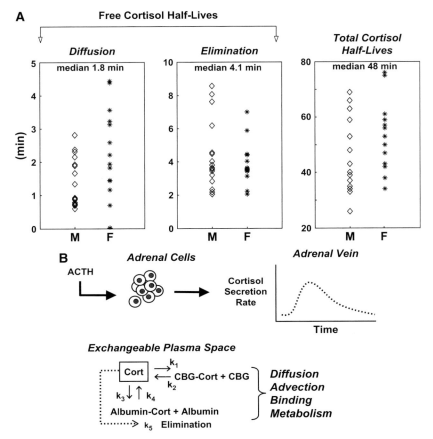

Fig. 3. (*A*) Estimated half-lives of the diffusion/advection of free cortisol (1.8 minutes), elimi-nation of free cortisol (4.1 minutes), and disappearance of total cortisol (48 minutes) from plasma in 32 healthy adults. Data are shown in men (M) and women (F). (*B*) Model of fate of secreted cortisol under ACTH drive (*top left*). An adrenal secretory burst (*top right*) results in rapid diffusion (random motion) and advection (linear flow) of free cortisol (CORT) mole-cules in plasma, reversible association of free cortisol with low-affinity albumin and high-affinity cortisol-binding globulin (CBG), and fractional elimination of free cortisol by the liver and kid-neys (*bottom*). (*From* Keenan DM, Roelfsema F, Veldhuis JD. Endogenous ACTH concentra-tion-dependent drive of pulsatile cortisol secretion in the human. Am J Physiol Endocrinol Metab 2004;287:E652–61; with permission.)

Adrenocorticotropic hormone pulsing mechanism

The timing of successive ACTH secretory bursts is apparently random (it is technically defined as a renewal process) [1,5,6]. Pulsatile secretion is quantitated as the mean rate of occurrence (frequency), intensity (amplitude and mass), and duration of secretory bursts [63]. Secretion comprises a finite admixture of pulsatile and basal (constitutive) hormone release [65]. Viewed from a pulsatility perspective, circadian rhythms in ACTH and cortisol concentrations can be accounted for primarily by 24-hour variations in ACTH and cortisol secretory-burst mass [15,63].

Model-free measures of feedback control

Feedback integrity of the ensemble corticotropic axis can be quantitated by the regularity of individual ACTH and cortisol secretory patterns and their joint synchrony using the univariate and bivariate (cross-) approximate entropy statistic [2,66–68]. Joint synchrony can be assessed in an ACTH → cortisol feedforward and cortisol → ACTH feedback direction (Fig. 4A). When applied to the corticotropic axis, regularity and synchrony analyses identify loss of cortisol → ACTH feedback but not ACTH → cortisol feedforward control in aging individuals (Fig. 4B) [69]. Such inferences extend the generality of inferred integrative failure of neurohormonal systems in the older human to include the corticotropic, somatotropic, and gonadotropic axes [2,70,71].

Hypothalamo-pituitary-adrenal adaptations in aging

Mean adrenocorticotropic hormone and glucocorticoid concentrations

In cohort-based studies, age does not consistently alter ACTH or cortisol concentrations. Waltman and colleagues [72] observed comparable mean overnight cortisol and ACTH concentrations in men 21 to 38 and 66 to 78 years of age. Pavlov and colleagues [14] reported similar 24-hour mean concentrations of ACTH and cortisol and cortisol/CBG ratios in three strata of healthy men 21 to 49, 50 to 69, and 70 to 85 years of age. In two other studies, cortisol concentrations in men and women did not vary over age spans as wide as 18 to 89 years [13].

In a metaanalysis, Van Cauter and colleagues [73] reported a positive correlation between unstimulated 24-hour mean cortisol concentrations and age in men and women. These authors reanalyzed data from 90 men (19–83 years of age) and 87 women (18–75 years of age). The linear age-related increase was attributable to gradual elevation of cortisol concentrations in the late day. This pattern mimics that elicited by fasting and by antagonism of negative feedback via MRs [33,34,74]. Analogously comprehensive data are not available for 24-hour mean free cortisol or ACTH concentrations.

Pulsatile secretion of adrenocorticotropic hormone and cortisol

Available studies of ACTH or cortisol do not identify consistent changes in pulsatile or basal hormone secretion in aging men or women [73,75]. A recent analysis by Keenan and colleagues [5] extended this inference to free cortisol secretion in 32 healthy adults whose ages spanned four decades

(Fig. 5). Because only three volunteers were older than 60 years of age, an unanswered question is how ACTH and cortisol dynamics change in later decades of life.

Feedforward drive by adrenocorticotropic hormone on adrenal cortisol secretion in aging

Recent analytic developments allow estimation of endogenously unfolding (implicit) dose-response properties without injecting hormones [3,5]. A requirement is frequent paired measurements of the coupled hormones. Dose-responsiveness is defined by efficacy (maximal response achievable), potency (one-half maximally effective concentration), and sensitivity (absolute slope of effector-response relationship) (Fig. 6). Implementation of such methodology in 32 adults 26 to 79 years of age identified no significant age-related adaptations in ACTH efficacy or potency or adrenal sensitivity [5].

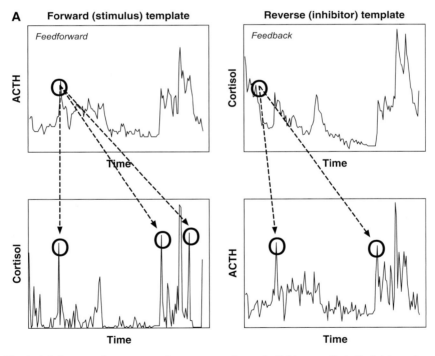

Fig. 4. (*A*) Concept of cross-approximate entropy (cross-ApEn) to quantitate the joint synchrony of ACTH's feedforward on cortisol patterns (forward cross-ApEn) (*left*) and cortisol's feedback on ACTH patterns (reverse cross-ApEn) (*right*). Hormonal input (effector) is rendered in concentration units and output (responses) as secretion rates, thus mirroring in vivo biologic coupling [65]. (*B*) Age selectively disrupts the quantifiable synchrony (elevates cross-ApEn) of cortisol-ACTH feedback patterns (*lower panel*) without altering joint ACTH-cortisol feedforward synchrony (*top*). Data are from 32 adults of the indicated ages. Time series were reanalyzed from Roelfsema and colleagues [65].

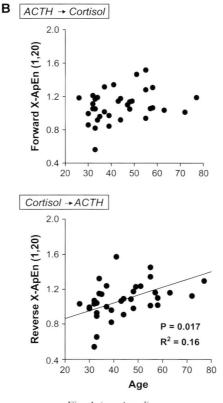

Fig. 4 (*continued*)

Nychthemeral adrenocorticotropic hormone and cortisol rhythms

A uniform inference is that diurnal nadir cortisol concentrations increase and occur earlier in the day in older than young adults [73]. Plausible mechanisms include an age-related reduction in the glucocorticoid distribution volume or metabolic clearance rate, heightened splanchnic drive to the adrenal gland, or diminished intra-adrenal restraint of cortisol synthesis in the late day. It is unknown whether the inferred phase advance reflects sociocultural behavioral differences (eg, earlier bedtime and arising) in older individuals or a true circadian shift. The distinction requires monitoring cortisol patterns under prolonged free-running conditions of so-called temporal isolation (ie, removal of all environmental Zeitgeber cues).

Stress-induced adrenocorticotropic hormone and cortisol secretion

The corticotropic axis responds to diverse physical (exercise), psychosocial (anxiety), and metabolic (fasting) stressors with increased output of ACTH,

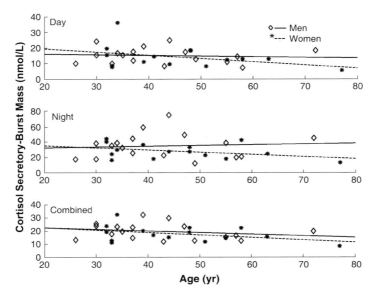

Fig. 5. Noninvasively estimated mass of cortisol secreted per burst in the day and night in 32 healthy adults 26 to 78 years of age. The regression slopes are not significant. To convert nmol/L to μg/L, multiply by 0.036. *Data from* Keenan DM, Roelfsema F, Veldhuis JD. Endogenous ACTH concentration-dependent drive of pulsatile cortisol secretion in the human. Am J Physiol Endocrinol Metab 2004;287:E652–61.

cortisol, epinephrine, and norepinephrine [76]. Hypothalamo-corticotropic-adrenal responses depend upon age; gender; and the severity, persistence, novelty, and type of stress imposed. Aging does not limit maximal ACTH and cortisol reserve (peak secretory capacity) (Box 3). In particular, older adults achieve normal maximal responses to injected CRH or ACTH [13,14,77], insulin-induced hypoglycemia [77,78], metyrapone administration [79], a cold-pressor test [80], and a 3.5-day fast [74]. It is important to clarify the time course of free-cortisol responses to each stressor in aging subjects as an index of integrated glucocorticoid exposure.

Age typically augments ACTH and cortisol responses to submaximal stimuli. An example is human CRH injected alone or with vasopressin (antidiuretic hormone) [83]. Heightened responsiveness persists in the presence of negative feedback imposed by a low dose of dexamethasone (Box 4) [84–86].

Feedback regulation of the hypothalamo-pituitary unit in aging subjects

Exaggerated acute pituitary responses to secretagogues in aging individuals point to reduced negative feedback or increased corticotrope ACTH stores (Fig. 1). Chronic glucocorticoid excess, recurrent stress, and age reduce the density of GRs and MRs in the limbic system, particularly in the hippocampus. A prediction of receptor impoverishment is impaired negative feedback by glucocorticoids and elevated adrenal glucocorticoid secretion

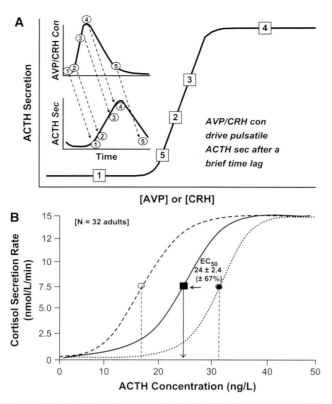

Fig. 6. (*A*) Schema of methodology for reconstructing in vivo dose-response relationships without infusing labeled or unlabeled hormones. The concept entails relating CRH or AVP concentrations within a pulse to calculated ACTH secretion rates after a time delay via a monotonic four-parameter interface function. (*B*) In 32 adults, analytic estimates of endogenous ACTH's concentration-dependent stimulation of cortisol secretion yielded a potency of 24 ± 2.4 (SEM) ng/L (ACTH concentration driving one half-maximal cortisol secretion, EC_{50}); efficacy of 14 ± 1.4 nmol/L/min (asymptotically maximal cortisol secretion); sensitivity of 0.17 ± 0.016 slope units (maximal positive slope of the feedforward relationship); and responsivity of 6.8 ± 0.7 nmol/L/min (cortisol secretory response associated with the ACTH EC_{50}). Interrupted curves are ± 1 SD of potency. In the same cohort of subjects, 24-hour plasma ACTH concentrations averaged 19 ± 0.71 ng/L. Age and gender did not affect any of the four measures of endogenous ACTH action. To convert nmol/L to μg/L, multiply by 0.036. (*From* Keenan DM, Roelfsema F, Veldhuis JD. Endogenous ACTH concentration-dependent drive of pulsatile cortisol secretion in the human. Am J Physiol Endocrinol Metab 2004;287:E652–61; with permission.)

[91]. In some contexts, impaired dexamethasone suppression correlated with age and reduced cognitive function in older adults [92,93]. Although inhibition of ACTH and cortisol concentrations by dexamethasone did not differ by age in men [72], infused cortisol is less effective in suppressing ACTH concentrations in older than young men [14,94,95]. One small study inferred diminished cortisol feedback in postmenopausal women compared with aged men [94]. In a large cohort, a low dose of dexamethasone reduced

---

Box 3. Conditions and stimuli yielding age-invariant hypothalamo-pituitary-adrenal responses

Unstressed cortisol concentrations [81]
Insulin-induced hypoglycemia [77]
Metyrapone-stimulated ACTH release [79]
ACTH-induced cortisol secretion [13,82]
Cold-immersion stress [80]
Fasting for 3.5 days [74]

---

cortisol more in 106 women than in 203 men (66–78 years of age) [96]. Cross-approximate entropy analysis, on the other hand, predicts comparable disruption of cortisol-ACTH feedback synchrony in middle-aged men and women (Fig. 4B) [68,69]. Further investigations are necessary to clarify the nature of age- and gender-related feedback adaptations.

Aging, gender, and stimulus type

Clinical studies of feedforward drive indicate that aging potentiates stress-induced ACTH and cortisol secretion in a gender-related and stimulus-selective fashion. A recent meta-analysis reviewed 45 parallel-cohort studies comprising 670 young and 625 older adults (28 $\pm$ 5 and 69 $\pm$ 6 years of age, respectively) [97]. Age accentuated stress-induced ACTH and cortisol responses by 2.4-fold, and female gender did so by 2.7-fold in older individuals. More detailed analyses indicate that age, gender, and type of stressor govern stimulated ACTH/cortisol secretion (Box 4).

Box 4. Age-related distinctions in hypothalamo-pituitary-adrenal responsivity

Increased CRH's stimulation of ACTH and cortisol secretion[a] [86]
Increased AVP/CRH (combined) stimulationa [85]
Decreased dexamethasone suppression of CRH's effect [86]
Increased paradoxic ACTH/cortisol response to somatostatin
    infusion [87]
Increased social-stress effect[b] [88]
Increased response to cognitive stress[a] [89]
Increased stimulation by 5HT-1A agonist (ipsapirone) [90]
Increased response to hypothermic stress [90]

---

[a] More prominent age contrast in women than in men.
[b] Especially cortisol vis-à-vis ACTH.

Compared with young men, premenopausal women respond more to paradigms of interpersonal rejection and to hypothermia and respond more prominently in the luteal than follicular phase of the menstrual cycle [31,86]. Compared with elderly men, postmenopausal women manifest higher ACTH and cortisol responses to ipsapirone (serotonin-1A agonist) or physostigmine (cholinergic agonist), lumbar puncture, driving simulations, and cognitive challenges (Box 4) [89]. Other stressors do not seem to depend upon gender and age (Box 3).

Gender differences in HPA regulation in the rodent arise from neuronal imprinting by sex steroids in the neonate and multisite actions of androgen and estrogen in the adult [98]. In particular, testosterone and nonaromatizable androgens repress hypothalamic AVP and CRH and induce GR gene expression [99]. Estrogens exert opposite effects [100] and increase CBG concentrations and decrease GR number in the pituitary gland [101,102].

Reported gender differences in humans do not necessarily mirror those in the rat. In young men, administration of estradiol for 48 hours amplified the ACTH response to cognitive-emotional stress [103]. This outcome is consistent with localization of estrogen-receptor α in central autonomic neurons and corticotropes [104]. On the other hand, young men exhibited higher-amplitude ACTH pulses and greater cortisol responses to reboxetine (a noradrenergic agonist) than young women [105,106], and combined estrogen withdrawal and testosterone administration potentiated ACTH-stimulated cortisol secretion in female-to-male trans-sexual patients [107]. Nonetheless, middle-aged and postmenopausal women manifested a greater cortisol response to ACTH than comparably aged men [96,108].

Analytical reconstruction of endogenous ACTH drive of cortisol pulses yielded no gender difference in middle-aged adults [5]. The last analyses evaluated ACTH efficacy, ACTH potency, and adrenal sensitivity (Fig. 6). A plausible proposition for disparate results of pharmacologic interventions is that age and gender influence GR and MR availability, the metabolism of testosterone by 5α-reductase and aromatase enzymes, and the local metabolism of glucocorticoids [109]. Box 5 gives some of the key changes proposed in aging.

Aging hypothesis

A general hypothesis is that time-integrated free cortisol availability, if determined over extended intervals in community-living adults, would be higher in older individuals. Free cortisol measurements have not been made accurately and repeatedly in a longitudinal fashion in healthy aging populations to test this notion, although urinary free cortisol excretion provides a surrogate estimate. Women who exhibited an increase in this measure over 2.5 years manifested greater memory loss than compeers [114]. In chronic stress models and in some cross-sectional studies, higher (free) cortisol concentrations forecast GR downregulation, hippocampal neuronal atrophy, osteopenia, sarcopenia, high blood pressure, visceral adiposity, and

---

Box 5. Proposed mechanisms of age-related HPA hyper-responsiveness

Decreased GR expression[a]
Decreased MR number[a,b]
Decreased adrenalectomy-induced upregulation of
    hippocampal GR
Increased colocalization of AVP and CRH (human)
Decreased hippocampal neuron number[a]
Decreased metabolic clearance of cortisol[b]

---

[a] Experiments in the rat (hypothalamus and hippocampus).
[b] Data in dog (amygdala and hippocampus).
Data from Refs. [110–113].

---

insulin resistance [59,94]. The same features typify aging. Nonetheless, a strict causal relationship between frequent incremental cortisol elevations and catabolic features of aging remains unproven.

A presumptive age-related increase in central CRH or AVP outflow could unify the tripartite features of heightened stress responsiveness, central hypogonadism, and hyposomatotropism in older adults [4,115]. In this regard, stress and injection of CRH or AVP reduce gonadotropin-releasing hormone secretion in the human, monkey, and rat, and CRH infusion blocks GH-releasing peptide stimulation of GH release in the human [116]. The relevance of increased central outflow of stress-adaptive signals to aging-associated hypogonadism and hyposomatotropism could be tested when potent, safe, and selective lipophilic (CNS-acting) CRH- and AVP-receptor antagonists become available for clinical use.

Summary

Aging is marked by depletion of adrenal androgens (DHEAs) in the face of elevated late-day total cortisol concentrations. CRH and AVP evoke greater ACTH and cortisol responses in older than young adults, especially in postmenopausal women. The joint synchrony and strength of cortisol$\rightarrow$ ACTH negative feedback decline with aging. Further studies are required to elucidate the precise mechanisms mediating and the long-term impact of impaired stress adaptations in aging.

Acknowledgments

We are grateful to Kris Nunez for preparing the manuscript.

References

[1] Keenan DM, Licinio J, Veldhuis JD. A feedback-controlled ensemble model of the stress-responsive hypothalamo-pituitary-adrenal axis. Proc Natl Acad Sci USA 2001;98: 4028–33.

[2] Pincus SM, Mulligan T, Iranmanesh A, et al. Older males secrete luteinizing hormone and testosterone more irregularly, and jointly more asynchronously, than younger males. Proc Natl Acad Sci USA 1996;93:14100–5.

[3] Keenan DM, Alexander SL, Irvine CHG, et al. Reconstruction of in vivo time-evolving neuroendocrine dose-response properties unveils admixed deterministic and stochastic elements in interglandular signaling. Proc Natl Acad Sci USA 2004;101:6740–5.

[4] Giustina A, Veldhuis JD. Pathophysiology of the neuroregulation of growth hormone secretion in experimental animals and the human. Endocr Rev 1998;19:717–97.

[5] Keenan DM, Roelfsema F, Veldhuis JD. Endogenous ACTH concentration-dependent drive of pulsatile cortisol secretion in the human. Am J Physiol Endocrinol Metab 2004; 287:E652–61.

[6] Keenan DM, Veldhuis JD. Cortisol feedback state governs adrenocorticotropin secretory-burst shape, frequency and mass in a dual-waveform construct: time-of-day dependent regulation. Am J Physiol 2003;285:R950–61.

[7] Orentreich N, Brind JL, Rizer RL, et al. Age changes and sex differences in serum dehydroepiandrosterone sulfate concentrations throughout adulthood. J Clin Endocrinol Metab 1984;59:551–5.

[8] Orentreich N, Brind JL, Vogelman JH, et al. Long-term longitudinal measurements of plasma dehydroepiandrosterone sulfate in normal men. J Clin Endocrinol Metab 1992;75: 1002–4.

[9] Orth DN, Kovacs WJ, Debold CR. The adrenal cortex. In: Wilson JD, Foster DW, editors. Williams textbook of endocrinology. 8th edition. Philadelphia: W.B. Saunders; 1992. p. 489–620.

[10] Staton BA, Mixon RL, Dharia S, et al. Is reduced cell size the mechanism for shrinkage of the adrenal zona reticularis in aging? Endocr Res 2004;30:529–34.

[11] Liu CH, Laughlin GA, Fischer UG, et al. Marked attenuation of ultradian and circadian rhythms of dehydroepiandrosterone in postmenopausal women: evidence for a reduced 17,20-desmolase enzymatic activity. J Clin Endocrinol Metab 1990;71:900–6.

[12] Schiebinger RJ, Albertson BD, Cassorla FG, et al. The developmental changes in plasma adrenal androgens during infancy and adrenarche are associated with changing activities of adrenal microsomal 17-hydroxylase and 17,20-desmolase. J Clin Invest 1981;67:1177–82.

[13] Vermeulen A, Deslypere JP, Schelfhout W, et al. Adrenocortical function in old age: response to acute adrenocorticotropin stimulation. J Clin Endocrinol Metab 1982;54:187–91.

[14] Pavlov EP, Harman SM, Chrousos GP, et al. Responses of plasma adrenocorticotropin, cortisol, and dehydroepiandrosterone to ovine corticotropin-releasing hormone in healthy aging men. J Clin Endocrinol Metab 1986;62:767–72.

[15] Veldhuis JD, Iranmanesh A, Lizarralde G, et al. Amplitude modulation of a burst-like mode of cortisol secretion subserves the circadian glucocorticoid rhythm in man. Am J Physiol 1989;257:E6–14.

[16] Nieschlag E, Loriaux DL, Ruder HJ, et al. The secretion of dehydroepiandrosterone and dehydroepiandrosterone sulphate in man. J Endocrinol 1973;57:123–34.

[17] Plotsky PM, Sawchenko PE. Hypophysial-portal plasma levels, median eminence content, and immunohistochemical staining of corticotropin-releasing factor, arginine vasopressin, and oxytocin after pharmacological adrenalectomy. Endocrinology 1987;120:1361–9.

[18] Canny BJ, Funder JW, Clarke IJ. Glucocorticoids regulate ovine hypophysial portal levels of corticotropin-releasing factor and arginine vasopressin in a stress-specific manner. Endocrinology 1989;125:2532–9.

[19] Redekopp C, Irvine CH, Donald RA, et al. Spontaneous and stimulated adrenocorticotropin and vasopressin pulsatile secretion in the pituitary venous effluent of the horse. Endocrinology 1986;118:1410–6.

[20] Lamberts SW, Verleun T, Oosterom R, et al. Corticotropin-releasing factor (ovine) and vasopressin exert a synergistic effect on adrenocorticotropin release in man. J Clin Endocrinol Metab 1984;58:298–303.

[21] Watanabe T, Orth DN. Detailed kinetic analysis of adrenocorticotropin secretion by dispersed anterior pituitary cells in a microperifusion system: effects of ovine corticotropin-releasing factor and arginine vasopressin. Endocrinology 1987;121:1133–45.

[22] Jia LG, Canny BJ, Orth DN, et al. Distinct classes of corticotropes mediate corticotropin-releasing hormone- and arginine vasopressin-stimulated adrenocorticotropin release. Endocrinology 1991;128:197–203.

[23] Jacobson L, Sapolsky R. The role of the hippocampus in feedback regulation of the hypothalamic-pituitary-adrenocortical axis. Endocr Rev 1991;12:118–34.

[24] Lentjes EG, Romijn F, Maassen RJ, et al. Free cortisol in serum assayed by temperature-controlled ultrafiltration before fluorescence polarization immunoassay. Clin Chem 1993; 39:2518–21.

[25] Yates FE, Leeman SE, Glenister DW, et al. Interaction between plasma corticosterone concentration and adrenocorticotropin-releasing stimuli in the rat: evidence for the reset of an endocrine feedback control. Endocrinology 1961;69:67–80.

[26] Fruchter O, Kino T, Zoumakis E, et al. The human glucocorticoid receptor (GR) isoform {beta} differentially suppresses GR{alpha}-induced transactivation stimulated by synthetic glucocorticoids. J Clin Endocrinol Metab 2005;90:3505–9.

[27] Kotelevtsev Y, Holmes MC, Burchell A, et al. 11beta-hydroxysteroid dehydrogenase type 1 knockout mice show attenuated glucocorticoid-inducible responses and resist hyperglycemia on obesity or stress. Proc Natl Acad Sci USA 1997;94:14924–9.

[28] Wust S, Van Rossum EF, Federenko IS, et al. Common polymorphisms in the glucocorticoid receptor gene are associated with adrenocortical responses to psychosocial stress. J Clin Endocrinol Metab 2004;89:565–73.

[29] Stevens A, Ray DW, Zeggini E, et al. Glucocorticoid sensitivity is determined by a specific glucocorticoid receptor haplotype. J Clin Endocrinol Metab 2004;89:892–7.

[30] Yau JL, Noble J, Kenyon CJ, et al. Lack of tissue glucocorticoid reactivation in 11beta-hydroxysteroid dehydrogenase type 1 knockout mice ameliorates age-related learning impairments. Proc Natl Acad Sci USA 2001;98:4716–21.

[31] Parker CR Jr, Rush AJ, MacDonald PC. Serum concentrations of deoxycorticosterone in women during the luteal phase of the ovarian cycle are not suppressed by dexamethasone treatment. J Steroid Biochem 1983;19:1313–7.

[32] Selye H. Compensatory atrophy of the adrenals. JAMA 1940;115:2246–52.

[33] Wellhoener P, Born J, Fehm HL, et al. Elevated resting and exercise-induced cortisol levels after mineralocorticoid receptor blockade with canrenoate in healthy humans. J Clin Endocrinol Metab 2004;89:5048–52.

[34] Gaillard RC, Riondel A, Muller AF, et al. RU 486: a steroid with antiglucocorticosteroid activity that only disinhibits the human pituitary-adrenal system at a specific time of day. Proc Natl Acad Sci USA 1984;81:3879–82.

[35] Erkut ZA, Pool C, Swaab DF. Glucocorticoids suppress corticotropin-releasing hormone and vasopressin expression in human hypothalamic neurons. J Clin Endocrinol Metab 1998;83:2066–73.

[36] Herman JP, Schafer MK, Young EA, et al. Evidence for hippocampal regulation of neuroendocrine neurons of the hypothalamo-pituitary-adrenocortical axis. J Neurosci 1989;9: 3072–82.

[37] Rubin RT, Mandell AJ, Crandall PH. Corticosteroid responses to limbic stimulation in man: localization of stimulus sites. Science 1966;153:767–8.

[38] Burke ZD, Ho MY, Morgan H, et al. Repression of vasopressin gene expression by gluco-corticoids in transgenic mice: evidence of a direct mechanism mediated by proximal 5′ flanking sequence. Neurosci 1997;78:1177–85.

[39] Van LP, Spengler DH, Holsboer F. Glucocorticoid repression of 3′,5′-cyclic-adenosine monophosphate-dependent human corticotropin-releasing-hormone gene promoter activity in a transfected mouse anterior pituitary cell line. Endocrinology 1990;127:1412–8.

[40] Giguere V, Labrie F, Cote J, et al. Stimulation of cyclic AMP accumulation and corticotropin release by synthetic ovine corticotropin-releasing factor in rat anterior pituitary cells: site of glucocorticoid action. Proc Natl Acad Sci USA 1982;79:3466–9.

[41] Loose DS, Do YS, Chen TL, et al. Demonstration of glucocorticoid receptors in the adrenal cortex: evidence for a direct dexamethasone suppressive effect on the rat adrenal gland. Endocrinology 1980;107:137–46.

[42] McEwen BS. Non-genomic and genomic effects of steroids on neural activity. Trends Pharmacol Sci 1991;12:141–7.

[43] Jones MT, Tiptaft EM, Brush FR. Evidence for dual corticosteroid-receptor mechanisms in the feedback control of adrenocorticotrophin secretion. J Endocrinol 1974;60:223–33.

[44] Watts AG, Tanimura S, Sanchez-Watts G. Corticotropin-releasing hormone and arginine vasopressin gene transcription in the hypothalamic paraventricular nucleus of unstressed rats: daily rhythms and their interactions with corticosterone. Endocrinology 2004;145: 529–40.

[45] Charlton BG. Adrenal cortical innervation and glucocorticoid secretion. J Endocrinol 1990;126:5–8.

[46] Saito M, Sugimoto T, Tahara A, et al. Molecular cloning and characterization of rat V1b vasopressin receptor: evidence for its expression in extra-pituitary tissues. Biochem Biophys Res Commun 1995;212:751–7.

[47] Preti A. CRF antagonists Dupont. Curr Opin Investig Drugs 2001;2:274–9.

[48] Habib KE, Weld KP, Rice KC, et al. Oral administration of a corticotropin-releasing hormone receptor antagonist significantly attenuates behavioral, neuroendocrine, and autonomic responses to stress in primates. Proc Natl Acad Sci USA 2000;97:6079–84.

[49] Serradeil-Le Gal C, Derick S, Brossard G, et al. Functional and pharmacological characterization of the first specific agonist and antagonist for the V1b receptor in mammals. Stress 2003;6:199–206.

[50] Davis ME, Pemberton CJ, Yandle TG, et al. Urocortin-1 infusion in normal humans. J Clin Endocrinol Metab 2004;89:1402–9.

[51] Slaunwhite WR Jr, Lockie GN, Back N, et al. Inactivity in vivo of transcortin-bound cortisol. Science 1962;135:1062–3.

[52] Schwarz S, Pohl P. Steroid hormones and steroid hormone binding globulins in cerebrospinal fluid studied in individuals with intact and with disturbed blood-cerebrospinal fluid barrier. Neuroendocrinology 1992;55:174–82.

[53] Viau V, Sharma S, Meaney MJ. Changes in plasma adrenocorticotropin, corticosterone, corticosteroid-binding globulin, and hippocampal glucocorticoid receptor occupancy/translocation in rat pups in response to stress. J Neuroendocrinol 1996;8:1–8.

[54] Kawai A, Yates FE. Interference with feedback inhibition of adrenocorticotropin release by protein binding of corticosterone. Endocrinology 1966;79:1040–6.

[55] Vogeser M, Groetzner J, Kupper C, et al. Free serum cortisol during the postoperative acute phase response determined by equilibrium dialysis liquid chromatography-tandem mass spectrometry. Clin Chem Lab Med 2003;41:146–51.

[56] Kraan GPB, Dullaart RPF, Pratt JJ, et al. The daily cortisol production reinvestigated in healthy men: the serum and urinary cortisol production rates are not significantly different. J Clin Endocrinol Metab 1998;83:1247–52.

[57] Bright GM. Corticosteroid-binding globulin influences kinetic parameters of plasma cortisol transport and clearance. J Clin Endocrinol Metab 1995;80:770–5.

[58] de Lacerda L, Kowarski A, Migeon CJ. Diurnal variation of the metabolic clearance rate of cortisol: effect on measurement of cortisol production rate. J Clin Endocrinol Metab 1973; 36:1043–9.

[59] Fernandez-Real JM, Pugeat M, Grasa M, et al. Serum corticosteroid-binding globulin concentration and insulin resistance syndrome: a population study. J Clin Endocrinol Metab 2002;87:4686–90.

[60] Besser GM, Orth DN, Nicholson WE, et al. Dissociation of the disappearance of bioactive and radioimmunoreactive ACTH from plasma in man. J Clin Endocrinol Metab 1971;32: 595–603.

[61] Iranmanesh A, Lizarralde G, Veldhuis JD. Coordinate activation of the corticotropic axis by insulin-induced hypoglycemia: simultaneous estimates of B-endorphin, ACTH, and cortisol secretion and disappearance in normal men. Acta Endocrinol (Copenh) 1993;128: 521–8.

[62] Iranmanesh A, Short D, Lizarralde G, et al. Intensive venous sampling paradigms disclose high-frequency ACTH release episodes in normal men. J Clin Endocrinol Metab 1990;71: 1276–83.

[63] Veldhuis JD, Iranmanesh A, Johnson ML, et al. Amplitude, but not frequency, modulation of ACTH secretory bursts gives rise to the nyctohemeral rhythm of the corticotropic axis in man. J Clin Endocrinol Metab 1990;71:452–63.

[64] Veldhuis JD, Iranmanesh A, Naftolowitz D, et al. Corticotropin secretory dynamics in humans under low glucocorticoid feedback. J Clin Endocrinol Metab 2001;86:5554–63.

[65] Keenan DM, Roelfsema F, Biermasz N, et al. Physiological control of pituitary hormone secretory-burst mass, frequency and waveform: a statistical formulation and analysis. Am J Physiol 2003;285:R664–73.

[66] Pincus SM, Singer BH. Randomness and degrees of irregularity. Proc Natl Acad Sci USA 1996;93:2083–8.

[67] Pincus SM, Hartman ML, Roelfsema F, et al. Hormone pulsatility discrimination via coarse and short time sampling. Am J Physiol 1999;277:E948–57.

[68] Liu PY, Pincus SM, Keenan DM, et al. Analysis of bidirectional pattern synchrony of concentration-secretion pairs: implementation in the human testicular and adrenal axes. Am J Physiol Regul Integr Comp 2005;288:R440–6.

[69] Roelfsema F, Pincus SM, Veldhuis JD. Patients with Cushing's disease secrete adrenocorticotropin and cortisol jointly more asynchronously than healthy subjects. J Clin Endocrinol Metab 1998;83:688–92.

[70] Pincus SM, Veldhuis JD, Mulligan T, et al. Effects of age on the irregularity of LH and FSH serum concentrations in women and men. Am J Physiol 1997;273:E989–95.

[71] Friend K, Iranmanesh A, Veldhuis JD. The orderliness of the growth hormone (GH) release process and the mean mass of GH secreted per burst are highly conserved in individual men on successive days. J Clin Endocrinol Metab 1996;81:3746–53.

[72] Waltman C, Blackman MR, Chrousos GP, et al. Spontaneous and glucocorticoid-inhibited adrenocorticotropin hormone and cortisol secretion are similar in healthy young and old men. J Clin Endocrinol Metab 1991;73:495–502.

[73] Van Cauter E, Leproult R, Kupfer DJ. Effects of gender and age on the levels and circadian rhythmicity of plasma cortisol. J Clin Endocrinol Metab 1996;81:2468–73.

[74] Bergendahl M, Iranmanesh A, Mulligan T, et al. Impact of age on cortisol secretory dynamics basally and as driven by nutrient-withdrawal stress. J Clin Endocrinol Metab 2000;85: 2203–14.

[75] Purnell JQ, Brandon DD, Isabelle LM, et al. Association of 24-hour cortisol production rates, cortisol-binding globulin, and plasma-free cortisol levels with body composition, leptin levels, and aging in adult men and women. J Clin Endocrinol Metab 2004;89:281–7.

[76] Bergendahl M, Vance ML, Iranmanesh A, et al. Fasting as a metabolic stress paradigm selectively amplifies cortisol secretory burst mass and delays the time of maximal nyctohemeral cortisol concentrations in healthy men. J Clin Endocrinol Metab 1996;81:692–9.

[77] Friedman M, Green MF, Sharland DE. Assessment of hypothalamic-pituitary-adrenal function in the geriatric age group. J Gerontol 1969;24:292–7.

[78] Muggeo M, Fedele D, Tiengo A, et al. Human growth hormone and cortisol response to insulin stimulation in aging. J Gerontol 1975;30:546–51.

[79] Blichert-Toft M, Hummer L. Serum immunoreactive corticotrophin and response to metyrapone in old age in man. Gerontology 1977;23:236–43.

[80] Casale G, Pecorini M, Cuzzoni G, et al. Beta-endorphin and cold pressor test in the aged. Gerontology 1985;31:101–5.

[81] Jensen HK, Blichert-Toft M. Serum corticotrophin, plasma cortisol and urinary excretion of 17-ketogenic steroids in the elderly (age group: 66–94 years). Acta Endocrinol (Copenh) 1971;66:25–34.

[82] West CD, Brown H, Simons EL, et al. Adrenocortical function and cortisol metabolism in old age. J Clin Endocrinol Metab 1961;21:1197–207.

[83] Born J, Ditschunet I, Schreiber M, et al. Effects of age and gender on pituitary-adrenocortical responsiveness in humans. Eur J Endocrinol 1995;132:705–11.

[84] Gotthardt U, Schweiger U, Fahrenberg J, et al. Cortisol, ACTH, and cardiovascular response to a cognitive challenge paradigm in aging and depression. Am J Physiol 1995; 268:R865–73.

[85] Born J, Ditschuneit I, Schreiber M, et al. Effects of age and gender on pituitary-adrenocortical responsiveness in humans. Eur J Endocrinol 1995;132:705–11.

[86] Heuser IJ, Gotthardt U, Schweiger U, et al. Age-associated changes of pituitary-adrenocortical hormone regulation in humans: importance of gender. Neurobiol Aging 1994;15: 227–31.

[87] Ambrosio MR, Campo M, Zatelli MC, et al. Unexpected activation of pituitary-adrenal axis in healthy young and elderly subjects during somatostatin infusion. Neuroendocrinology 1998;68:123–8.

[88] Kudielka BM, Buske-Kirschbaum A, Hellhammer DH, et al. HPA axis responses to laboratory psychosocial stress in healthy elderly adults, younger adults, and children: impact of age and gender. Psychoneuroendocrinology 2004;29:83–98.

[89] Seeman TE, Singer B, Charpentier P. Gender differences in patterns of HPA axis response to challenge: Macarthur studies of successful aging. Psychoneuroendocrinol 1995;20:711–25.

[90] Gelfin Y, Lerer B, Lesch KP, et al. Complex effects of age and gender on hypothermic, adrenocorticotrophic hormone and cortisol responses to ipsapirone challenge in normal subjects. Psychopharmacology (Berl) 1995;120:356–64.

[91] Sapolsky RM, Krey LC, McEwen BS. The adrenocortical axis in the aged rat: impaired sensitivity to both fast and delayed feedback inhibition. Neurobiol Aging 1986;7:331–5.

[92] O'Brien JT, Schweitzer I, Ames D, et al. Cortisol suppression by dexamethasone in the healthy elderly: effects of age, dexamethasone levels, and cognitive function. Biol Psychiatry 1994;36:389–94.

[93] Oxenkrug GF, Pomara N, McIntyre IM, et al. Aging and cortisol resistance to suppression by dexamethasone: a positive correlation. Psychiatry Res 1983;10:125–30.

[94] Wilkinson CW, Peskind ER, Raskind MA. Decreased hypothalamic-pituitary-adrenal axis sensitivity to cortisol feedback inhibition in human aging. Neuroendocrinology 1997;65: 79–90.

[95] Boscaro M, Paoletta A, Scarpa E, et al. Age-related changes in glucocorticoid fast feedback inhibition of adrenocorticotropin in man. J Clin Endocrinol Metab 1998;83:1380–3.

[96] Reynolds RM, Walker BR, Syddall HE, et al. Is there a gender difference in the associations of birthweight and adult hypothalamic-pituitary-adrenal axis activity? Eur J Endocrinol 2005;152:249–53.

[97] Otte C, Hart S, Neylan TC, et al. A meta-analysis of cortisol response to challenge in human aging: importance of gender. Psychoneuroendocrinology 2005;30:80–91.

[98] Arai Y, Gorski RA. Critical exposure time for androgenization of the developing hypothalamus in the female rat. Endocrinology 1968;82:1010–4.

[99] Seale JV, Wood SA, Atkinson HC, et al. Organisational role for testosterone and estrogen on adult HPA axis activity in the male rat. Endocrinology 2005;146:1973–82.

[100] Vamvakopoulos NC, Chrousos GP. Evidence of direct estrogenic regulation of human corticotropin-releasing hormone gene expression: potential implications for the sexual dimorphism of the stress response and immune/inflammatory reaction. J Clin Invest 1993;92: 1896–902.

[101] Peiffer A, Lapointe B, Barden N. Hormonal regulation of type II glucocorticoid receptor messenger ribonucleic acid in rat brain. Endocrinology 1991;129:2166–74.

[102] Peiffer A, Barden N. Estrogen-induced decrease of glucocorticoid receptor messenger ribonucleic acid concentration in rat anterior pituitary gland. Mol Endocrinol 1987;1:435–40.

[103] Kirschbaum C, Schommer N, Federenko I, et al. Short-term estradiol treatment enhances pituitary-adrenal axis and sympathetic responses to psychosocial stress in healthy young men. J Clin Endocrinol Metab 1996;81:3639–43.

[104] Bao AM, Hestiantoro A, Van Someren EJ, et al. Colocalization of corticotropin-releasing hormone and oestrogen receptor-{alpha} in the paraventricular nucleus of the hypothalamus in mood disorders. Brain 2005;128:1301–13.

[105] Horrocks PM, Jones AF, Ratcliffe WA, et al. Patterns of ACTH and cortisol pulsatility over twenty-four hours in normal males and females. Clin Endocrinol (Oxf) 1990;32: 127–34.

[106] Tse WS, Bond AJ. Sex differences in cortisol response to reboxetine. J Psychopharmacol 2005;19:46–50.

[107] Polderman KH, Gooren LJ, Van der Veen EA. Testosterone administration increases adrenal response to adrenocorticotrophin. Clin Endocrinol (Oxf) 1994;40:595–601.

[108] Clark PM, Neylon I, Raggatt PR, et al. Defining the normal cortisol response to the short Synacthen test: implications for the investigation of hypothalamic-pituitary disorders. Clin Endocrinol (Oxf) 1998;49:287–92.

[109] Wagner CK, Morrell JI. Distribution and steroid hormone regulation of aromatase mRNA expression in the forebrain of adult male and female rats: a cellular-level analysis using in situ hybridization. J Comp Neurol 1996;370:71–84.

[110] Hassan AH, Patchev VK, von Rosenstiel P, et al. Plasticity of hippocampal corticosteroid receptors during aging in the rat. FASEB J 1999;13:115–22.

[111] Issa AM, Rowe W, Gauthier S, et al. Hypothalamic-pituitary-adrenal activity in aged, cognitively impaired and cognitively unimpaired rats. J Neurosci 1990;10:3247–54.

[112] Rothuizen J, Reul JM, van Sluijs FJ, et al. Increased neuroendocrine reactivity and decreased brain mineralocorticoid receptor-binding capacity in aged dogs. Endocrinology 1993;132:161–8.

[113] Sapolsky RM, Krey LC, McEwen BS. Prolonged glucocorticoid exposure reduces hippocampal neuron number: implications for aging. J Neurosci 1985;5:1222–7.

[114] Seeman TE, McEwen BS, Singer BH, et al. Increase in urinary cortisol excretion and memory declines: MacArthur studies of successful aging. J Clin Endocrinol Metab 1997;82: 2458–65.

[115] Veldhuis JD, Iranmanesh A, Keenan DM. An ensemble perspective of aging-related hypoandrogenemia in men. In: Winters SJ, editor. Male hypogonadism: basic, clinical, and theoretical principles. Totowa (NJ): Humana Press; 2004. p. 261–84.

[116] Rivier C, Vale W. Corticotropin-releasing factor (CRF) acts centrally to inhibit growth hormone secretion in the rat. Endocrinology 1984;114:2409–11.

ELSEVIER
SAUNDERS

Endocrinol Metab Clin N Am
34 (2005) 1015–1030

ENDOCRINOLOGY
AND METABOLISM
CLINICS
OF NORTH AMERICA

Pathophysiology of Age-Related Bone Loss and Osteoporosis

Sundeep Khosla, MD*, B. Lawrence Riggs, MD

*Division of Endocrinology, Metabolism, and Nutrition,
Mayo Clinic College of Medicine, Rochester, MN, USA*

Aging is associated with significant bone loss in women and in men [1]. Fig. 1, which draws on numerous cross-sectional and longitudinal studies using areal bone mineral density (aBMD) by dual energy x-ray absorptiometry (DXA), depicts the overall pattern of bone loss in both sexes. The menopause in women is associated with a rapid loss of trabecular bone, as is present in the vertebrae, pelvis, and ultra-distal forearm. There is a less dramatic loss of cortical bone (present in the long bones of the body and as a thin rim around the vertebrae and other sites of trabecular bone) following the menopause. Approximately 8 to 10 years following menopause, slow, age-related phase of bone loss in trabecular and cortical bone becomes apparent and continues throughout life. Because men lack the equivalent of a menopause, they generally do not exhibit this rapid phase of bone loss. Men, however, have a very similar pattern of slow, age-related bone loss as is present in women.

Although DXA has provided important insights into the patterns of age-related bone loss, its utility is limited by the fact that it cannot clearly separate trabecular from cortical bone or provide information on possible changes in bone size/geometry with age. In recent studies, Riggs and colleagues [2] used central and peripheral quantitative CT (QCT) along with new image analysis software [3] to better define age-associated changes in bone volumetric density, geometry, and structure at different skeletal sites. As shown in Fig. 2, there were large decreases in volumetric BMD (vBMD) at the spine over life (predominantly trabecular bone), which

---

This work was supported by Grants AG004875 and AR027065 from the National Institutes of Health.

* Corresponding author. Division of Endocrinology, Metabolism, and Nutrition, Mayo Clinic College of Medicine, 200 First Street Southwest, Rochester, MN 55905.

E-mail address: khosla.sundeep@mayo.edu (S. Khosla).

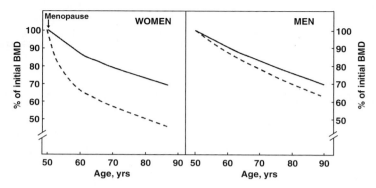

Fig. 1. Patterns of age-related bone loss in women and in men. Dashed lines represent trabecular bone and solid lines, cortical bone. The figure is based on multiple cross-sectional and longitudinal studies using DXA.

seemed to begin even before middle life. These decreases were greater in women (approximately 55%) than in men (approximately 45%, $P <$ .001). Even in this cross-sectional study, there was an apparent small midlife acceleration in the slope of the decrease in women that accounted for much of their significantly greater decrease in vertebral vBMD over life compared with men. In contrast to this pattern of changes in trabecular vBMD at the spine, cortical vBMD at the radius showed little change until midlife in either women or men (see Fig. 2). Thereafter, there were linear decreases in both sexes, but the decreases were greater in women (28%) than in men

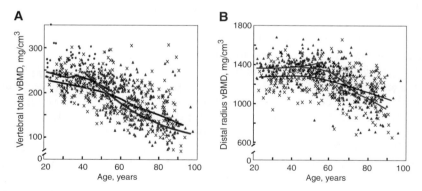

Fig. 2. (A) Values for vBMD (mg/cm3) of the total vertebral body in a population sample of Rochester, Minn., women and men between the ages of 20 and 97 years. Individual values and smoother lines are given for premenopausal women in red, for postmenopausal women in blue, and for men in black. (B) Values for cortical vBMD at the distal radius in the same cohort. Color code is as in (A). All changes with age were significant ($P < .05$). (*Reproduced from* Riggs BL, Melton LJ 3rd, Robb RA, et al. A population-based study of age and sex differences in bone volumetric density, size, geometry, and structure at different skeletal sites. J Bone Miner Res 2004;19:1950; with permission.)

(18%, P < .001). Aging also was associated with increases in bone cross-sectional area at various sites because of continued periosteal apposition throughout life. Bone marrow space, however, increased even more because of ongoing bone resorption. Thus, because endocortical resorption increased even more than periosteal apposition, there was a net decrease in cortical area and thickness [2]. This process, however, also resulted in outward displacement of the cortex, which increased the strength of bone to bending stresses and partially offset the decrease in bone strength resulting from decreased cortical area.

These age-associated changes in bone mass and structure lead, in turn, to a marked increase in the incidence of osteoporotic fractures in both sexes. As shown in Fig. 3, distal forearm (Colles) fractures increase sharply in women soon after menopause and then plateau after 10 to 15 years postmenopausally. The increase in incidence of vertebral fractures after menopause is more gradual but, in contrast to Colles' fractures, vertebral fractures continue to increase throughout life. The rise in hip fractures follows that in vertebral fractures, and hip fractures increase markedly late in life. Men do not appear to have a measurable increase in Colles' fractures with age (see Fig. 3), which may, in part, be because of their larger bones. With increasing age, however, there is a clear increase in the incidence of vertebral and hip fractures in men, although the onset of these fractures is delayed by about 10 years as compared with women, likely because of the absence of menopause and the associated accelerated bone loss present in women.

Based on these types of data, it has been estimated that 4 out of every 10 white women aged 50 years or older in the United States will experience a hip, spine, or wrist fracture sometime during the remainder of their lives; 13% of white men in this country also will suffer one of these fractures [4].

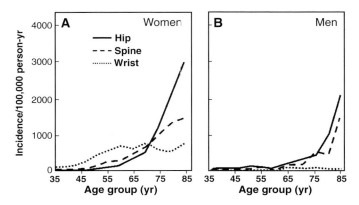

Fig. 3. Age-specific incidence rates for proximal femur (hip), vertebral (spine). and distal forearm (wrist) fractures in Rochester, Minnesota, women (A) and men (B). (*Adapted from* Cooper C, Melton LJ. Epidemiology of osteoporosis. Trends Endocrinol Metab 1992;3:225; with permission.)

Although the risk of these fractures is lower in nonwhite women and men, it remains substantial. Collectively, osteoporotic fractures result in a significant financial burden on society, with estimated direct care expenditures of $12.2 to $17.9 billion each year, measured in 2002 dollars [5].

Pathogenesis of age-related bone loss in women

Menopause triggers a rapid phase of bone loss in women that can be prevented by estrogen replacement [6,7] and clearly results from loss of ovarian function. During the menopausal transition, serum estradiol levels fall to 10% to 15% of the premenopausal level, although levels of serum estrone, a fourfold weaker estrogen, fall to about 25% to 35% of the premenopausal level [8]. Serum testosterone levels also decrease following the menopause [9] although to a lesser extent, since testosterone continues to be produced by the adrenal cortex and by the ovarian interstitium. Bone resorption, as assessed by biochemical markers, increases by 90% at menopause, whereas bone formation markers increase by only 45% [10]. This imbalance between bone resorption and bone formation leads to accelerated bone loss. The rapid bone loss in this phase produces an increased outflow of calcium from bone into the extracellular pool, but hypercalcemia is prevented by compensatory increases in urinary calcium excretion [11], decreases in intestinal calcium absorption [12], and by a partial suppression of parathyroid hormone (PTH) secretion [13].

The cellular and molecular mechanisms by which estrogen mediates its effects on bone resorption are being worked out. Fig. 4 provides summarizes the cellular and molecular factors involved in osteoclast differentiation and function. The key, essential molecule for osteoclast development is the receptor activator of NF-κB ligand (RANKL) [14], which is expressed on the surface of bone marrow stromal/osteoblast precursor cells, T cells, and B cells [15]. RANKL binds its cognate receptor, RANK, on osteoclast lineage cells [16], and is neutralized by the soluble, decoy receptor osteoprotegerin (OPG), which also is produced by osteoblastic lineage cells [17]. Combined in vitro and in vivo studies have demonstrated that estrogen suppresses RANKL production by osteoblastic, T cells, and B cells [15] and also increases OPG production [18,19]. In addition to the effects of estrogen on RANKL and OPG expression, estrogen also regulates production of additional cytokines in osteoblasts or bone marrow mononuclear cells, thus modulating osteoclastic activity in a paracrine fashion [20]. There is an increasing body of evidence that bone-resorbing cytokines, such as interleukin (IL)-1, IL-6, tumor necrosis factor-α (TNF-α), macrophage colony-stimulating factor (M-CSF), and prostaglandins may be potential candidates for mediating the bone loss following estrogen deficiency. IL-1 and M-CSF production are increased in estrogen-deficient model systems [21,22]; this can be inhibited using specific antagonists [23–25]. Additionally, the

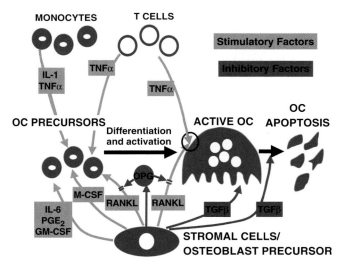

Fig. 4. Summary of stimulatory and inhibitory factors involved in osteoclast development and apoptosis.

bone resorptive effects of TNF-α are documented and can be reversed using a soluble type I TNF receptor [26]. Numerous other studies indicate that IL-6 plays a key role in mediating bone loss following estrogen deficiency [27,28]. It is likely, however, that, in vivo, multiple cytokines act cooperatively in inducing bone resorption following sex steroid deficiency, and that a single cytokine may account only partially for the effects of sex steroid deficiency on the skeleton. Finally, in addition to suppressing the production of proresorptive cytokines, estrogen also stimulates production of transforming growth factor (TGF)-β by osteoblastic cells [29]. TGF-β, in turn, has been shown to induce apoptosis of osteoclasts [30]. Estrogen also has direct effects on osteoclast lineage cells. Thus, it induces apoptosis of these cells [30] and can suppress RANKL-induced osteoclast differentiation by blocking RANKL/M-CSF-induced activator protein-1-dependent transcription through a reduction of c-jun activity [31,32]. The latter is caused by reduced c-jun expression and decreased phosphorylation. Moreover, estrogen also has been shown to inhibit the activity of mature osteoclasts through direct, receptor-mediated mechanisms [33].

Loss of these multiple actions of estrogen on restraining bone resorption thus triggers the rapid phase of bone loss, which generally subsides after 4 to 8 years. It has been suggested that estrogen deficiency alters the sensing of mechanical loading by the skeleton, perhaps through effects on osteocytes in bone [34]. Thus, for a given level of mechanical loading, bone mass may be perceived by these cells as being excessive in the setting of estrogen deficiency, leading to bone loss. Once sufficient bone is lost, however, increased mechanical loading on the remaining bone may serve to limit additional bone loss, accounting for the cessation of the rapid phase of bone loss following estrogen deficiency.

In contrast to the trend for suppression of PTH levels during the rapid phase of bone loss, the late, slow phase of bone loss is associated with progressive increases in levels of serum PTH and in biochemical markers of bone turnover. These increases correlate with each other [13]. Moreover, when serum PTH levels were suppressed by a 24-hour calcium infusion in groups of young premenopausal and elderly postmenopausal women, the increases in biochemical markers in the postmenopausal women that were present on the control day were no longer present in the calcium infusion day, strongly suggesting that the increased serum PTH was the cause of the increase in bone turnover [35].

The increase in serum PTH with age represents secondary hyperparathyroidism, which likely has multiple etiologies. Certainly, vitamin D deficiency is common in elderly women [36] and leads to increases in PTH levels. In addition, however, it appears that longstanding estrogen deficiency may lead to chronic negative calcium balance because of loss of effects of estrogen on enhancing intestinal calcium absorption [12,37] and renal tubular calcium reabsorption [38,39]. It appears that unless this negative calcium balance is compensated for by very large increases in dietary calcium intake, it will result in secondary hyperparathyroidism and will contribute to the slow phase of bone loss.

In addition to increases in bone resorption, estrogen deficiency and aging are associated with impaired compensatory bone formation. The latter generally has been attributed to age-related factors, particularly to decreases in paracrine production of growth factors [40] or to decreases in circulating levels of growth hormone [41,42] and insulin-like growth factor (IGF)-I [43–45]. If estrogen stimulates bone formation, however, postmenopausal estrogen deficiency could be a contributing cause. Indeed, impaired bone formation becomes apparent soon after menopause [46]. Estrogen increases production of IGF-I [47], TGF-β [29], and procollagen synthesis by osteoblastic cells in vitro [47] and increases osteoblast life span by decreasing osteoblast apoptosis [48,49]. Direct evidence that estrogen can stimulate bone formation after cessation of skeletal growth was provided by Khastgir and colleagues [50], who obtained iliac biopsies for histomorphometry in 22 elderly women (mean age of 65 years) before and 6 years after percutaneous administration of high dosages of estrogen. They found a 61% increase in cancellous bone volume and a 12% increase in the wall thickness of trabecular packets. Tobias and Compston [51] have reported similar results. It is unclear whether these results represent only pharmacologic effects or are an augmentation of physiologic effects of estrogen that are ordinarily not large enough to detect. Thus, accumulating data implicate estrogen deficiency as a contributing cause of decreased bone formation with aging. Still, there is not a clear consensus on whether estrogen stimulates osteoblast function, and, if it does, what is the relative contribution of increased proliferation function and decreased apoptosis.

Pathogenesis of age-related bone loss in men

Although osteoporosis is more common in women, men lose half as much bone with aging and have one third as many fragility fractures as women [13]. Because most men do not develop overt hypogonadism with aging, the prevailing opinion has been that sex steroid deficiency is not a major cause of age-related bone loss in men. It now is clear, however, that the failure of earlier studies to find major decreases in serum levels of total sex steroids was caused by the fact that they did not account for the confounding effect of a greater than twofold age-related rise in levels of serum sex hormone-binding globulin (SHBG) [52]. It generally is believed that circulating sex steroids that are bound to SHBG have restricted access to target tissues, whereas the 1% to 3% fraction that is free and the 35% to 55% fraction that is bound loosely to albumin are readily accessible. Although there are various methods to assess the bioavailable or non–SHBG-bound sex steroids, several groups have reported substantial decreases in serum levels of free or bioavailable sex steroid levels with aging [52,53]. Data from a population of 346 men from Rochester, Minn., are shown in Table 1. The precise cause of the age-related increase in serum SHBG levels and the failure of the hypothalamic-pituitary-testicular axis to compensate for this and maintain free or bioavailable sex steroids at young normal levels is unclear and the focus of ongoing studies.

As shown in Table 1, aging is associated with substantial decreases in bioavailable testosterone and estrogen levels. The traditional notion had been that because testosterone is the major sex steroid in men, it was the decrease in bioavailable testosterone levels that would be associated most closely with bone loss in men. The initial attempts to address this issue came from

Table 1
Changes in serum sex steroids and gonadotropins over life in a random sample of 346 men (Rochester, MN) aged 23–90 years

Hormone	Percent change*
Bioavailable estrogen	−47
Bioavailable testosterone	−64
SHBG	+124
Luteinizing hormone	+285
Follicle-stimulating hormone	+505

  * $P < 0.005$.
  Adapted from Khosla S, Melton LJI, Atkinson EJ, et al. Relationship of serum sex steroid levels and bone turnover markers with bone mineral density in men and women: a key role for bioavailable estrogen. J Clin Endocrinol Metab 1998;83:2268; with permission.

cross-sectional observational studies in which sex steroid levels were related to BMD at various sites in cohorts of adult men. Slemenda and colleagues [54] found that BMD at various sites in 93 healthy men over age 55 years correlated with serum estradiol levels (correlation coefficients, depending on the site, of +0.21 to +0.35, $P = 0.01$ to 0.05) and, in fact, inversely with serum testosterone levels (correlation coefficients of -0.20 to -0.28, $P = 0.03$ to 0.10). Subsequent to this report, other similar cross-sectional studies have demonstrated significant positive associations between BMD and estrogen levels in men [52,53,55–59], particularly circulating bioavailable estradiol levels.

Although these findings are compatible with the hypothesis that estrogen plays an important role in maintaining bone mass in men, they suffer from two potential weaknesses. First, cross-sectional analyses cannot clearly dissociate the effects of estrogen to maintain or prevent bone loss from the effects of estrogen to achieve peak bone mass. For example, a particular individual with a relatively low bone mass at age 50 and low estradiol levels (relative to his age-matched peers) could have had life-long low estradiol levels going back to childhood. In this case, the low estradiol levels would reflect a deficiency in achieving peak bone mass, not necessarily an effect of estrogen to maintain or prevent bone loss. A second weakness of cross-sectional observational data is that correlation never proves causality.

To circumvent the first of these problems, Khosla and colleagues [60] studied, in a longitudinal manner, young (22 to 39 years) and older (60 to 90 years) men in whom rates of change in BMD at various sites over 4 years were related to sex steroid levels. These two different age groups permitted a separate comparison of the possible effects of estrogen on the final stages of skeletal maturation versus age-related bone loss. Forearm sites (distal radius and ulna) provided the clearest data, perhaps because of the greater precision of peripheral site measurements as compared with central sites such as the spine or hip. In the younger men, BMD at the forearm sites increased by 0.42% to 0.43% per year, whereas in the older men, BMD at these sites declined by 0.49% to 0.66% per year. Both the increase in BMD in the younger men and the decrease in BMD in the older men were associated with serum bioavailable estradiol levels more closely than with testosterone levels (Table 2). Moreover, further analysis of the data suggested that there may be a threshold bioavailable estradiol level of approximately 40 pmol/L (11 pg/mL), below which the rate of bone loss in the older men clearly was associated with bioavailable estradiol levels. Above this level, there did not appear to be any relationship between the rate of bone loss and bioavailable estradiol levels (Fig. 5). In these older men, the bioavailable estradiol level of 40 pmol/L (11 pg/mL) represented the median bioavailable estradiol level in these men and corresponded to a total estradiol level of approximately 114 pmol/L (31 pg/mL), which is close to the middle of the reported normal range for estradiol levels in men (10 to 50 pg/mL). Similar findings were reported by Gennari and

Table 2
Spearman correlation coefficients relating rates of change in bone mineral density at the radius and ulna to serum sex steroid levels among a sample of men (Rochester, MN) stratified by age

Spearman correlation coefficients	Young		Middle-aged		Elderly	
	Radius	Ulna	Radius	Ulna	Radius	Ulna
T	−0.02	−0.19	−0.18	−0.25*	0.13	0.14
E_2	0.33**	0.22*	0.03	0.07	0.21*	0.18*
E_1	0.35***	0.34**	0.17	0.23*	0.16	0.14
Bio T	0.13	−0.04	0.07	0.01	0.23**	0.27**
Bio E_2	0.30**	0.20	0.14	0.21*	0.29**	0.33***

Abbreviations: Bio, bioavailable; E_1, estrone; E_2, estradiol; T, testosterone.
* $P < 0.05$; ** $P < 0.01$; *** $P < 0.001$.
Reproduced from Khosla S, Melton LJ, Atkinson EJ, et al. Relationship of serum sex steroid levels to longitudinal changes in bone density in young versus elderly men. J Clin Endocrinol Metab 2001;86:3558; with permission.

colleagues [61], where, in a cohort of elderly Italian men, those subjects with serum free estradiol levels below the median value lost bone over 4 years at the lumbar spine and femur neck, whereas the men with free estradiol levels above the median did not lose bone.

Although these studies helped to establish that estrogen levels are associated with skeletal maintenance in males, they could not establish causal relationships definitively. To address this issue, Falahati-Nini and colleagues [62] performed a direct interventional study to distinguish between the relative contributions of estrogen versus testosterone in regulating bone

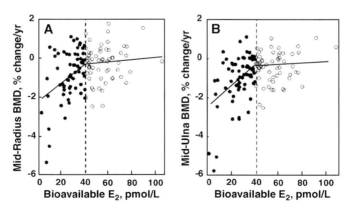

Fig. 5. Rate of change in midradius BMD (*A*) and midulna BMD (*B*) as a function of bioavailable estradiol levels in elderly men. Model R^2 values were 0.20 and 0.25 for the radius and ulna, respectively, both less than 0.001 for comparison with a one-slope model. Solid circles correspond to subjects with bioavailable estradiol levels below 40 pmol/L (11 pg/mL) and open circles those with values above 40 pmol/L. (*Reproduced from* Khosla S, Melton LJ 3rd, Atkinson EJ, et al. Relationship of serum sex steroid levels to longitudinal changes in bone density in young versus elderly men. J Clin Endocrinol Metab 2001;86(8):3558; with permission.)

resorption and formation in normal elderly men. Endogenous estrogen and testosterone production were suppressed in 59 elderly men using a combination of a long-acting gonadotropin-releasing hormone (GnRH) agonist and an aromatase inhibitor. Physiologic estrogen and testosterone levels were maintained by simultaneously placing the men on estrogen and testosterone patches delivering doses of sex steroids that mimicked circulating estradiol and testosterone levels in this age group. After baseline measurements of bone resorption (urinary deoxypyridinoline [Dpd] and N-telopeptide of type I collagen [NTx]) and bone formation (serum osteocalcin and amino–terminal propeptide of type I collagen [PINP]) markers, the subjects were randomized to one of four groups. Group A (−T, −E) discontinued both the testosterone and estrogen patches; group B (−T, +E) discontinued the testosterone patch but continued the estrogen patch. Group C (+T, −E) discontinued the estrogen patch but continued the estrogen patch, and group D (+T, +E) continued both patches. Because gonadal and aromatase blockade was continued throughout the 3-week period, separate effects of estrogen versus testosterone (in the absence of aromatization to estrogen) on bone metabolism could be delineated.

As shown in Fig. 6A, significant increases in both urinary Dpd and NTx excretion, (group A [−T, −E]), were prevented completely by continuing testosterone and estrogen replacement (group D [+T, +E]). Estrogen alone (group B) was almost completely able to prevent the increase in bone resorption, whereas testosterone alone (group C) was much less effective. Using a two-factor analysis of variance (ANOVA) model, the effects of estrogen on urinary Dpd and NTx excretion were highly significant ($P = .005$ and .0002, respectively). Estrogen accounted for 70% or more of the total effect of sex steroids on bone resorption in these older men, while testosterone could account for no more than 30% of the effect. Using a somewhat different design, Leder and colleagues [63] confirmed an independent effect of testosterone on bone resorption, although the data in the aggregate clearly favor a more prominent effect of estrogen for controlling bone resorption in men.

Fig. 6B shows the corresponding changes in the bone formation markers, serum osteocalcin and PINP. The reductions in both osteocalcin and PINP levels with the induction of sex steroid deficiency (group A) were prevented with continued estrogen and testosterone replacement (group D). Interestingly, serum osteocalcin, which is a marker of function of the mature osteoblast and osteocyte [64], was maintained by either estrogen or testosterone (ANOVA, $P = 0.002$ and 0.013, respectively). By contrast, serum PINP, which represents type I collagen synthesis throughout the various stages of osteoblast differentiation [64], was maintained by estrogen (ANOVA, $P = 0.0001$), but not testosterone.

Collectively, these findings provided conclusive proof of an important (and indeed, dominant) role for estrogen in bone metabolism in the mature skeleton of adult men. Similar findings were reported by Taxel colleagues

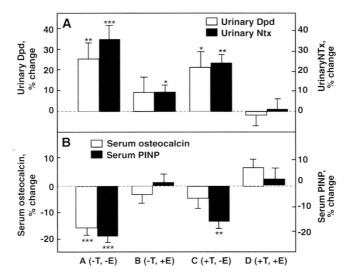

Fig. 6. Percent changes in (*A*) bone resorption markers (urinary deoxypyridinoline [Dpd] and N-telopeptide of type I collagen [NTx]) and (*B*) bone formation markers (serum osteocalcin and N-terminal extension peptide of type I collagen [PINP]) in a group of elderly men (mean age 68 years) made acutely hypogonadal and treated with an aromatase inhibitor (group A), treated with estrogen alone (group B), testosterone alone (group C), or both (group D). Significance for change from baseline: * *P* < .05; ** *P* < .01; *** *P* < .001. (*Adapted from* Falahati-Nini A, Riggs, BL, Atkinson EJ, et al. Relative contributions of testosterone and estrogen in regulating bone resorption and formation in normal elderly men. J Clin Invest 2000;106: 1556–7; with permission.)

[65] in a study of 15 elderly men treated with an aromatase inhibitor for 9 weeks. Suppression of estrogen production resulted in significant increases in bone resorption markers and a suppression of bone formation markers.

It appears, therefore, that similar to women, declining bioavailable estrogen levels in men may play a significant role in mediating age-related bone loss. Declining bioavailable testosterone levels may also contribute, however, because testosterone has some antiresorptive effects and is important for maintaining bone formation. Moreover, it provides the substrate for aromatization to estradiol. In addition, at least in rodents, testosterone has been shown to enhance periosteal apposition [66]. Because larger bones are more resistant to fracture, effects of testosterone on increasing bone size in men may provide important protection against fracture risk.

As in aging women, serum PTH levels also increase with age in men [13]. Because the higher ambient sex steroid levels in aging men as compared with elderly women may protect partially against the bone-resorbing effects of PTH, it has been more difficult to demonstrate a direct role for PTH in contributing to age-related increases in bone resorption in men [67]. Thus, while secondary hyperparathyroidism likely also contributes to age-related bone loss in men, the data in support of this are not as clear as in women.

Other factors contributing to age-related bone loss in both sexes

The previous discussion focused on the role of declining sex steroid and increasing serum PTH levels in the pathogenesis of bone loss in women and in men. Multiple other factors, however, also contribute to age-related bone loss. The role of vitamin D deficiency in aggravating the secondary hyperparathyroidism of aging has been noted. In addition, although declining sex steroid levels may contribute to the age-related impairment in bone formation, this may be caused by other, sex steroid-independent factors, such as intrinsic reductions in the production of key growth factors important for osteoblast differentiation/function. Also, aging decreases the amplitude and frequency of growth hormone secretion [42], which leads to decreased hepatic production of IGF-I. Indeed, serum IGF-I levels decrease markedly with age, and there are also smaller decreases in serum IGF-II levels [43,44]. Thus, decreased systemic and skeletal production of IGFs may contribute to decreases in bone formation with aging.

Other changes in endocrine function with aging appear to make smaller contributions to bone loss. Among the weak adrenal androgens, levels of serum dehydroepiandrosterone (DHEA) and dehydroepiandrosterone sulfate (DHEA-SO_4) decrease by about 80% [68]. Because cortisol secretion remains constant or increases throughout life, the decrease in adrenal androgenic steroids leads to an increase in the catabolic/anabolic ratio of circulating adrenal steroid hormones with aging that could contribute to bone loss.

Peak bone mass also contributes to the risk of osteoporotic fractures later in life. Thus, those persons who achieve a higher peak bone mass are less likely to develop osteoporosis as age-related bone loss ensues, whereas those with low levels are at greater risk [69]. In addition, numerous sporadic factors that affect some, but not other, members of the aging population may contribute to fracture risk in 40% of men and 20% of women [70]. These include use of drugs such as corticosteroids; diseases such as malabsorption, anorexia nervosa, and idiopathic hypercalciuria; and behavioral factors such as smoking, alcohol abuse, and inactivity.

Finally, age-related osteopenia and sarcopenia are parallel processes. Frost [71,72] has suggested that the loss of muscle mass with aging is the principal cause of age-related bone loss. Although this contention remains controversial, it is likely that age-related decreases in muscle loading on bone may contribute to age-related bone loss.

Summary

Age-related bone loss in women and in men is driven, in large part, by changes in sex steroid production or availability and by secondary hyperparathyroidism. Superimposed on these mechanisms, other factors such as vitamin D deficiency, intrinsic defects in osteoblast function, impairments in the growth hormone/IGF axis, reduced peak bone mass, age-associated sarcopenia, and various sporadic factors also contribute to bone loss and increased fracture risk in the elderly. An improved understanding of the relative importance of these various factors in the causation of bone loss should lead to enhanced preventive and therapeutic approaches for involutional osteoporosis, which, if left unchecked, is likely to impose an increasing health care burden on society.

References

[1] Riggs BL, Khosla S, Melton LJ. Sex steroids and the construction and conservation of the adult skeleton. Endocr Rev 2002;23:279–302.

[2] Riggs BL, Melton LJ III, Robb RA, et al. A population-based study of age and sex differences in bone volumetric density, size, geometry and structure at different skeletal sites. J Bone Miner Res 2004;19:1945–54.

[3] Camp JJ, Karwoski RA, Stacy MC, et al. A system for the analysis of whole bone strength from helical CT images. Proceedings of the International Society for Optical Engineering (SPIE) 2004;5369:74–88.

[4] Cummings SR, Melton LJ. Epidemiology and outcomes of osteoporotic fractures. Lancet 2002;359:1761–7.

[5] Tosteson AN, Hammond CS. Quality-of-life assessment in osteoporosis: health-status and preference-based measures. Pharmagenomics 2002;20:289–303.

[6] Lindsay R, Aitken JM, Anderson JB, et al. Long-term prevention of postmenopausal osteoporosis by oestrogen: evidence for an increased bone mass after delayed onset of oestrogen treatment. Lancet 1976;1:1038–41.

[7] Genant HK, Cann CE, Ettinger B, et al. Quantitative computed tomography of vertebral spongiosa: A sensitive method for detecting early bone loss after oophorectomy. Ann Intern Med 1982;97:699–705.

[8] Khosla SK, Atkinson EJ, Melton LJ III. Effects of age and estrogen status on serum parathyroid hormone levels and biochemical markers of bone turnover in women: a population-based study. J Clin Endocrinol Metab 1997;82:1522–7.

[9] Horton R, Romanoff E, Walker J. Androstenedione and testosterone in ovarian venous and peripheral plasma during ovariectomy for breast cancer. J Clin Endocrinol Metab 1966;26:1267–9.

[10] Garnero P, Sornay-Rendu E, Chapuy M, et al. Increased bone turnover in late postmenopausal women is a major determinant of osteoporosis. J Bone Miner Res 1996;11:337–49.

[11] Young MM, Nordin BEC. Effects of natural and artificial menopause on plasma and urinary calcium and phosphorus. Lancet 1967;2:118–20.

[12] Gennari C, Agnusdei D, Nardi P, et al. Estrogen preserves a normal intestinal responsiveness to 1,25-dihydroxyvitamin D3 in oophorectomized women. J Clin Endocrinol Metab 1990;71:1288–93.

[13] Riggs BL, Khosla S, Melton LJI. A unitary model for involutional osteoporosis: estrogen deficiency causes both type I and type II osteoporosis in postmenopausal women and contributes to bone loss in aging men. J Bone Miner Res 1998;13:763–73.

[14] Lacey DL, Timms E, Tan HL, et al. Osteoprotegerin ligand is a cytokine that regulates osteoclast differentiation and activation. Cell 1998;93:165–76.

[15] Eghbali-Fatourechi G, Khosla S, Sanyal A, et al. Role of RANK ligand in mediating increased bone resorption in early postmenopausal women. J Clin Invest 2003;111:1221–30.

[16] Hsu H, Lacey DL, Dunstan CR, et al. Tumor necrosis factor receptor family member RANK mediates osteoclast differentiation and activation induced by osteoprotegerin ligand. Proc Natl Acad Sci U S A 1999;96:3540–5.

[17] Simonet WS, Lacey DL, Dunstan CR, et al. Osteoprotegerin: a novel secreted protein involved in the regulation of bone density. Cell 1997;89:309–19.

[18] Hofbauer LC, Khosla S, Dunstan CR, et al. Estrogen stimulates gene expression and protein production of osteoprotegerin in human osteoblastic cells. Endocrinology 1999;140: 4367–70.

[19] Khosla S, Atkinson EJ, Dunstan CR, et al. Effect of estrogen versus testosterone on circulating osteoprotegerin and other cytokine levels in normal elderly men. J Clin Endocrinol Metab 2002;87:1550–4.

[20] Manolagas SC, Jilka RL. Bone marrow, cytokines, and bone remodeling: emerging insights into the pathophysiology of osteoporosis. N Engl J Med 1995;332:305–11.

[21] Pacifici R, Brown C, Puscheck E, et al. Effect of surgical menopause and estrogen replacement on cytokine release from human blood mononuclear cells. Proc Natl Acad Sci U S A 1991;88:5134–8.

[22] Tanaka S, Takahashi N, Udagawa N, et al. Macrophage colony-stimulating factor is indispensable for both proliferation and differentiation of osteoclast progenitors. J Clin Invest 1993;91:257–63.

[23] Kimble RB, Vannice JL, Bloedow DC, et al. Interleukin-1 receptor antagonist decreases bone loss and bone resorption in ovariectomized rats. J Clin Invest 1994;93:1959–67.

[24] Ammann P, Rizzoli R, Bonjour J, et al. Transgenic mice expressing soluble tumor necrosis factor-receptor are protected against bone loss caused by estrogen deficiency. J Clin Invest 1997;99:1699–703.

[25] Kimble RB, Srivastava S, Ross FP, et al. Estrogen deficiency increases the ability of stromal cells to support murine osteoclastogenesis via an interleukin-1-and tumor necrosis factor-mediated stimulation of macrophage colony-stimulating factor production. J Biol Chem 1996;271:28890–7.

[26] Kitazawa R, Kimble RB, Vannice JL, et al. Interleukin-1 receptor antagonist and tumor necrosis factor binding protein decrease osteoclast formation and bone resorption in ovariectomized mice. J Clin Invest 1994;94:2397–406.

[27] Girasole G, Jilka RL, Passeri G, et al. 17 beta-estradiol inhibits interleukin-6 production by bone marrow-derived stromal cells and osteoblasts in vitro: a potential mechanism for the antiosteoporotic effect of estrogens. J Clin Invest 1992;89:883–91.

[28] Jilka RL, Hangoc G, Girasole G, et al. Increased osteoclast development after estrogen loss: Mediation by interleukin-6. Science 1992;257:88–91.

[29] Oursler MJ, Cortese C, Keeting PE, et al. Modulation of transforming growth factor-beta production in normal human osteoblast-like cells by 17 beta-estradiol and parathyroid hormone. Endocrinology 1991;129:3313–20.

[30] Hughes DE, Dai A, Tiffee JC, et al. Estrogen promotes apoptosis of murine osteoclasts mediated by TGF-beta. Nat Med 1996;2:1132–6.

[31] Shevde NK, Bendixen AC, Dienger KM, et al. Estrogens suppress RANK ligand-induced osteoclast differentiation via a stromal cell independent mechanism involving c-Jun repression. Proc Natl Acad Sci U S A 2000;97:7829–34.

[32] Srivastava S, Toraldo G, Weitzmann MN, et al. Estrogen decreases osteoclast formation by down-regulating receptor activator of NF-kB ligand (RANKL)-induced JNK activation. J Biol Chem 2001;276:8836–40.

[33] Oursler MJ, Pederson L, Fitzpatrick L, et al. Human giant cell tumors of the bone (osteoclastomas) are estrogen target cells. Proc Natl Acad Sci U S A 1994;91:5227–31.

[34] Frost HM. On the estrogen-bone relationship and postmenopausal bone loss: a new model. J Bone Miner Res 1999;14(9):1473–7.

[35] Ledger GA, Burritt MF, Kao PC, et al. Role of parathyroid hormone in mediating nocturnal and age-related increases in bone resorption. J Clin Endocrinol Metab 1995;80:3304–10.

[36] Eastell R, Riggs BL. Vitamin D and osteoporosis. San Diego (CA): Academic Press; 1997.

[37] Gallagher JC, Riggs BL, DeLuca HF. Effect of estrogen on calcium absorption and serum vitamin D metabolites in postmenopausal osteoporosis. J Clin Endocrinol Metab 1980;51: 1359–64.

[38] Nordin BEC, Need AG, Morris HA, et al. Evidence for a renal calcium leak in postmenopausal women. J Clin Endocrinol Metab 1991;72:401–7.

[39] McKane WR, Khosla S, Burritt MF, et al. Mechanism of renal calcium conservation with estrogen replacement therapy in women in early postmenopause - a clinical research center study. J Clin Endocrinol Metab 1995;80:3458–64.

[40] Marie PJ, Hott M, Launay JM, et al. In vitro production of cytokines by bone surface-derived osteoblastic cells in normal and osteoporotic postmenopausal women: relationship with cell proliferation. J Clin Endocrinol Metab 1993;77:824–30.

[41] Giustina A, Veldhuis JD. Pathophysiology of the neuroregulation of growth hormone secretion in experimental animals and the human. Endocr Rev 1998;19:717–97.

[42] Ho KY, Evans WS, Blizzard RM, et al. Effects of sex and age on the 24-hour profile of growth hormone secretion in man: importance of endogenous estradiol concentrations. J Clin Endocrinol Metab 1987;64:51–8.

[43] Bennett A, Wahner HW, Riggs BL, et al. Insulin-like growth factors I and II, aging and bone density in women. J Clin Endocrinol Metab 1984;59:701–4.

[44] Boonen S, Mohan S, Dequeker J, et al. Down-regulation of the serum stimulatory components of the insulin-like growth factor (IGF) system (IGF-I, IGF-II, IGF binding protein [BP]-3, and IGFBP-5) in age-related (type II) femoral neck osteoporosis. J Bone Miner Res 1999;14:2150–8.

[45] Pfeilschifter J, Diel I, Kloppinger T, et al. Concentrations of insulin-like growth factor (IGF)-I, -II, and IGF binding protein-4, and -5 in human bone cell conditioned medium do not change with age. Mech Aging Dev 2000;117:109–14.

[46] Heaney RP, Recker RR, Saville PD. Menopausal changes in calcium balance performance. J Lab Clin Med 1978;92:953–63.

[47] Ernst M, Heath JK, Rodan GA. Estradiol effects on proliferation, messenger ribonucleic acid for collagen and insulin-like growth factor-I, and parathyroid hormone-stimulated adenylate cyclase activity in osteoblastic cells from calvariae and long bones. Endocrinology 1989;125:825–33.

[48] Manolagas SC. Birth and death of bone cells: basic regulatory mechanisms and implications for the pathogenesis and treatment of osteoporosis. Endocr Rev 2000;21: 115–37.

[49] Gohel A, McCarthy MB, Gronowicz G. Estrogen prevents glucocorticoid-induced apoptosis in osteoblasts in vivo and in vitro. Endocrinology 1999;140:5339–47.

[50] Khastgir G, Studd J, Holland N, et al. Anabolic effect of estrogen replacement on bone in postmenopausal women with osteoporosis: histomorphometric evidence in a longitudinal study. J Clin Endocrinol Metab 2001;86:289–95.

[51] Tobias JH, Compston JE. Does estrogen stimulate osteoblast function in postmenopausal women? Bone 1999;24:121–4.

[52] Khosla S, Melton LJI, Atkinson EJ, et al. Relationship of serum sex steroid levels and bone turnover markers with bone mineral density in men and women: a key role for bioavailable estrogen. J Clin Endocrinol Metab 1998;83:2266–74.

[53] Greendale GA, Edelstein S, Barrett-Connor E. Endogenous sex steroids and bone mineral density in older women and men: the Rancho Bernardo study. J Bone Miner Res 1997;12: 1833–43.

[54] Slemenda CW, Longcope C, Zhou L, et al. Sex steroids and bone mass in older men: positive associations with serum estrogens and negative associations with androgens. J Clin Invest 1997;100:1755–9.

[55] Center JR, Nguyen TV, Sambrook PN, et al. Hormonal and biochemical parameters in the determination of osteoporosis in elderly men. J Clin Endocrinol Metab 1999;84:3626–35.

[56] Ongphiphadhanakul B, Rajatanavin R, Chanprasertyothin S, et al. Serum oestradiol and oestrogen-receptor gene polymorphism are associated with bone mineral density independently of serum testosterone in normal males. Clin Endocrinol (Oxf) 1998;49:803–9.

[57] van den Beld AW, de Jong FH, Grobbee DE, et al. Measures of bioavailable serum testosterone and estradiol and their relationships with muscle strength, bone density, and body composition in elderly men. J Clin Endocrinol Metab 2000;85:3276–82.

[58] Amin S, Zhang Y, Sawin CT, et al. Association of hypogonadism and estradiol levels with bone mineral density in elderly men from the Framingham study. Ann Intern Med 2000; 133:951–63.

[59] Szulc P, Munoz F, Claustrat B, et al. Bioavailable estradiol may be an important determinant of osteoporosis in men: the MINOS study. J Clin Endocrinol Metab 2001;86:192–9.

[60] Khosla S, Melton LJ, Atkinson EJ, et al. Relationship of serum sex steroid levels to longitudinal changes in bone density in young versus elderly men. J Clin Endocrinol Metab 2001;86: 3555–61.

[61] Gennari L, Merlotti D, Martini G, et al. Longitudinal association between sex hormone levels, bone loss, and bone turnover in elderly men. J Clin Endocrinol Metab 2003;88:5327–33.

[62] Falahati-Nini A, Riggs BL, Atkinson EJ, et al. Relative contributions of testosterone and estrogen in regulating bone resorption and formation in normal elderly men. J Clin Invest 2000;106:1553–60.

[63] Leder BZ, LeBlanc KM, Schoenfeld DA, et al. Differential effects of androgens and estrogens on bone turnover in normal men. J Clin Endocrinol Metab 2003;88:204–10.

[64] Lian JB, Stein GS, Canalis E, et al. Bone formation: osteoblast lineage cells, growth factors, matrix proteins, and the mineralization process. Primer on the Metabolic Bone Diseases and Disorders of Mineral Metabolism 1999;3:14–29.

[65] Taxel P, Kennedy DG, Fall PM, et al. The effect of aromatase inhibition on sex steroids, gonadotropins, and markers of bone turnover in older men. J Clin Endocrinol Metab 2001;86: 2869–74.

[66] Turner RT, Wakley GK, Hannon KS. Differential effects of androgens on cortical bone histomorphometry in gonadectomized male and female rats. J Orthop Res 1990;8:612–7.

[67] Kennel KA, Riggs BL, Achenbach SJ, et al. Role of parathyroid hormone in mediating age-related changes in bone resorption in men. Osteoporos Int 2003;14:631–6.

[68] Labrie F, Belanger A, Cusan L, et al. Marked decline in serum concentrations of adrenal C19 sex steroid precursors and conjugated androgen metabolites during aging. J Clin Endocrinol Metab 1997;82:2396–402.

[69] Seeman E. From density to structure: growing up and growing old on the surfaces of bone. J Bone Miner Res 1997;12:509–21.

[70] Riggs BL, Melton LJ. Medical progress series: Involutional osteoporosis. N Engl J Med 1986;314:1676–86.

[71] Frost HM. On our age-related bone loss: insights from a new paradigm. J Bone Miner Res 1997;12:1539–46.

[72] Frost HM. Why the ISMNI and the Utah paradigm? Their role in skeletal and extraskeletal disorders. J Musculoskelet Neuronal Interact 2000 Sep;1(1):5–9.

ELSEVIER
SAUNDERS

Endocrinol Metab Clin N Am
34 (2005) 1031–1046

ENDOCRINOLOGY
AND METABOLISM
CLINICS
OF NORTH AMERICA

Abnormalities of Water Homeostasis in Aging

Steven P. Hodak, MD[1], Joseph G. Verbalis, MD*

*Division of Endocrinology and Metabolism, Georgetown University Medical Center,
Washington, DC, USA*

Findley [1] first proposed the presence of age-related dysfunction of the hypothalamic-neurohypophyseal-renal axis more than 50 years ago. His hypothesis was based on clinical observations and occurred well in advance of the first assays for arginine vasopressin (AVP). Since then, the evolution of more sophisticated scientific methodologies has resulted in a corroboration of Findley's suspicion and has revealed many aspects of the physiology that underlies this manifestation of the aging process. It is now clear that perturbations in water homeostasis occur commonly with aging. This article summarizes the distinct points along the hypothalamic-neurohypophyseal-renal axis where these changes have been characterized.

Physiologic overview of disturbances of water metabolism

The ratio of solute content to body water determines the osmolality of body fluids, including plasma. As the most abundant extracellular electrolyte, serum sodium concentration is the single most important determinant of plasma osmolality under normal circumstances. Although the regulation of water and sodium balance is interrelated, it is predominantly the homeostatic control of water, rather than of sodium, that is the main determinant of serum sodium concentration and therefore plasma osmolality. Homeostatic controls of sodium metabolism and obligate shifts in extracellular fluids driven by sodium flux more directly regulate the volume status of body fluid compartments rather than their osmolality. Isolated shifts in body water, when unaccompanied by simultaneous shifts in body solute, do not

---

* Corresponding author.

[1] *Present address:* Division of Endocrinology and Metabolism, University of Pittsburgh, Pittsburgh, PA.

E-mail address: verbalis@georgetown.edu (J.G. Verbalis).

0889-8529/05/$ - see front matter © 2005 Elsevier Inc. All rights reserved.
doi:10.1016/j.ecl.2005.09.002   *endo.theclinics.com*

typically result in clinically relevant changes in volume status. However, such isolated changes in total body water can have a dramatic impact on serum sodium concentration and plasma osmolality [2]. For example, in a 70-kg adult, a 10% increase in total body water would cause a significant decrease in serum sodium concentration ($[Na^+]$) of approximately 14 mmol/L. Such a change could easily cause clinically significant hyponatremia and hypo-osmolality. Yet this same 10% gain of total body water would only cause an increase of approximately 400 mL in intravascular volume. It is unlikely that such a mild increase in circulating volume would cause observable clinical findings. The reverse situation (ie, water loss causing a similar increase in serum $[Na^+]$) would similarly produce clinically significant hyperosmolality without clinically significant hypovolemia [2]. Such is the case in uncompensated diabetes insipidus.

Aging produces changes in water metabolism and sodium balance, leading to alterations in plasma osmolality and the volume of body fluid compartments. The consequence of such changes is an increase in the frequency and the severity of hypo- and hyperosmolality, typically manifested as hypo- and hypernatremia and hypo- and hypervolemia in the elderly. Although the processes of water and sodium metabolism cannot be completely separated from each other, this article concentrates mainly on how water balance, and thus plasma osmolality, is affected by aging.

Clinical overview of disturbances of water metabolism

Hyponatremia

Hyponatremia is the most common electrolyte disorder encountered in clinical practice [3]. However, hyponatremia is of clinical significance only when it reflects corresponding hypo-osmolality of the plasma. If hyponatremia is defined as a serum $[Na^+]$ of less than 135 mmol/L, the inpatient incidence is reported to be between 15% and 22%. Studies that define hyponatremia as a serum $[Na^+]$ less than 130 mmol/L demonstrate a lower, but still significant, incidence of 1% to 4% [4]. Hyponatremia remains an important clinical entity because it is a strong independent predictor of mortality, reported to be as high as 60% in some series [5,6]. Recent data also suggest that even mild chronic hyponatremia, not typically thought to be clinically significant, may in fact be associated with significant neurocognitive effects and possibly increased falls in the elderly [7].

Determination of a true incidence and prevalence of hyponatremia in the elderly is problematic. Several excellent observational studies examining this issue have been published, but the literature has lacked a uniform threshold for defining hyponatremia. Similarly, the term *elderly* has also been used somewhat arbitrarily in these studies. Study criteria, including age, stratification by serum $[Na^+]$, medication use, and clinical setting, also have varied widely. Thus, direct comparisons among such clinical series are difficult.

One recent review illustrates the disparate nature of the existing literature. This review suggests that, depending on the study, the incidence of hyponatremia in elderly populations has been reported to vary widely between 0.2% and 29.8%, depending on the criteria used to define *hyponatremia* and *elderly* [8].

Miller and colleagues [9] published numerous observational studies on the elderly and hyponatremia. In a retrospective study of 405 ambulatory elderly patients who had a mean age of 78 years, the incidence of serum [Na$^+$] less than 135 mmol/L was 11% over a 24-month observational period. These results are analogous to an earlier study by Caird and colleagues [10], which reported that among healthy patients aged 65 years or older living at home, the incidence of serum [Na$^+$] less than 137 mmol/L was 10.5%. Miller [11] has also observed that the incidence of hyponatremia doubled to approximately 22% among elderly who reside in long-term institutional settings. He further noted that during a 1-year observational period, 53% of such institutional populations experienced one or more hyponatremic episodes [11]. A more recent study by Anpalahan [12] found similar results; 25% of patients aged 65 years and older who resided in an acute geriatric rehabilitation hospital had hyponatremia, defined as a serum [Na$^+$] less than 135 mmol/L. Although it may be impossible to accurately define the true incidence of hyponatremia among the elderly, these studies demonstrate that the problem is not uncommon.

The syndrome of inappropriate antidiuretic hormone secretion (SIADH) is a common cause of hyponatremia in elderly populations. SIADH was first described by Schwartz and colleagues [13] in 1957. The defining criteria presented in this landmark publication from almost 50 years ago still remain valid and clinically relevant today [4]. SIADH can be caused by many types of diseases and injuries common in the elderly. Central nervous system injury, pulmonary disease, paraneoplastic malignancy, nausea, and pain are all known to cause SIADH. However, SIADH can also occur in an idiopathic form, unassociated with any of the previously listed conditions. Several studies have demonstrated that SIADH accounts for approximately half (50%–58.7%) of the hyponatremia observed in some elderly populations [9,12,14], and roughly one quarter to one half (26%–60%) of elderly patients who have SIADH appear to have an idiopathic form of this disorder [9,12,14].

Hypernatremia

Hypernatremia always reflects an increase in plasma osmolality. Cross-sectional studies of hospitalized elderly patients and elderly residents of long-term care facilities show incidences of hypernatremia that vary between 0.3% to 8.9% [5,8]. Hypernatremia is a common presenting diagnosis in the elderly; however, 60% to 80% of the hypernatremia in elderly populations has been noted to occur following hospital admission [5]. In elderly nursing home patients, up to 30% may become hypernatremic following hospital admission [15].

The implications of hypernatremia in elderly patients who are hospitalized are significant. Snyder and colleagues [16] retrospectively reviewed outcomes in 162 hypernatremic elderly patients, representing 1.1% of all elderly patients admitted for acute hospital care to a community teaching hospital. All patients were at least 60 years of age with a serum [Na$^+$] greater than 148 mmol/L. Of these patients, 43% presented with hypernatremia at admission and the remaining 57% developed hypernatremia after admission. All-cause mortality in this group of hypernatremic elderly patients was 42%, which was seven times greater than age-matched normonatremic patients. Furthermore, 38% of the hypernatremic patients who survived to discharge had a significantly decreased ability to provide self-care. Mortality among patients who presented with hypernatremia on admission was lower (29%) than mortality among patients who developed hypernatremia after admission (52%), despite higher peak serum [Na$^+$] in the former compared with the latter group. Hypernatremia discovered at the time of admission was associated with greater age (mean age of 81 years) and female gender, and was more common in patients admitted from a nursing home.

As hypernatremia (ie, hyperosmolality) develops, the normal physiologic response integrates renal water conservation through osmotically stimulated secretion of AVP and an accompanying potent stimulation of thirst [17]. Although renal water conservation can forestall the development of severe hyperosmolality, only appropriate stimulation of thirst, with subsequent increases in water ingestion, can replace lost body fluid and reverse existing hyperosmolality [2]. This entire physiologic response is typically impaired with aging. Thus, the elderly have a greatly increased susceptibility to various situations that can induce hypernatremia and hyperosmolality, with the attendant increases in mortality and morbidity associated with this disorder [16,18].

Mechanisms involved with disturbances of water metabolism in the elderly

Alterations in the regulation of water homeostasis in the elderly, listed in Box 1, result from changes in body composition, alterations in renal function, and changes in hypothalamic–pituitary regulation of thirst and AVP secretion. The cumulative effect of these changes is a diminution of homeostatic reserve and loss of appropriate corrective responses to environmental and metabolic stressors [19,20]. Each of these potential mechanisms are considered separately, and then combined into an integrated explanation of the origin of water metabolism disorders in the elderly.

Changes in body composition with aging

Aging typically leads to a 5% to 10% increase in total body fat, and a decrease in total body water of an equal magnitude. In an elderly 70-kg man,

---

Box 1. Effects of aging on body fluid homeostasis

Altered body composition
Reduced plasma volume
Increased osmolal "flux"

Kidney
Impaired free water excretion
Decreased urine concentrating ability

Brain
Decreased thirst perception
Increased AVP secretion

---

this can account for a reduction of total body water of as much as 7 to 8 L compared with a young man of the same weight [19]. With aging, plasma volume has also been shown to decrease by as much as 21% relative to body weight and surface area in older men when compared with younger controls [21]. The consequence of these changes is that an equivalent acute gain, or loss, of body water will cause a greater degree of flux in osmolality in elderly compared with younger individuals. Thus, in the elderly, states of mild dehydration or volume overload are more likely to cause clinically significant shifts in the concentration of body solutes, such as sodium. Rolls and Phillips [20] unequivocally demonstrated this in a study that compared plasma osmolality in elderly and young subjects before and after fluid deprivation. Despite identical weight loss and similar changes in plasma volume indices, the elderly clearly sustained a significantly greater increase in plasma osmolality than did younger controls (Fig. 1).

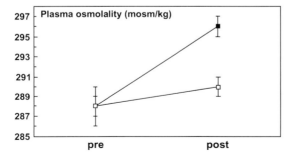

Fig. 1. Mean changes, pre- and postfluid deprivation in young (*open boxes*) and elderly (*closed boxes*) subjects after equivalent degrees of induced weight loss. (*From* Rolls BJ, Phillips PA. Aging and disturbances of thirst and fluid balance. Nutr Rev 1990;48:137–44; with permission.)

Changes in renal function with aging

Many aspects of renal function related to water homeostasis are under neu-rohormonal control through secretion of AVP from the posterior pituitary. However, intrinsic renal mechanisms that play a key role in the derangement of water balance in aging also exist. Typical age-associated changes in the kid-ney include loss of parenchymal mass, progressive glomerulosclerosis, tubul-opathy, interstitial fibrosis, and the development of afferent–efferent arteriolar shunts [22]. By age 80, the normal kidney loses up to 25% of its mass and develops a histopathologic appearance similar to that seen in chronic tubulointerstitial disease [18]. Beck [18,19] has described the resulting func-tional changes as an "inelasticity" in fluid homeostasis. Such defects may not be of immediate consequences during states of health, but in the elderly—especially under conditions of stress, disease, dehydration, or volume over-load—such moderate impairments in normal renal physiology may cause significant imbalances in water and solute homeostasis [18]. The clinical result is the development of depletional or dilutional states such as hyper- and hypo-osmolality.

Age-associated changes in glomerular filtration rate

The Baltimore Longitudinal Study of Aging showed that up to 30% of healthy aged adults maintain a normal glomerular filtration rate (GFR). However, with few exceptions, in the remaining 70% of subjects, the study noted that GFR decreased by approximately $1 \text{ mL/min}/1.73\text{m}^2/\text{y}$ after age 40. A further acceleration in the rate of decline after age 65 was also noted [18,22,23]. Whether these changes are an inevitable consequence of aging or are the result of subtle pathologic states remains uncertain. However, the consequences of such changes are well established. Reductions in GFR in-crease proximal renal tubular fluid absorption, which leads to a decrease in tubular delivery of free water to the distal diluting segments of the neph-ron [5]. The result is a loss of the dilutional capacity of the kidney, mani-fested by an impaired ability to excrete a free water load [15,20]. Faull and colleagues [24] studied free-water excretion among elderly subjects (mean age 68 years) compared with young controls. That study showed that although the older group was able to achieve normal excretion follow-ing a standard water load of 20-mL/kg body weight, a significant decrement in maximal free-water clearance in the older group was present. Clark and colleagues [25] suggest that this may be partly because of decreased distal renal tubular delivery of water caused by reduced prostaglandin production in the elderly. Such an impairment in the ability to excrete excess body water has direct implications in the susceptibility of the elderly to dilutional states that predispose to hypo-osmolality and hyponatremia.

Loss of urinary concentrating ability

Concomitant with the loss of diluting capacity, the aging kidney also loses the ability to maximally conserve body water during states of dehydration [26]. In such a volume-depleted state, in the absence of fluid ingestion, maximal urinary concentration is the only means by which further losses of body water can be reduced. By age 80, maximal urinary concentration typically declines from a youthful peak of 1100 to 1200 mOsm/kg H_2O, to the range of 400 to 500 mOsm/kg H_2O [15]. Phillips and colleagues [27] established that following 24 hours of water deprivation, older subjects demonstrated significantly less urinary concentrating ability compared with younger controls despite higher levels of plasma osmolality. This effect was also noted to occur despite higher plasma AVP levels in the elderly, suggesting that the concentrating defect is predominantly caused by intrinsic renal factors. The clinical implications of this age-acquired defect in the maintenance of normal plasma osmolality are clear: loss of urinary concentrating ability contributes to the exacerbation of numerous conditions common in the elderly, such as diarrhea, vomiting, decreased thirst, and poor oral intake, thus worsening the resulting dehydration, hyperosmolality, and hypovolemia.

Changes in centrally mediated control of water homeostasis with aging

Central neuroendocrine control of AVP secretion and thirst are the major regulators of normal water balance in subjects who have normal renal function. Despite large variations in fluid intake, plasma osmolality is maintained within narrow limits through the secretion of AVP, the renal response to AVP secretion, and the appropriate control of thirst. Each of these processes is significantly affected by aging.

Regulation of arginine vasopressin secretion in aging

AVP has a central role in the regulation of renal water excretion through its control of membrane insertion and abundance of the water channel aquaporin-2 (AQP-2) in the distal nephron [28]. These effects are mediated through AVP interaction with the type 2 vasopressin receptor (V2R) expressed in the renal collecting ducts. Increased membrane-bound AQP-2 increases water permeability of the collecting duct, and thereby induces a decrease in renal free-water excretion or antidiuresis. AVP is a nonapeptide synthesized by the cell bodies of the supraoptic and paraventricular nuclei of the hypothalamus. AVP is packaged in granules with its carrier protein neurophysin, and transported down axons terminating in the posterior pituitary where it is stored and ultimately secreted in response to specific stimuli [17]. The secretion of AVP is under exquisite, moment-to-moment control of osmoreceptors located in and around the organum vasculosum of the lamina terminalis and the anterior wall of the third ventricle. For any given individual, an osmotic threshold, or set point, for AVP release typically exists within a narrow normal range. An increase in plasma osmolality as small as 1% is sufficient to cause an increase in plasma AVP concentration of 1 pg/mL. Such an increase is able to rapidly and significantly decrease free-water excretion and reduce urine flow [17]. Any increase in plasma osmolality above the set point induces a linear increase in the secretion of AVP [5], with maximum antidiuresis occurring with plasma AVP concentrations above 5 pg/mL [17]. This extraordinarily sensitive mechanism is able to maintain plasma osmolality within the range of 275 to 295 mOsm/kg H_2O. A secondary hemodynamic and volume-dependant regulatory mechanism for AVP secretion also exists. This mechanism is controlled by baroreceptors located in the cardiac atria and large arteries. In contrast to the exquisitely sensitive osmotic regulation of AVP secretion, the AVP response to a volume or hemodynamic stimulus does not occur until effective arterial volume is decreased by at least 8% to 10% [5,17]. The interaction of osmoreceptor and baroreceptor regulation of AVP secretion produces an integrated AVP secretory profile that is linear, with a slope that is modulated by changes in volume and hemodynamic status [5].

Secretion and end organ effects of AVP are also affected by aging. Most studies have found that basal AVP levels in healthy elderly subjects are at least equal to, or more typically greater than, those of young controls. However, a few studies have reported no differences in basal AVP levels in the elderly [29], and at least one study has suggested that basal AVP levels may be lower in older subjects [30].

Regardless of basal AVP levels, most of the literature regarding water homeostasis has demonstrated that the elderly have a greater augmentation of AVP secretion per unit change in plasma osmolality than do younger subjects. This finding is consistent with an increase in osmoreceptor sensitivity in the elderly [30]. Helderman and colleagues [26] first made this observation over 25 years ago in studies of dehydrated elderly patients subjected to hypertonic saline infusions (Fig. 2). Subsequent studies have repeatedly confirmed this observation [26,27,30,31]. However, despite general agreement, a few notable exceptions exist. The early work of Phillips and colleagues [27] showed a threefold increase in secretion of AVP per unit change in osmolality in the elderly, but later work by the same group indicated that AVP secretion in response to osmolar stimulus is maintained rather than augmented [32,33]. There is also one isolated study that demonstrates the absence of a correlation between AVP secretion and osmolality in the elderly [34]. Nonetheless, preservation, or more commonly augmentation, of osmoreceptor sensitivity has been repeatedly confirmed in the elderly.

Several mechanistic explanations for observed age-associated changes in AVP secretion have been proposed. Rowe and colleagues [35] studied AVP secretory responses to orthostatic maneuvers in young and elderly subjects. That group found that 11 of 12 young subjects augmented AVP secretion in response to a position change from supine to erect. However, only 8 of 15, or just over half, of the elderly patients had a similar response [35]. The study also demonstrated an appropriate increase in sympathetic nervous system discharge of norepinephrine in response to positional changes in the elderly subjects regardless of AVP secretory status. This observation

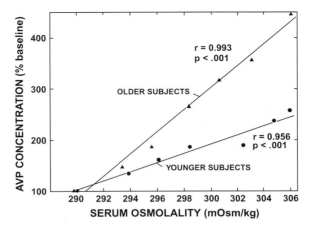

Fig. 2. Correlation between serum osmolality and AVP concentration in eight young and eight older subjects during 2-hour 3% saline infusion following mild dehydration. The older subjects have significantly higher plasma levels of AVP per unit increase in plasma osmolality, strongly suggesting an enhanced osmotically stimulated secretion. (*From* Helderman JH, Vestal RE, Rowe JW, et al. The response of arginine vasopressin to intravenous ethanol and hypertonic saline in man: the impact of aging. J Gerontol 1978;33(1):39–47; with permission.)

suggests that aging may not affect AVP secretion through impairment of the baroreceptor afferent–efferent loop; rather, the study concluded that aging may result in a loss of appropriate transmission of postural stimuli from the vasomotor centers of the brainstem where these stimuli are received, to the hypothalamus where secretion of AVP is controlled. Such a defect would thereby impair normal secretion of AVP in response to position changes. Based on these results, Rowe and colleagues [35] speculated that the increased AVP secretion in response to osmolar stimuli, which has been verified in most studies performed in the elderly, may represent a compensatory response to the loss of normal baroreceptor-mediated control of AVP secretion resulting from hemodynamic changes.

Although Rowe and colleagues [35] suggest that the loss of baroreceptor influence on AVP secretion occurs because of the loss of a neurologic pathway between the vasomotor center and the hypothalamus, Stachenfeld and colleagues [31] more recently made an argument for a role of atrial natriuretic peptide (ANP) as an important mediator of AVP secretion. This group employed studies of isosmotic central blood volume expansion during head-out water immersion (HOI) and measured AVP responses in healthy elderly and young cohorts. They found that in addition to the loss of normal baroreceptor response to increases in central pressure, the elderly also demonstrated more exuberant secretion of ANP. They postulate that increased secretion of ANP may directly suppress AVP secretion during HOI [31]. This hypothesis is consistent with earlier reports that exogenous ANP infusion suppresses osmotically stimulated AVP release in young and elderly subjects [36]. However, other recent work has cast doubt over whether ANP infusion does in fact have any effect on AVP secretion [37]. Thus, it is unclear whether ANP exerts any significant meaningful physiologic control over AVP secretion in the elderly.

Regulation of arginine vasopressin function in aging

AVP V2Rs, the site of AVP action in the kidney, are members of the seven-transmembrane domain G-protein coupled receptor family. Activation of the receptor by AVP induces production of the intracellular second messenger cyclic-AMP (cAMP) through activation of adenylyl cyclase. Through activation of the cAMP pathway, new AQP2 water channels are synthesized and existing AQP2s are shuttled from intracellular storage vesicles and inserted into the apical plasma membrane of the renal collecting duct cells [38]. Once inserted into the apical membrane, AQP2s form channels through which water molecules can be absorbed from the lumen of the collecting duct into the renal medullary interstitium driven by the medullary osmotic gradient. The resulting antidiuresis is capable of concentrating urine to an osmolality equivalent to that at the tip of inner renal medulla [17].

Because AVP levels are generally found to be elevated in the elderly, a pituitary secretory defect is unlikely to explain the decreased renal response to AVP noted in aging. A more likely explanation is a decrease in normal renal responsivity to AVP. Decreased V2R receptor expression or decreased second messenger response to AVP-V2R signaling would result in loss of maximal urinary concentration. Both defects have been suggested in rat models of aging. A recent study of F344BN rats demonstrated an age-related impairment of renal concentrating ability after a moderate water restriction, despite a normal AVP secretory response [39]. This study found lower basal levels of AQP-2 water channel expression in aging rats, and an inability of aging rats to normally upregulate AQP-2 synthesis and mobilization despite appropriate AVP secretion. Other animal studies have suggested that decreased AVP-V2R signaling in the thick ascending limb and collecting ducts may also have deleterious effects on generation of the medullary concentrating gradient required for maximal urine concentration [40,41]. Unfortunately, no correlating human studies have yet been possible. Consequently, the presence of such changes in the human kidney—although a provocative hypothesis—currently must be considered speculative.

Regulation of thirst in aging

Stimulation of thirst osmoreceptors produce signals that are conveyed to the higher cerebral cortex, resulting in the perception of thirst and water-seeking behavior [2]. The osmotic threshold for thirst is 5 to 10 mOsm/kg H_2O above that for AVP release. This small difference in the set points regulating AVP secretion and manifestation of the thirst response has important physiologic consequences. Small osmolar excursions relative to an individual's osmotic set point induce changes only in AVP secretion and

AVP-mediated changes in renal water excretion to maintain normal plasma osmolality. Only larger osmolar excursions are able to trigger the robust thirst response that either increases or decreases thirst to restore normal plasma osmolality. The important behavioral consequence of this mechanism is that the primary and earliest response to increased plasma osmolality involves an unconscious increase in AVP-mediated augmentation of renal concentration that occurs below the level of awareness. Only a more pronounced increase in plasma osmolality from more significant hydration is able to induce the potent and potentially disruptive behavioral response of water-seeking.

Intrinsic defects in thirst develop with aging. A study by Phillips and colleagues [27] showed that older men deprived of hydration for 24 hours showed no subjective increase in thirst or mouth dryness, and drank less water than young controls despite significant increases in serum [Na$^+$] and plasma osmolality. Furthermore, when allowed free access to drinking water, in contrast to the young controls, elderly subjects drank less and did not restore serum [Na$^+$] to predeprivation levels (Fig. 3). These data suggest a blunted thirst response to osmotic changes in the elderly [42]. Mack and colleagues [43] offer one explanation for these findings. Their study showed that although a blunted thirst response was present in the elderly, the rate of fluid intake in healthy elderly and young controls was equivalent for equivalent degrees of thirst. Thus, elderly subjects appeared to have a higher osmolar set point for thirst, resulting in a decrease in the degree of perceived thirst for any given level of plasma osmolality. This leads to a net decrease in

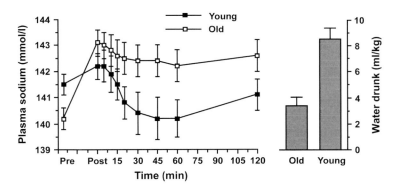

Fig. 3. Plasma sodium concentration and total water intake in healthy elderly and young subjects following 24 hours of dehydration. Baseline sodium concentration before dehydration (*pre-*) and after dehydration (*post-*) are noted. Free access to water was allowed for 60 minutes following dehydration starting at time of 0 minutes. Cumulative water intake during the free drinking period by young and old subjects is depicted in the bar graph. Despite a greater initial increase in serum [Na$^+$], elderly subjects drank significantly less water, resulting in lesser correction of the elevated serum [Na$^+$]. (*From* Phillips PA, Johnston CI, Gray L. Disturbed fluid and electrolyte homeostasis following dehydration in elderly people. Age and Ageing 1993;22:26–33; with permission.)

the amount of fluid ingested due to a decrease in the thirst response [43]. However, more recent studies of thirst in the elderly, using hypertonic saline infusions and HOI, have suggested that the response of thirst to an osmotic stimulus unaccompanied by a change in plasma volume is not affected by normal aging [30,31]. Instead, these studies demonstrated a diminution of baroreceptor-mediated regulation of thirst in response to changes in plasma volume [44]. Studies employing HOI have supported the concept that control of thirst by volume shifts may actually take priority and override contradictory osmotic stimuli, at least in young subjects [45]. Using this same method, Stachenfeld and colleagues [31] demonstrated that in carefully selected healthy dehydrated participants, HOI caused a greater suppression of thirst and drinking response in the young compared with the elderly subjects. This study found that although net thirst was not different between the elderly and the young, the lack of difference was due to greater baroreceptor-mediated suppression of more exuberant thirst in the young compared with the elderly subjects. These combined data therefore provide further evidence of an intrinsic defect in thirst with normal aging.

The subjective sensation of thirst requires unimpaired transmission of efferent signals from hypothalamic osmoreceptors to the cerebral cortex where thirst is perceived. Although the neural pathways that conduct these signals are not well characterized, it is likely that one of the major factors responsible for age-related changes in thirst is impairment of these poorly defined efferent pathways [32]. Subtle and cumulative brain injury caused by age-associated illness, rather than aging per se, may play an active role in such a process. It has been suggested that elderly patients with many types of mild chronic illness may not have been adequately excluded from study populations previously described as "healthy." How the possible inclusion of such patients may have colored early studies of aging is difficult to assess [29,30]. Nonetheless, recent well-controlled studies of highly selected groups of healthy elderly subjects appear to corroborate the early findings of the presence of intrinsic defects in thirst with normal aging. Most studies confirm that aging is accompanied by decreased thirst. However, how osmolar changes, volume status, and other stimuli interact to mediate thirst, and how these are affected by aging, remain incompletely understood. Thirst is a complex response to multiple and frequently interrelated physiologic stimuli. The literature provides observations of numerous stimulus-response mechanisms involved in the generation and perception of thirst, and changes associated with aging. The exact mechanisms by which these changes occur, and whether they are an unavoidable consequence of normal aging, remain to be ascertained.

Integration of changes in arginine vasopressin secretion, thirst, and kidney function with aging

Laurence Beck's [18] conceptualization of homeostatic inelasticity aptly describes the consequences of the spectrum of physiologic changes that occur with aging. Aging causes distinct changes that impact normal water homeostasis at several discreet locations along the neuro-renal axis responsible for maintaining normal water balance. The net result of these changes is that the elderly experience a loss of homeostatic reserve and increased susceptibility to pathologic and iatrogenic causes of disturbed water homeostasis.

The sensation of thirst and the appropriate drinking response to thirst is compromised with aging. As Phillips and colleagues [33] have suggested, it is likely that part of this defect is caused by loss of normal neural pathways that convey sensory input to the higher cortical centers where thirst is perceived and from which the thirst response emanates. Recent studies have also demonstrated that there is a change in baroreceptor-mediated control of thirst in the elderly. Stachenfeld and colleagues [31] have clearly demonstrated that plasma volume expansion in elderly subjects does not generate the normal suppression of thirst found in the young. Whether the reverse case (ie, whether aging decreases activation of thirst in response to volume contraction) is less clearly established.

A clear age-related deficit in the thirst response appears to arise from decreased sensitivity to osmolar stimulation. The early work of Phillips and colleagues [42] demonstrated the presence of such a defect. More recent studies by Mack and colleagues [43] suggest that this defect is caused by a higher osmotic set point leading to a blunted thirst response in the elderly. The loss of an appropriate thirst response compromises this critical compensatory mechanisms responsible for the drive to replace lost body fluid, and the only true physiologic means of correcting a hyperosmolar state.

Impaired GFR and resultant loss of maximal urinary concentrating ability appear common, if not certain, consequences of aging [23,46]. Although it appears that the development of such deficits is not inevitable, how to discern which elderly are most likely to suffer such losses is not easily determined. Because most otherwise "normal" elderly patients manifest a decrement in renal function, the argument regarding whether such a change is inevitable may be overly academic. It may, on the other hand, be appropriate to assume that such a defect is probable, though some elderly who age more "successfully" than others may maintain reasonably normal renal function. The consequence of such a defect is clear: decreased GFR causes an inability to maximally conserve free water and favors development of inappropriate body-water deficits. This outcome can lead to clinically relevant hyperosmolality, and is also a likely cause of the observed increase in the frequency of hypernatremia in the elderly.

Paradoxically, a decrement in maximal water excretion also occurs in the elderly [24,25]. Such a defect would have consequences in situations of overhydration. The elderly are at a higher risk for developing diseases, such as congestive heart failure, that are associated with volume overload. So, too, are the elderly at risk for inadvertent iatrogenic overhydration from intravenous and enteral hydration therapy. The inability to appropriately excrete an unnecessary fluid load would predispose to hypo-osmolality.

The secretion and end-organ effects of AVP account for two of the most interesting and perhaps least well-understood aspects of water regulation in the elderly. Although a few exceptions exist, most investigators have found that basal AVP secretion is at least maintained, and more likely increased, with normal aging [17]. Further, the AVP secretory response (ie, the osmo-receptor sensitivity to osmolar stimuli) is also increased in normal aging [30]. Thus, AVP secretion represents one of the few endocrine responses that increases rather than decreases with age. Animal studies have unequivocally indicated an accompanying age-acquired end organ insensitivity to the effects of AVP [39]. Though renal responsiveness to AVP may be reduced with aging, these studies show that it is not entirely eliminated. This finding may underlie the increased incidence of idiopathic SIADH that occurs in the elderly that often cannot be explained by identifiable pathology [9]. We hypothesize that enhanced secretion of AVP in the elderly and the inability to appropriately suppress AVP secretion during fluid intake [33], combined with an intrinsic inability to excrete free water [25,47], increase the likelihood that SIADH will occur in this group of patients. We believe these factors may explain the unusually high incidence of idiopathic SIADH noted in elderly populations. Direct experimental proof of this hypothesis is still required. Nonetheless, the preponderance of existing experimental data suggest that this assumption is well founded.

Summary

Much has been learned in the 5 decades since Findley's original reflections about the effects of aging on water homeostasis. Clearly demonstrated deficits in renal function, thirst, and responses to osmotic and volume stimulation have been repeatedly demonstrated in the elderly population. Although much is already known about the renal actions of AVP at the V2R, it remains an active area of study regarding age-induced changes in renal concentrating ability. The lessons learned over the past 5 decades of work serve to emphasize the fragile nature of water balance characteristic of aging. The elderly are at increased risk for disturbances of water homeostasis caused by intrinsic disease and iatrogenic causes. It is therefore incumbent on all those who care for the elderly to realize the more limited nature of the compensatory and regulatory mechanisms that occur with aging, and to incorporate this understanding into the diagnosis and clinical interventions that are made in the care of this unique group of patients.

References

[1] Findley T. Role of the neurohypophysis in the pathogenesis of hypertension and some allied disorders associated with aging. Am J Med 1949;7:70–84.

[2] Palevsky PM, editor. Hypernatremia. 2nd edition. San Diego (CA): Academic Press; 1998.

[3] Janicic N, Verbalis JG. Evaluation and management of hypo-osmolality in hospitalized patients. Endocrinol Metab Clin North Am 2003;32(2):459–81 [vii.].

[4] Verbalis JG, editor. Hyponatremia and hypoosmolar disorders. 3rd edition. San Diego (CA): Academic Press; 2001.

[5] Fried LF, Palevsky PM. Hyponatremia and hypernatremia. Med Clin North Am 1997;81(3): 585–609.

[6] Terzian C, Frye EB, Piotrowski ZH. Admission hyponatremia in the elderly: factors influencing prognosis. J Gen Intern Med 1994;9(2):89–91.

[7] Musch WX, Hedeshi O, Decaux AG. Fall is a frequent motif of admission in patients with chronic hyponatremia. In: Annual Meeting of the American Society of Nephrology. San Diego, California, November 14–16, 2003. San Diego (CA); 2003. p. 748A.

[8] Hawkins RC. Age and gender as risk factors for hyponatremia and hypernatremia. Clin Chim Acta 2003;337(1–2):169–72.

[9] Miller M, Hecker MS, Friedlander DA, et al. Apparent idiopathic hyponatremia in an ambulatory geriatric population. J Am Geriatr Soc 1996;44(4):404–8.

[10] Caird FI, Andrews GR, Kennedy RD. Effect of posture on blood pressure in the elderly. Br Heart J 1973;35(5):527–30.

[11] Miller M. Hyponatremia: age-related risk factors and therapy decisions. Geriatrics 1998; 53(7):32–42.

[12] Anpalahan M. Chronic idiopathic hyponatremia in older people due to syndrome of inappropriate antidiuretic hormone secretion (SIADH) possibly related to aging. J Am Geriatr Soc 2001;49(6):788–92.

[13] Schwartz WB, Bennett W, Curelop S, et al. A syndrome of renal sodium loss and hyponatremia probably resulting from inappropriate secretion of antidiuretic hormone. 1957. J Am Soc Nephrol 2001;12(12):2860–70.

[14] Hirshberg B, Ben-Yehuda A. The syndrome of inappropriate antidiuretic hormone secretion in the elderly. Am J Med 1997;103(4):270–3.

[15] Beck LH. Changes in renal function with aging. Clin Geriatr Med 1998;14(2):199–209.

[16] Snyder NA, Feigal DW, Arieff AI. Hypernatremia in elderly patients. A heterogeneous, morbid, and iatrogenic entity. Ann Intern Med 1987;107(3):309–19.

[17] Wong LL, Verbalis JG. Systemic diseases associated with disorders of water homeostasis. Endocrinol Metab Clin North Am 2002;31(1):121–40.

[18] Beck LH. The aging kidney. Defending a delicate balance of fluid and electrolytes. Geriatrics 2000;55(4):26–32.

[19] Beck LH, Lavizzo-Mourey R. Geriatric hypernatremia. Ann Intern Med 1987;107(5):768–9.

[20] Rolls BJ, Phillips PA. Aging and disturbances of thirst and fluid balance. Nutr Rev 1990; 48(3):137–44.

[21] Davy KP, Seals DR. Total blood volume in healthy young and older men. J Appl Physiol 1994;76(5):2059–62.

[22] Lamb EJ, O'Riordan SE, Delaney MP. Kidney function in older people: pathology, assessment and management. Clin Chim Acta 2003;334(1–2):25–40.

[23] Lindeman RD. Assessment of renal function in the old. Special considerations. Clin Lab Med 1993;13(1):269–77.

[24] Faull CM, Holmes C, Baylis PH. Water balance in elderly people: is there a deficiency of vasopressin? Age Ageing 1993;22(2):114–20.

[25] Clark BA, Shannon RP, Rosa RM, et al. Increased susceptibility to thiazide-induced hyponatremia in the elderly. J Am Soc Nephrol 1994;5(4):1106–11.

[26] Helderman JH, Vestal RE, Rowe JW, et al. The response of arginine vasopressin to intravenous ethanol and hypertonic saline in man: the impact of aging. J Gerontol 1978; 33(1):39–47.

[27] Phillips PA, Rolls BJ, Ledingham JG, et al. Reduced thirst after water deprivation in healthy elderly men. N Engl J Med 1984;311(12):753–9.

[28] Abramow M, Beauwens R, Cogan E. Cellular events in vasopressin action. Kidney Int Suppl 1987;21:S56–66.

[29] Duggan J, Kilfeather S, Lightman SL, et al. The association of age with plasma arginine vasopressin and plasma osmolality. Age Ageing 1993;22(5):332–6.

[30] Davies I, O'Neill PA, McLean KA, et al. Age-associated alterations in thirst and arginine vasopressin in response to a water or sodium load. Age Ageing 1995;24(2):151–9.

[31] Stachenfeld NS, DiPietro L, Nadel ER, et al. Mechanism of attenuated thirst in aging: role of central volume receptors. Am J Physiol 1997;272(1 Pt 2):R148–57.

[32] Phillips PA, Bretherton M, Risvanis J, et al. Effects of drinking on thirst and vasopressin in dehydrated elderly men. Am J Physiol 1993;264(5 Pt 2):R877–81.

[33] Phillips PA, Johnston CI, Gray L. Disturbed fluid and electrolyte homoeostasis following dehydration in elderly people. Age Ageing 1993;22(1):S26–33.

[34] Johnson AG, Crawford GA, Kelly D, et al. Arginine vasopressin and osmolality in the elderly. J Am Geriatr Soc 1994;42(4):399–404.

[35] Rowe JW, Minaker KL, Sparrow D, et al. Age-related failure of volume-pressure-mediated vasopressin release. J Clin Endocrinol Metab 1982;54(3):661–4.

[36] Clark BA, Elahi D, Fish L, et al. Atrial natriuretic peptide suppresses osmostimulated vasopressin release in young and elderly humans. Am J Physiol 1991;261(2 Pt 1):E252–6.

[37] Wanza-Wesly JM, Meranda DL, Carey P, et al. Effect of atrial natriuretic hormone on vasopressin and thirst response to osmotic stimulation in human subjects. J Lab Clin Med 1995;125:734–42.

[38] Nielsen S, Fror J, Knepper MA. Renal aquaporins: key roles in water balance and water balance disorders. Curr Opin Nephrol Hypertens 1998;7(5):509–16.

[39] Tian Y, Serino R, Verbalis JG. Downregulation of renal vasopressin V2 receptor and aquaporin-2 expression parallels age-associated defects in urine concentration. Am J Physiol Renal Physiol 2004;287(4):F797–805.

[40] Catudioc-Vallero J, Sands JM, Klein JD, et al. Effect of age and testosterone on the vasopressin and aquaporin responses to dehydration in Fischer 344/Brown-Norway F1 rats. J Gerontol A Biol Sci Med Sci 2000;55(1):B26–34.

[41] Combet S, Geffroy N, Berthonaud V, et al. Correction of age-related polyuria by dDAVP: molecular analysis of aquaporins and urea transporters. Am J Physiol Renal Physiol 2003; 284(1):F199–208.

[42] Phillips PA, Bretherton M, Johnston CI, et al. Reduced osmotic thirst in healthy elderly men. Am J Physiol 1991;261(1 Pt 2):R166–71.

[43] Mack GW, Weseman CA, Langhans GW, et al. Body fluid balance in dehydrated healthy older men: thirst and renal osmoregulation. J Appl Physiol 1994;76(4):1615–23.

[44] Stachenfeld NS, Mack GW, Takamata A, et al. Thirst and fluid regulatory responses to hypertonicity in older adults. Am J Physiol 1996;271(3 Pt 2):R757–65.

[45] Wada F, Sagawa S, Miki K, et al. Mechanism of thirst attenuation during head-out water immersion in men. Am J Physiol 1995;268(3 Pt 2):R583–9.

[46] Lindeman RD, Tobin J, Shock NW. Longitudinal studies on the rate of decline in renal function with age. J Am Geriatr Soc 1985;33(4):278–85.

[47] Faull CM, Holmes C, Baylis PH. Water balance in elderly people: is there a deficiency of vasopressin? Age Ageing 1993;22(2):114–20.

ELSEVIER
SAUNDERS

Endocrinol Metab Clin N Am
34 (2005) 1047

ENDOCRINOLOGY
AND METABOLISM
CLINICS
OF NORTH AMERICA

Addendum

Early Diabetes-Related Complications in Children and Adolescents with Type 1 Diabetes: Implications for Screening and Intervention

I, Franco Chiarelli, published a chapter entitled, "Angiopathy in Children with Diabetes" in the book *Pediatric and Adolescent Diabetes*, edited by Stuart J. Brink and Viorel Serban and published by Brumar Publishers, Timisoara, Romania in 2004.

My chapter was inadvertently copied almost entirely from an article by Drs. Etienne Sochett and Denis Daneman entitled, "Early Diabetes-Related Complications in Children and Adolescents with Type 1 Diabetes: Implications for Screening and Intervention" that appeared in the December 1999 issue of *Endocrinology and Metabolism Clinics of North America*, Volume 28, issue 4, pages 865–82.

I, Franco Chiarelli, take full responsibility for this action and apologize to all affected parties.

Franco Chiarelli*
Professor
Paediatrics and Paediatric Endocrinology
University of Chieti
Chieti, Italy

Ospedale Policlinico
Chieti, Italy

E-mail address: chiarelli@unich.it

The publisher, Elsevier, views violations of our plagiarism policy seriously.

* Ospedale Policlinico, Via dei Vestini 5, 66013 Chieti, Italy.

0889-8529/05/$ - see front matter © 2005 Elsevier Inc. All rights reserved.
doi:10.1016/j.ecl.2005.09.001   *endo.theclinics.com*

ELSEVIER
SAUNDERS

Endocrinol Metab Clin N Am
34 (2005) 1049–1113

ENDOCRINOLOGY
AND METABOLISM
CLINICS
OF NORTH AMERICA

Cumulative Index 2005

Note: Page numbers of article titles are in **boldface** type.

A

A Study of Cardiovascular Events in Diabetes (ASCEND), 227, 229

A1c level. See *Hemoglobin A1c level.*

Abdominal obesity, in Cushing's syndrome. See *Central (abdominal) obesity.*

Aberrant hormone receptors, adrenal Cushing's syndrome associated with, 446–449

Absolute insulin deficiency, 140

Acanthosis nigricans, in polycystic ovary syndrome, 678, 680

Acarbose, antihyperglycemic mechanisms of, 77
    for type 2 diabetes mellitus, 207–209
    medical benefit evidence, 82

ACCORD (Action to Control Cardiovascular Risk in Diabetes) Trials, 32, 39, 221–223, 227–229

Acid-labile subunit (ALS), in growth hormone insensitivity, 582, 590

Acne, in polycystic ovary syndrome, 677–678, 685, 687
    as screening indication, 689
    hyperandrogenism, 707–708
    oral contraceptive therapy impact on, 714

ACT NOW (Actos Now for the Prevention of Type 2 Diabetes), 211, 213

ACTH-independent adrenal Cushing's syndrome, bilateral macronodular hyperplasia in, 443–445
    clinical manifestations of, 444
    diagnosis of, 444–445
    pathophysiology of, 443–444
    treatment of, 449, 490, 497
    etiologies of, 441–443
        frequencies of, 403–404
    invasive testing for, 408–413

primary pigmented nodular adrenocortical disease, 450–451
    treatment of, 451, 490, 497

ACTH-independent macronodular adrenal hyperplasia (AIMAH), bilateral, 443–445
    etiologies of, 441–443
    treatment of, 449, 490, 497
    unilateral, 442

ACTH-releasing hormone. See *Corticotropin-releasing hormone (CRH).*

Action for Health in Diabetes (Look AHEAD) Study, 227, 229

Action in Diabetes and Vascular Disease (ADVANCE) Trial, 221–222, 227, 229

Action to Control Cardiovascular Risk in Diabetes (ACCORD) Trial, 32, 39, 221–223, 227–229

Activity level, for type 2 diabetes mellitus prevention, 214–215
    dyslipidemia and, 11
    hypertension and, 65–66

Actos Now for the Prevention of Type 2 Diabetes (ACT NOW), 211, 213

Acute lymphoblastic leukemia (ALL), treatment of, bone mineral density and, 779–782
    endocrinopathies with, 769–770, 775
    obesity associations, 783

Addison, Thomas, 258

Adenomas, adrenal. See *Adrenal mass.*
    incidental. See *Adrenal incidentalomas.*

Adiponectin, insulin sensitizers and, 124

Adipose tissue. See *Body fat.*

Adolescents, intrauterine growth retardation consequences in, 601–608.

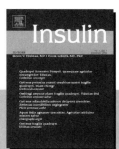

United States Postal Service
Statement of Ownership, Management, and Circulation

1. Publication Title	2. Publication Number										3. Filing Date
Endocrinology and Metabolism Clinics of North America	0	8	8	9	-	8	5	2	9		9/15/05

4. Issue Frequency	5. Number of Issues Published Annually	6. Annual Subscription Price
Mar, Jun, Sep, Dec	4	$170.00

7. Complete Mailing Address of Known Office of Publication (Not printer) (Street, city, county, state, and ZIP+4)

Elsevier, Inc.
6277 Sea Harbor Drive, Orlando, FL 32887-4800, Orange County

Contact Person
Gwen C. Campbell

Telephone
215-239-3685

8. Complete Mailing Address of Headquarters or General Business Office of Publisher (Not printer)

Elsevier, Inc., 360 Park Avenue South, New York, NY 10010-1710

9. Full Names and Complete Mailing Addresses of Publisher, Editor, and Managing Editor (Do not leave blank)

Publisher (Name and complete mailing address)

Tim Griswold, Elsevier, Inc., 1600 John F. Kennedy Blvd., Suite 1800, Philadelphia, PA 19103-2899

Editor (Name and complete mailing address)

Joe Rusko, Elsevier, Inc., 1600 John F. Kennedy Blvd., Suite 1800, Philadelphia, PA 19103-2899

Managing Editor (Name and complete mailing address)

Heather Cullen, Elsevier, Inc., 1600 John F. Kennedy Blvd., Suite 1800, Philadelphia, PA 19103-2899

10. Owner (Do not leave blank. If the publication is owned by a corporation, give the name and address of the corporation immediately followed by the names and addresses of all stockholders owning or holding 1 percent or more of the total amount of stock. If not owned by a corporation, give the names and addresses of the individual owners. If owned by a partnership or other unincorporated firm, give its name and address as well as those of each individual owner. If the publication is published by a nonprofit organization, give its name and address.)

Full Name	Complete Mailing Address
Wholly owned subsidiary of	4520 East-West Highway
Reed/Elsevier, US Holdings	Bethesda, MD 20814

11. Known Bondholders, Mortgagees, and Other Security Holders Owning or Holding 1 Percent or More of Total Amount of Bonds, Mortgages, or Other Securities. If none, check box ▶ ☐ None

Full Name	Complete Mailing Address
N/A	

12. Tax Status (For completion by nonprofit organizations authorized to mail at nonprofit rates) (Check one)
The purpose, function, and nonprofit status of this organization and the exempt status for federal income tax purposes:
☐ Has Not Changed During Preceding 12 Months
☐ Has Changed During Preceding 12 Months (Publisher must submit explanation of change with this statement)

(See Instructions on Reverse)

PS Form 3526, October 1999

---

13. Publication Title		14. Issue Date for Circulation Data Below
Endocrinology and Metabolism Clinics of North America		June 2005

15.		Extent and Nature of Circulation	Average No. Copies Each Issue During Preceding 12 Months	No. Copies of Single Issue Published Nearest to Filing Date
a.		Total Number of Copies (Net press run)	4025	3900
b. Paid and/or Requested Circulation	(1)	Paid/Requested Outside-County Mail Subscriptions Stated on Form 3541. (Include advertiser's proof and exchange copies)	1897	1800
	(2)	Paid In-County Subscriptions Stated on Form 3541 (Include advertiser's proof and exchange copies)		
	(3)	Sales Through Dealers and Carriers, Street Vendors, Counter Sales, and Other Non-USPS Paid Distribution	1114	1185
	(4)	Other Classes Mailed Through the USPS		
c.		Total Paid and/or Requested Circulation [Sum of 15b. (1), (2), (3), and (4)] ▶	3011	2985
d. Free Distribution by Mail (Samples, complimentary, and other free)	(1)	Outside-County as Stated on Form 3541	77	94
	(2)	In-County as Stated on Form 3541		
	(3)	Other Classes Mailed Through the USPS		
e.		Free Distribution Outside the Mail (Carriers or other means)		
f.		Total Free Distribution (Sum of 15d. and 15e.) ▶	77	94
g.		Total Distribution (Sum of 15c. and 15f.) ▶	3088	3079
h.		Copies not Distributed	937	821
i.		Total (Sum of 15g. and h.) ▶	4025	3900
j.		Percent Paid and/or Requested Circulation (15c. divided by 15g. times 100)	98%	97%

16. Publication of Statement of Ownership
☐ Publication required. Will be printed in the **December 2005** issue of this publication. ☐ Publication not required

17. Signature and Title of Editor, Publisher, Business Manager, or Owner

[signature] John Panucci – Executive Director of Subscription Services

Date 9/15/05

I certify that all information furnished on this form is true and complete. I understand that anyone who furnishes false or misleading information on this form or who omits material or information requested on the form may be subject to criminal sanctions (including fines and imprisonment) and/or civil sanctions (including civil penalties).

Instructions to Publishers

1. Complete and file one copy of this form with your postmaster annually on or before October 1. Keep a copy of the completed form for your records.
2. In cases where the stockholder or security holder is a trustee, include in items 10 and 11 the name of the person or corporation for whom the trustee is acting. Also include the names and addresses of individuals who are stockholders who own or hold 1 percent or more of the total amount of bonds, mortgages, or other securities of the publishing corporation. In item 11, if none, check the box. Use blank sheets if more space is required.
3. Be sure to furnish all circulation information called for in item 15. Free circulation must be shown in items 15d, e, and f.
4. Item 15h., Copies not Distributed, must include (1) newsstand copies originally stated on Form 3541, and returned to the publisher, (2) estimated returns from news agents, and (3), copies for office use, leftovers, spoiled, and all other copies not distributed.
5. If the publication had Periodicals authorization as a general or requester publication, this Statement of Ownership, Management, and Circulation must be published; it must be printed in any issue in October or, if the publication is not published during October, the first issue printed after October.
6. In item 16, indicate the date of the issue in which this Statement of Ownership will be published.
7. Item 17 must be signed.

Failure to file or publish a statement of ownership may lead to suspension of Periodicals authorization.

PS Form 3526, October 1999 (Reverse)

Changing Your Address?

Make sure your subscription changes too! When you notify us of your new address, you can help make our job easier by including an exact copy of your Clinics label number with your old address (see illustration below.) This number identifies you to our computer system and will speed the processing of your address change. Please be sure this label number accompanies your old address and your corrected address—you can send an old Clinics label with your number on it or just copy it exactly and send it to the address listed below.

We appreciate your help in our attempt to give you continuous coverage. Thank you.

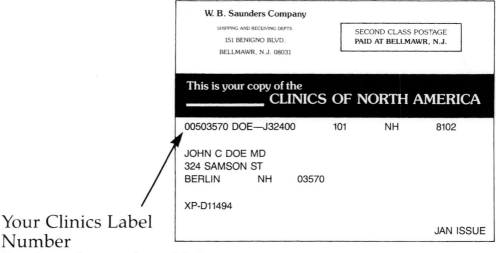

Your Clinics Label Number

Copy it exactly or send your label
along with your address to:
W.B. Saunders Company, Customer Service
Orlando, FL 32887-4800
Call Toll Free 1-800-654-2452

Please allow four to six weeks for delivery of new subscriptions and for processing address changes.